Wife, Widow, Now What?
How I Navigated the Cancer World and
How You Can, Too

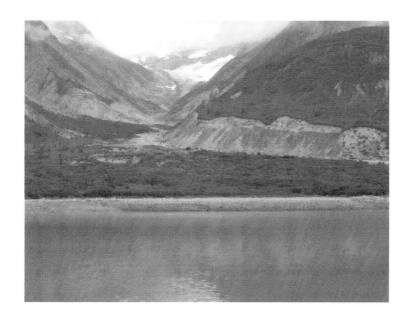

Rachel Engstrom, M.S.W., C.H.E.S.

This book is my story, along with suggestions and ideas of what I found to be most helpful and work best in my situation along the cancer journey. Please contact your medical professionals regarding diagnosis, treatments, medical needs and any other questions, as this is not intended to replace the advice or instructions of these professionals and experts.

Rachel Engstrom/Wife, Widow, Now What? How I Navigated the Cancer World and How You Can, Too

The Holy Bible, New International Version. (1986) by the Moody Bible Institute of Chicago.

This book is not affiliated with Facebook or Instagram nor does it attempt to replicate or promote products or material on behalf of Facebook or Instagram.

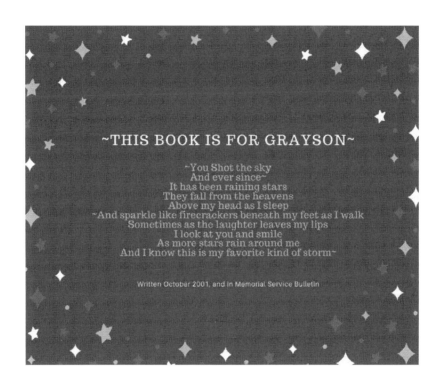

~THIS BOOK IS FOR GRAYSON~

~You Shot the sky
And ever since~
It has been raining stars
They fall from the heavens
Above my head as I sleep
~And sparkle like firecrackers beneath my feet as I walk
Sometimes as the laughter leaves my lips
I look at you and smile
As more stars rain around me
And I know this is my favorite kind of storm~

Written October 2001, and in Memorial Service Bulletin

Acknowledgements

I want to thank my mom and dad for joining me for the rollercoaster ride of this cancer journey. You provided me with more security, comfort and peace than I could ever ask for. I will be forever grateful to you both for giving Grayson and me your unlimited and unconditional love and support. I love you to the moon and back. To my sisters Felicity and Diana, and brother Jack— Thank you for believing in me, supporting me, holding me up, and always being there when I'd call and need to hear your voices to feel less alone. To my entire family, immediate and extended—I value you all more than you'll ever know.

Thank you to all of the Team Grayson supporters, the Rachel supporters and those who have stuck by me through it all. You know who you are, and if we don't talk anymore as life has moved on or gotten in the way, always know how much you meant to me during it all and still do. To my family of friends in the life I created in my twenty years here in Minneapolis, thank you for standing by me, continuing to listen when I needed/need it most. Thinking back on all of it, I could just bawl my eyes out in thankfulness that you were there with me during those years, when I needed it most– I love and appreciate you more than words can say.

To the medical staff who kept me informed, supported and afloat during Grayson's health journey—thank you from the bottom of my heart for every minute you worked to give him the best quality of life possible. I am forever grateful to you for that and for what you have done, do and will do for future patients.

To Greta, you are one heck of a lady– I love you so.

To Ethan and Bridget— thank you for being you and loving me as I am. You are the moon and stars in my nighttime sky.

I am grateful to the Lord for His faithfulness, grace and strength through the many storms I faced.

In the hundreds of hours it took me to write and format this book, I learned levels of patience I didn't know I had. Just like with cancer, I had to give myself grace with whatever was thrown at me. I wanted perfection in this text, but had to learn to let the precision placement of each chapter title go, due to the fact that if I spaced it all equally-this book would be another 50+ pages long. Life is full of imperfections and that is what makes each and every one of you beautiful and unique!

Introduction

Becoming a cancer wife then widow changed my life in more ways than I'd ever imagine. In the years that my late husband was ill, I believe that I added another master's degree to my education, in cancer life and culture, as well as a PhD in survival and adapting to what life threw at me. The combination of knowledge, faith, love and support from my friends and family were my air and water, when I'd been involuntarily signed up for the biggest marathon and warrior challenge of my life.

I was only twenty-eight when my thirty-five year old husband was diagnosed with cancer. At the time I knew no one else that was going through what I was, so I had to research and dig deep until I found the resources to adequately meet my needs regarding diagnosis and treatment decisions, time off of work, disability, navigating insurance, finding support groups, and resources to provide additional funding. It was through this that I became a future resource that would connect friends, family and those I came across to these cancer resources as well.

I found that C-A-N-C-E-R became less haunting when I educated myself more, often staying up late at night to read "Cure Magazine," the American Cancer Society's website, and other sites I'd find online to feel more connected to the cancer community. Just because I didn't know anyone within my circle that had cancer, didn't mean millions of people in the world weren't in my same shoes as well. Throughout my husband's illness I became acquaintances or friends with so many people in the oncology medical community in the hospital, clinics, support groups and online arenas, that when he died, I felt such a loss in losing the positive people who added sunshine to my days. The oncology community isn't one that anyone wishes to be a part of as a patient or spouse/significant other, but in my experience, once you are a part of it, you're fully embraced, honored and well taken care of and supported.

I learned by trial and error how to care less about plans, more about letting the chips fall where they may, and living in the moment. I didn't always get what needed to be done finished, but my husband felt supported, I took care of household chores, I showed up at work and I had slept, dressed, made sure I ate and strove to survive another day.

This is my story, and only mine. It's how I got from point A to B while still staying on the map, despite the many, many detours I'd face. It's my hope you find something within this that keeps you company in knowing you aren't alone in your journey. I speak of my faith in God, which is a big part of me, but have a great respect for every person to be who they are, individuals with differing beliefs and walks of life. I have written my experience on navigating the cancer journey with inclusion of all peoples and have changed the names of everyone in this book, except myself, in order to provide my raw and honest truths and to protect and honor my loved ones.

From the bottom of my heart, I wish you health, wellness, laughter and love.   Rachel Engstrom, 2020

Table of Contents:

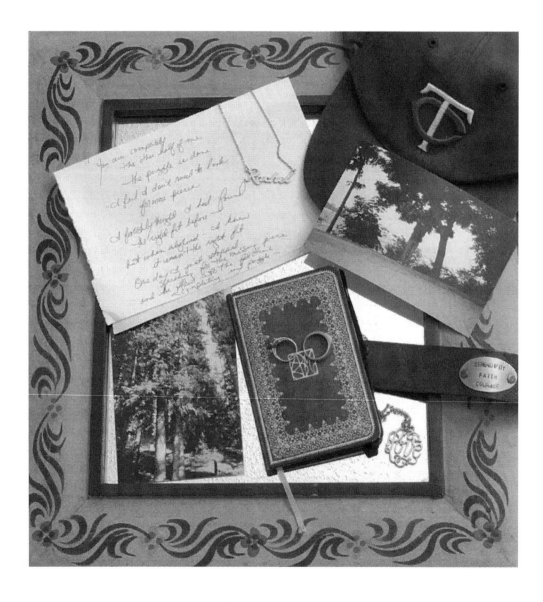

M‌usic has always been a lighthouse in the storm for me. These songs are a compilation of what I listened to during each year of my cancer wife then widow journey. I wanted to give you the option to make a playlist or reference the songs while you're reading along. Enjoy!

2011:

- ☐ "Fast Car" Tracy Chapman
- ☐ "When You Say Nothing at All" Alison Krauss
- ☐ "Better" Regina Spektor
- ☐ "Closet" Pete Yorn
- ☐ "Even Better Than the Real Thing" U2
- ☐ "Time is Love" Josh Turner
- ☐ "Dog Days are Over" Florence and the Machine
- ☐ "Dare You to Move" Switchfoot
- ☐ "Heart Like Mine" Miranda Lambert
- ☐ "Friday I'm in Love" The Cure
- ☐ "Dancing Lessons" Sinead O'Connor
- ☐ "September" Earth, Wind & Fire
- ☐ "Escapade" Janet Jackson
- ☐ "Empty Sky" Bruce Springsteen
- ☐ "Keep Ya Head Up" 2Pac
- ☐ "Goodnight and Go" Imogen Heap
- ☐ "Fire and Rain" James Taylor
- ☐ "Everything is Everything" Lauren Hill
- ☐ "I Shall Believe" Sheryl Crow
- ☐ "Float On" Modest Mouse
- ☐ "Hungry Heart" Bruce Springsteen
- ☐ "Chasing Cars" Snow Patrol
- ☐ "The Story" Brandi Carlile
- ☐ "In My Place" Coldplay

- ☐ "Samson" Regina Spektor
- ☐ "I Walk The Line" Johnny Cash
- ☐ "Be Mine" David Gray
- ☐ "Tutti Frutti," Little Richard
- ☐ "Blue Suede Shoes," Carl Perkins
- ☐ "Santa Monica" Everclear
- ☐ "Sad But True" Metallica
- ☐ "Mona Lisa" Nat King Cole
- ☐ "Drive" The Cars
- ☐ "Midnight City" M83
- ☐ "Bigger Than My Body" John Mayer
- ☐ "Better Life" Keith Urban
- ☐ "Another Day in Paradise" Phil Collins
- ☐ "Jesus, Etc." Wilco
- ☐ "Queen of the Supermarket" Bruce Springsteen
- ☐ "Enjoy the Silence" Depeche Mode
- ☐ "Kashmir" Led Zeppelin
- ☐ "Kids" MGMT
- ☐ "Bring Me Some Water" Melissa Etheridge
- ☐ "Meant to Live" Switchfoot
- ☐ "Changes" 2Pac
- ☐ "In Your Eyes" Peter Gabriel
- ☐ "Crazy Little Thing Called Love" Queen
- ☐ "This Charming Man" The Smiths
- ☐ "Untitled "Interpol
- ☐ "Jolene" Ray LaMontagne
- ☐ "Thieves in the Temple "Prince
- ☐ "Baby Please Come Home" Death Cab for Cutie (cover)

2012:

- [ ] "Everlong" Foo Fighters
- [ ] "Far Behind" Candlebox
- [ ] "Feel So Close" Calvin Harris
- [ ] "Malibu" Hole
- [ ] "Me and Julio Down by the Schoolyard" Paul Simon
- [ ] "What I Am" Edie Brickell
- [ ] "Use Me" Bill Withers
- [ ] "Forever My Friend" Ray LaMontagne
- [ ] "Good Times Roll" The Cars
- [ ] "Mercy, Mercy Me" Marvin Gaye
- [ ] "Pardon Me" Incubus
- [ ] "Good Feeling" Flo Rida
- [ ] "Springsteen" Eric Church
- [ ] "What's the Frequency Kenneth?" R.E.M.
- [ ] "We Are Young" Fun
- [ ] "Hunger Strike" Temple of the Dog
- [ ] "Maggie May" Rod Stewart
- [ ] "What's Going On" Marvin Gaye
- [ ] "Fade Into You" Mazzy Star
- [ ] "Ain't Got You" Bruce Springsteen
- [ ] "We Float" P.J. Harvey
- [ ] "Calendar Girl" Stars
- [ ] "Every Little Step" Bobby Brown
- [ ] "Don't Do Me Like That" Tom Petty
- [ ] "Blue in Green" Miles Davis
- [ ] "Interstate Love Song" Stone Temple Pilots
- [ ] "Elsewhere" Sarah McLachlan
- [ ] "Each Coming Night" Iron & Wine

- ☐ "This is Your Life" Switchfoot
- ☐ "Heroes" David Bowie
- ☐ "Numb" Linkin Park
- ☐ "Dream On" Depeche Mode
- ☐ "Sign O' the Times" Prince
- ☐ "Fidelity" Regina Spektor
- ☐ "Cheek to Cheek" Ella Fitzgerald & Louis Armstrong
- ☐ "Relator" Pete Yorn & Scarlett Johansson
- ☐ "Jackie's Strength" Tori Amos
- ☐ "Positively 4th Street" Bob Dylan
- ☐ "Back When" Tim McGraw
- ☐ "Close to Me" The Cure
- ☐ "On Your Side" Sade
- ☐ "Sweet Jane" Cowboy Junkies
- ☐ "Maps" Yeah Yeah Yeahs
- ☐ "Unsingable Name" Mike Doughty
- ☐ "Man in the Mirror" Michael Jackson
- ☐ "I'm on Fire" Bruce Springsteen
- ☐ "Matter of Trust" Billy Joel
- ☐ "Shelter from the Storm" Bob Dylan
- ☐ "Red Rain" Peter Gabriel
- ☐ "Eyes Open" Snow Patrol
- ☐ "Shadow of the Day" Linkin Park
- ☐ "Another Lonely Christmas" Prince
- ☐ "Count Your Blessings (Instead of Sheep" Bing Crosby
- ☐ "Last Christmas" Wham

2013:

- ☐ "Blackbird" Sarah McLachlan
- ☐ "Human Nature" Michael Jackson

- ☐ "How Come" Ray LaMontagne
- ☐ "Folsom Prison Blues" Johnny Cash
- ☐ "Jane Says" Jane's Addiction
- ☐ "Lazuli" Beach House
- ☐ "Mint Car" The Cure
- ☐ "Bicycle Race" Queen
- ☐ "Eyes Open" Snow Patrol
- ☐ "Don't Fear the Reaper" Blue Oyster Cult
- ☐ "Carry Me Ohio" Sun Kil Moon
- ☐ "One of These Things First" Nick Drake
- ☐ "Elsewhere" Sarah McLachlan
- ☐ "I and You and Love" The Avett Brothers
- ☐ "You Are So Beautiful" Joe Cocker
- ☐ "Love Will Tear Us Apart" Joy Division
- ☐ "Yellow" Coldplay
- ☐ "Porcelain" Moby
- ☐ "Jesus Was an Only Son" Bruce Springsteen
- ☐ "Ceremony" Joy Division
- ☐ "Bizarre Love Triangle" New Order
- ☐ "Heartbeats" Jose Gonzalez
- ☐ "Freedom! '90" George Michael
- ☐ "I'll Remember" Madonna
- ☐ "Be Here Now" Mason Jennings
- ☐ "The Mother We Share" Chvrches
- ☐ "Just Can't Get Enough" Depeche Mode
- ☐ "Recover" Chvrches
- ☐ "Waiting on an Angel" Ben Harper
- ☐ "Ice Age" Pete Yorn
- ☐ "Learning to Fly" Tom Petty
- ☐ "All These Things That I Have Done" The Killers

- ☐ "No Rain" Blind Melon
- ☐ "Unemployed Boyfriend" Everclear
- ☐ "Blank Sheet of Paper" Tim McGraw
- ☐ "Once in a Lifetime" Talking Heads
- ☐ "Come Pick Me Up" Ryan Adams
- ☐ "Walking on Sunshine" Katrina & the Waves
- ☐ "Ho Hey" The Lumineers
- ☐ "Shadowboxer" Fiona Apple
- ☐ "I'm Like a Bird" Nelly Furtado
- ☐ "Breathe" Melissa Etheridge
- ☐ "Overwhelming" Everclear
- ☐ "Breathe Me" Sia
- ☐ "Oh My God, Whatever, Etc." Ryan Adams
- ☐ "Welcome to Paradise" Green Day
- ☐ "Something Pretty" Patrick Park
- ☐ "Ageless Beauty" Stars
- ☐ "Golden Slumbers" the Beatles
- ☐ "Raspberry Beret" Prince
- ☐ "Taxi Ride" Tori Amos
- ☐ "Too Close" Alex Clare
- ☐ "Wildflowers" Tom Petty
- ☐ "Can't Hold Us" Macklemore & Ryan Lewis
- ☐ "Fell on Black Days" Chris Cornell/Soundgarden
- ☐ "Christmas Wrapping" The Waitresses

2014:

- ☐ "All I Wanna Do" Sheryl Crow
- ☐ "I Miss You Blink 182
- ☐ "American Girl" Tom Petty
- ☐ "Lips Like Sugar" Echo and the Bunnymen
- ☐ "Spiderwebs" No Doubt

- "Nothing Man" Bruce Springsteen
- "Beat of the Music" Brett Eldredge
- "Enter Sandman" Metallica
- "Last Goodbye" Jeff Buckley
- "Watch Me" Labi Siffre
- "It Had to Be You" Harry Connick Jr.
- "Personal Jesus" Depeche Mode
- "Wake Me Up" Avicii feat. Aloe Black
- "Back in Black" AC/DC
- "West End Girls" Pet Shop Boys
- "Come Over" Kenny Chesney
- "Even if it Breaks Your Heart" Eli Young Band
- "Babylon" David Gray
- "Hard to Love "Lee Brice
- "Diamonds on the Inside" Ben Harper
- "Helluva Life" Frankie Ballard
- "O-o-h Child" The Five Stairsteps
- "Poison" Bel Biv DeVoe
- "Tupelo Honey" Van Morrison
- "Chain of Fools" Aretha Franklin
- "Ride" Cary Brothers *
- "Superstition" Stevie Wonder
- "Five" Dierks Bentley
- "Midnight Train to Georgia "Gladys Knight & the Pips
- "Gather the Horses" Charlie Mars
- "One in a Million" Aaliyah
- "1901" Phoenix
- "The Distance" Cake
- "Help I'm Alive" Metric
- "Burrito" Pete York

- [ ] "Astair" Matt Costa
- [ ] "Blue Sky" Common
- [ ] "Against the Wind" Bob Seger and the Silver Bullet Band
- [ ] "Cinnamon Girl" Prince
- [ ] "Yeah" Joe Nichols
- [ ] "Maybe Tomorrow" Stereophonics
- [ ] "Runnin' Out of Moonlight Randy Houser
- [ ] "Riser" Dierks Bentley
- [ ] "Music" Madonna
- [ ] "Tranatlanticism" Death Cab for Cutie
- [ ] "Please Forgive Me" David Gray
- [ ] "Oxford Camera" Vampire Weekend
- [ ] "Bad Law" Sondre Lerche
- [ ] "Someday That I Used to Know" Gotye
- [ ] "I Wanna Dance with Somebody" Bootstraps (cover)
- [ ] "32 Flavors" Alana Davis (cover)
- [ ] "Sleeping Giant" Bootstraps
- [ ] "Operator" Jim Croce
- [ ] "Someone Else's Girl" The Olms
- [ ] "Life's Been Good" Joe Walsh
- [ ] "Orange Sky" Alexi Murdoch
- [ ] "I Hold On" Dierks Bentley
- [ ] "Trap Door" Stars
- [ ] "A Sorta Fairytale" Tori Amos
- [ ] "Same Old Lang Syne" Dan Fogelberg

2015:

- [ ] "Your Misfortune" Mike Doughty
- [ ] "3005" Childish Gambino
- [ ] "Casimir Pulaski Day" Sufjan Stevens
- [ ] "Carolina" Eric Church

- [ ] "Pennies from Heaven "Bing Crosby
- [ ] "The Hi De Ho Man" Cab Calloway
- [ ] "Milord" Edith Piaf
- [ ] "Drifting" Sarah McLachlan
- [ ] "Ain't No Sunshine" Bill Withers
- [ ] "Bad" Michael Jackson
- [ ] "Grandma's Hands" Bill Withers
- [ ] "Sir Duke" Stevie Wonder
- [ ] "Die a Happy Man" Thomas Rhett
- [ ] "Pink Toes" Childish Gambino
- [ ] "Loving You is Easy" Sarah McLachlan
- [ ] "I'm the Man Who Loves You" Wilco
- [ ] "Try Again" Aaliyah
- [ ] "Kodachrome" Paul Simon
- [ ] "Landslide" Dixie Chicks (cover)
- [ ] "Little Lies" Fleetwood Mac
- [ ] "Ain't That A Kick In The Head" Dean Martin
- [ ] "Only Living Boy in New York" Simon and Garfunkel
- [ ] "Lovely Day" Bill Withers
- [ ] "Gimme Something Good" Ryan Adams
- [ ] "Say It Ain't So" Weezer
- [ ] "Home and Dry" Pet Shop Boys
- [ ] "Hard to Handle" Otis Redding
- [ ] "Sing Me to Sleep" Fran Healy feat. Neko Case *
- [ ] "A Whiter Shade of Pale" Procol Harum
- [ ] "The Shade" Metric
- [ ] "Army of Me" Bjork
- [ ] "Stolen Dance" Milky Chance
- [ ] "Fever Dream" Iron & Wine
- [ ] "Hey Pretty Girl" Kip Moore

- ☐ "Cool Kids" Echosmith
- ☐ "A Little Respect" Erasure
- ☐ "Polichinelle" Edith Piaf
- ☐ "Walking in Memphis" Marc Cohn
- ☐ "Bad, Bad Leroy Brown" Jim Croce
- ☐ "In the Meantime" Spacehog
- ☐ "Fallen" Sarah McLachlan
- ☐ "Listen to the Darkside" Charlie Mars
- ☐ "La Vie en Rose" Edith Piaf
- ☐ "Happy" Pharrell Williams
- ☐ "All of Me" John Legend
- ☐ "Me and Tequila" Kenny Chesney feat. Grace Potter
- ☐ "Heart Shaped Box" Nirvana
- ☐ "The Wolves" Ben Howard
- ☐ "I'm Gonna Be (500 Miles)" the Proclaimers
- ☐ "Hell on the Heart" Eric Church
- ☐ "When You Became King" Alana Davis
- ☐ "Higher Ground" Stevie Wonder
- ☐ "Keep Your Head Up" Ben Howard
- ☐ "OH CA" Bootstraps
- ☐ "Come Fly With Me" Frank Sinatra
- ☐ "Upside Down" Diana Ross
- ☐ "Big Me" Foo Fighters
- ☐ "Bloom" Paper Kites
- ☐ "Don't Lose My Number" Phil Collins
- ☐ "Breathe" Télépopmusik *
- ☐ "Honey and the Moon" Joseph Arthur *
- ☐ "Royals" Lorde
- ☐ "Satellite" Guster
- ☐ "Old Pine" Ben Howard

~Part 1~

Chapter 1:
Fairy Tales and Dreams Unravel

I often think my story is like that of Humpty Dumpty falling off the wall, then egg spilling on the pavement. Other times I think it's like that song we learned as small children about the meatball that rolled off the spaghetti plate onto the floor, out the door, past the dog and all over the neighborhood. So many times I felt I was alone in my experience because I didn't know any other young cancer spouses back in 2011. It was only when I began to seek out cancer groups and knowledge online that I found out how common my circumstance was.

Nowadays everyone posts photos of every holiday, outing, meal and updates on nearly every burp online. Through the "likes" we feel supported and connected, but that only lasts momentarily. The rawness of life's pains and trials is often not displayed publicly, often resulting in insincere support. I was fortunate to have an authentic group of supporters that backed me from day one as I spilled my guts via Facebook and CaringBridge, asking for support when the landslide that would become my next two and a half years started with a fortune cookie on New Year's Eve 2010.

I'd just gotten over my own health issues and was focusing on a healthy and happy New Year with Grayson over Chinese food. We read aloud our fortune cookies. His said, "You are about to have a major life change." Little did we know that life change was going to be less like a new job or exciting vacation, but the most difficult challenge we would ever face. Some days it was like the scene from "Twister" where Helen Hunt and Bill Paxton are trying to run from the tornado and end up in the confines of a barn with shovels, hatchets and knives flying overhead. Other days it was more like Tom Hanks as Forrest Gump, in his beige suit and blue plaid shirt peacefully sitting on the bus bench watching the feather float above his head. Either way, I knew I was on this journey and like it or not, it was time to buckle up!

~The Story of Grayson and Rachel~

In the fall of 2000 I moved to Minneapolis, Minnesota, as a doe-eyed eighteen-year-old who had dreamed of living in a place with more diversity and cultural opportunities. My smaller Michigan hometown was filled with kind and loving people, but it just didn't have the freedoms I craved as a liberal teen who wanted to break free out on her own. I attended the University of Minnesota for undergrad to study cultural anthropology, thanks to the support of my generous and amazing parents. It was here in "The Cities," that I fell in love with the cities themselves, the music scene

where I'd attend countless concerts each year on the stomping grounds of Prince, the weather (yes, even the insanely cold winters of -24 degrees at times) and people. I had no idea

I'd create a family of friends when I moved here all those years ago, not knowing one person, and certainly had no idea I'd meet someone seven years older than me when I was only nineteen that would later become my husband.

I met Grayson at my friend Maria's boyfriend's birthday party the fall of 2001. I'd heard about this Everett guy from Maria and August, and was told that he was older, tall, kind, and funny and I just had to meet him. That Friday night around 11:30 p.m., the tall, handsome stranger with dark hair walked in and immediately calmed my nerves as he smiled, stuck out his hand and said, "Hi Rachel, nice to meet you, I'm Grayson. I go by Everett at work, my first name, but my friends call me Grayson."

I want to say that our first date was super romantic or pretty epic, but that would be a lie. That is, aside from the kiss. Grayson picked me up at the dorm carrying a single red rose then walked me to his car. I stifled a laugh as I saw the tiny little white Honda CRX and wondered how this 6'2 guy fit into this little car. He opened the door for me to my surprise, then gracefully folded himself into his seat. We met Maria and August at Chili's where I nervously chatted over chicken fingers and soda. Afterwards we went back to our friends' apartment only to leave shortly thereafter due to their bickering.

Grayson drove me to Rosemount to see the industrial factory that when lit up at night, looks like a magical little fairyland, much like the factory in Willy Wonka, sans the Oompa Loompas and candy. He purchased coffee for himself and hot chocolate for me from a nearby truck stop that we drank in the car as we talked for an hour, waiting for the daylight to fade. When it became dark we got out and stood in the nearby field in slightly awkward silence as we gazed at the lights. After a couple minutes I looked up at him and blurted out, "Are you ever going to kiss me?" He threw his coffee cup to the wind and kissed me. In my mind it was cute, funny and movie-worthy with a sweeping musical score behind us. Yes, he did pick up his trash later, and from that night we were together until his literal last breath.

Grayson worked from 3-11 p.m. in an industrial factory as a technician creating ink colors to be printed on flexible packaging. His role was to mix gigantic drums of ink that kept him busy and in peak physical shape while the rest of the world enjoyed evenings out or at home, going to bed at normal sleeping times. His odd hours were always something that frustrated him, but we made it work. We were inseparable on weekends and he'd come get me around midnight from the dorm every Tuesday then take me to school the next morning. He told me right away he had a cat named Puddin' he adored and I knew that he must a good guy to have something he could keep alive and give a name that silly. On the weekends we'd take day trips where we'd stop for photo-ops or stay in for movie marathons. I was pretty busy in my later college years, balancing school and a part time job helping a disabled adult, but we made sure we had time to see each other regularly.

By the time I was twenty-one and he was nearly twenty-eight, we started talking about marriage. One night in the fall of 2003 as he was sitting on my blue sofa in my little studio apartment on Grand Avenue in St. Paul, I decided to propose. I took his Sam Adams out of his hand, climbed onto his lap, looked into his eyes and said, "Will you marry me?," to which he replied, "What?, are you sure this is the way you want it?" I said, "Yes, I don't want you to have to come up with some romantic scheme or spent a lot of money. I love you, let's get married!" I jumped off his lap then ran to the kitchen, grabbed two Tootsie Rolls, had us each bite into one then swap the other half with each other, solidifying our engagement. The next morning we called our parents, as I couldn't have a boy over of course, telling my mom that Grayson proposed over breakfast. Sorry, Mom, but it did all turn out for the best and you adored Grayson!

We got married on a hot summer night in August 2004 at the Wabasha Street Caves in front of a fireplace gouged with bullet holes from gangster Prohibition days. The previous spring I'd graduated with my bachelors from the University of Minnesota, got a job at a local zoo in the education department, and moved into Grayson's apartment. Life was good. Over the next seven years we traveled, spent time with family and friends, loved our pets, bought our first house and got a dog together.

We were as close as you can get to perfect. We had what I called a "space age marriage." We rarely had a big fight, only once or twice a year, and when we did bicker it was over small things like household chores. I'd nag him endlessly to take better care of himself as I'd often find him still gaming at 7 a.m. when I'd wake for work, causing me to get so mad at his lack of self-care. I'd later learn he hated his job so much; this activity was one of the only things he enjoyed during the week. We were only able to see each other on the weekends.

In our old apartment in the Cathedral Hill area in St. Paul, he'd always promise to do dishes but often didn't get them done as he'd stayed up too late the night before, then woke up too late to do them before work. I got so mad at times I'd stack them on a cookie sheet on the stove and leave them there in my passive aggressive way. He'd tell me when he did want to do them he couldn't because the kitchen was by the bedroom and he'd wake me up if he did them when he got home from work. It was an endless cycle that makes me smile to think about how trivial it all was.

He was perpetually late and a serial procrastinator. It drove me up the walls. I even witnessed him going to work in wet jeans a couple times because he was running late and the dryer wasn't done before he had to go. He was my rock and I was his roll. We fit and that was all that I needed. He loved me through the growing pains of my twenties and I his mid-to-late twenties and early-to-mid-thirties. He was the kindest person I'd ever known, goody-two-shoes nice, and I was so proud to be his girlfriend then wife.

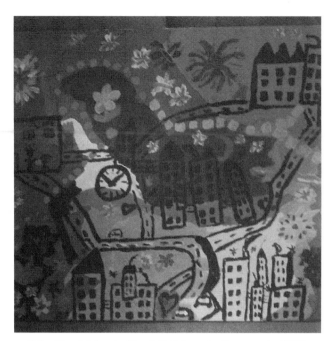

"The Road Map to Our Life" I made Grayson in 2007.

Chapter 2:
The Text: aka- the Target Parking Lot

On a cold windy Wednesday in January as I was loading the residents of the mental health assisted living facility I worked at and their purchases into the large maroon twelve-passenger van in the Target parking lot, my phone buzzed. I reached into my coat to find a text from Grayson that read, "Went to doctor. Now have to go to North Memorial for a blood transfusion." I tried not to panic and thought back to the night before, as I drove the twenty minutes back to work.

I had awakened around 2:30 a.m. to go to the bathroom and had found Grayson sitting on the kitchen mat in front of the sink with his head in his hands. When I asked what was going on, he replied in a tired voice, "I don't know, I am so tired, I can't even stand up while waiting for my food to heat in the friggin' microwave!" His forehead felt normal to me, but he was pale and I knew he'd been overextending himself lately with the mandatory extra late hours he was working, sometimes as late as 1:30 a.m. I gave him the business card of my doctor, telling him to go in the next day, thinking he might have a virus or the flu.

Back at work, I told my boss what was going on and that I had to go home. I jetted out of there like my feet were on fire. I tried to call Grayson on the two-mile ride home but got his voicemail. I prepared myself to track him down at the hospital if I had to.

On gut instinct I decided to go home first and was relieved when I saw his car in the driveway when I arrived. I opened the front door yelling his name, only to surprise him as he exited the bathroom and asked why I was home so early. He caught me up, telling me that he'd had his blood taken and was told his hemoglobin was only 7, to the normal adult male range of 13.5-17.5, resulting in the need for a blood transfusion to help with what the doctor thought might be anemia, hence his lethargy. We drove to the hospital in silence as he closed his eyes in sheer exhaustion, resting his head. I parked in the cold concrete structure and I wondered what was next as we walked through an adjoining tunnel, seeing our breaths in front of us. Once we found the right area, we were told to head to the lab for what we thought was the transfusion, only to find out that he was only getting a "type-cross" to find out his blood type. The transfusion was scheduled for the next day.

The next day I worked a half day then drove him to the hospital again. The entire transfusion process took four hours, two hours per bag of blood, which flew by as we talked and looked at magazines. Just as the last bag was finishing, we were told that they were talking to his doctor from the day before and we needed to wait. After sitting for ten minutes in the fluorescent lights that seemed to be getting brighter as my paranoia and worry grew, a nurse told us that something of concern had been found in his blood tests from the prior day, and to head down the street to the Humphrey Center. I told Grayson not to worry as I attempted to remain calm, but as we pulled into the parking lot, I felt like I had to eat my words as I saw the sign that said "Humphrey Cancer Center." We held hands walking through the darkly-lit lobby, then were quickly led to an empty patient room with uncomfortable ugly chairs and a large fish tank. We waited nearly twenty-five minutes in silence that no words could fill. I put my arm around his back, squeezing him to me as he wiped a tear from his left eye. After what seemed like forever, a doctor came in and told us he had TTP: Thrombotic Thrombocytopenic Purpura, a rare blood disorder that could present like anemia and would require him to come in seven days a week for three weeks to have his blood cycled out, cleaned, then cycled back into his body so his system could properly work as it normally should be. We were assured that although it was rare, it was treatable and he would feel better in no time.

After the doctor left the room, we put on our coats to leave. Grayson stopped at the bathroom as I called my work to update them, asking for prayers. As my husband walked out of the bathroom and down the hallway towards me, he shot his long arms above his head and said "At least it isn't the Big C!" I gave him a kiss and a hug and sighed, "Yes!" then drove us home.

That night we rested downstairs on our comfy sofas with only one light on, trying to forget the last few hours. Being the research nerd that I am, I looked online for anything I could find on TTP. I read academic and scientific article after article, assuring Grayson that TTP seemed very doable and that he would be fine. He began to softly cry, telling me he was so tired and asking why this had to happen to him. Just as I was comforting him with a hug, his phone rang. It was the doctor we'd just seen. He put it on speakerphone on the table in front of us.

"Everett?"

"Yes, this is him."

"It turns out we misdiagnosed you with TTP, based on a few more tests we ran after you left."

I felt myself sink into the large brown couch and wrapped my arms around Grayson's back and middle. What in the world was going on? How was this happening? I felt like I was floating in the room, yet anchored to my sweet husband.

"That's good then, right?"

"Actually, Everett, no. We need you to come in tomorrow so we can do a bone marrow biopsy, we think it may be something more serious. Please come to the clinic at North Memorial at 9:30 a.m."

"Ok, thank you, bye."

At this point I had no words….I had no idea what to say. This was scary enough as this was happening to my husband…but yikes! I had no idea what to tell him! I couldn't be crying, sobbing, yelling, and going out of my freaking mind! Stay calm Rachel, be soothing and no matter what you do, do not mention cancer. We immediately began to pray. We asked God for peace, guidance and comfort, not knowing what was going to happen.

I went upstairs to our little wooden cabin-looking office and called my parents to catch them up on the events of the day, asking them to pray. They told me not to get too upset until I knew more. At that point Grayson didn't want his parents to know anything yet so they wouldn't worry. That night we slept restlessly, worrying about what the next day would bring.

Chapter 3:
Biopsies and Cheese Crackers

The next morning, Grayson and I arrived for his appointed 9:30 a.m. intake for the bone marrow biopsy. We were placed in a brightly-lit room, with an examination table covered with sheet paper and a gown on top. Grayson began to cry with nervousness as we waited in the freezing room. I rubbed his back and sang Sarah McLachlan songs, my favorite go-to since age thirteen.

A nurse came in and told him to take off all of his clothes in exchange for the gown. In another seven or eight minutes the nurse returned and we dropped the hands we'd been holding together as he was told to lie down. The nurse pulled his gown open in the back and began to prep the site for the procedure. Within a couple minutes, a doctor came in to explain what the biopsy would entail and that local and general anesthesia would be used. Within five minutes Grayson was laying on his stomach, loopy, looked up and asked, "Are you going to do a tattoo of Sarah Palin on my ass?" then laid his head back down and conked out.

As they turned the metal torture-looking device in his lower back over his hip, I double checked to make sure he was out then began asking questions as they told me he most likely had leukemia. I was told that people go through chemo and radiation treatments and go on to become marathon runners, doctors, nurses, lawyers and live long and successful lives. I kept shifting uncomfortably on the small metal stool I sat on near his head, while I took in the information. At one point he woke up again, raised his head and said "Having fun back there?" then went back under again. In that moment I felt in my bones that my husband had cancer and there was nothing I could do to stop our impending fate. I was oddly calm and credited it to God's grace being upon me.

As Grayson rested after the procedure, I went out into the lobby and called his superior to tell him Everett (Grayson) would not be coming back to work anytime soon. His boss, Adam, told me that the guys at work had thought that Everett was anemic and probably just needed to eat a few steaks, that they were planning on pooling their money to get him some Outback Steakhouse gift cards. After that I updated my parents and Grayson's. His dad had died when Grayson was sixteen after his second stroke and cystic fibrosis that was thought to be caused from asbestos in the warehouse he used to work in, had made him very ill. Grayson's mom Victoria and step-dad Bernard lived in his hometown of St. Cloud, about seventy-five miles away.

Grayson and I went home both feeling nervous and somber. We had to wait until the following Monday to find out the biopsy results. I had no idea how we'd make it all weekend without knowing his fate, our fate. After I parked in our driveway, I took Grayson's hand and said a quick prayer when I saw he was reluctant to get out of the car or to move. We spent the next few hours attempting to distract ourselves with TV and our pets, until the doorbell rang at 4 p.m.

My brother Jack was on the porch. He'd talked to my parents the night before and told his wife Maddie that he needed to drop everything to come support us through this uncertain time. I was so elated to have Jack there to ease the tension we felt on that difficult weekend. He is fourteen years older than me, the oldest of the four of us, who lived seven hours away in northern Wisconsin at the time, with his wife and three little girls. Shortly thereafter, Victoria and Bernard arrived, which I thought was a good time to take a break and head to Target to get the groceries I'd planned to get that night before any of this happened. Victoria was shocked I was going to the store at a time like that, but we needed food, so off Jack and I went to hunt and gather.

On the five-mile drive there we talked about my nieces as a light snow fell around us. As I sat in the darkly lit cab of Jack's green truck, I felt a sense of relief to be distanced from my reality, if only for an hour. Jack and I had always gotten along well, but I hadn't been as close to him as my sisters, Felicity who was twelve years older than me, and Diana, two years older.

We walked into Target and as I began to fill my cart with produce and non-perishable foods, I found Jack in a state of wonderment seeing the available treasures that were not sold at the smaller merchants where he lived. I watched him put box after box of pepper jack cheese crackers into his cart while saying, "They don't have these things where I live! This is great!" I laughed and said "Whatever floats your boat, dude!" When we made our way around the back of the store to the cold cases, I saw an arm chair on an end display and decided to take a seat to call Grayson's sister Natasha in Louisiana to update her. I told her I was pretty sure that her brother had cancer and that I'd call again when we had definite news. She sounded concerned yet even keeled and was thankful for my call. As we walked outside, we were enveloped in a winter wonderland of fast and heavy falling snowflakes that filled my mind and senses with peace and serenity as I put my purchases into the truck. Later that night after Victoria and Bernard left, and Jack was settled on our couch downstairs and the pets were all taken care of, Grayson and I prayed and talked about what our future might hold.

The next morning Victoria, Bernard, Jack, Grayson and I all tried to remain patient and calm over the pancakes I'd made, as we sat around our dining room table. Time felt like molasses seeping out of a tipped jar. Around 10:30 a.m., Grayson received a call from an unknown number. He went into the office, shut the door and emerged after ten minutes, asking me to come in and to close the door.

Time stood still as he looked at me with sad eyes and said, "I have to tell you something. I have Acute Lymphoblastic Leukemia and have to be admitted to the hospital at 1 p.m. to start treatment right away. I have cancer." His eyes enlarged as he looked at me for guidance and reassurance. I looked at my beautiful husband in front of me, looking so small in that moment in our little wooden office. I wished we could have stayed cocooned in there and that what he'd just said was only a bad dream. I snapped back to reality within seconds, reassuring him that no matter what happened we were a team, in it together. I took his hand and led him to our bedroom where we laid on our pillows and prayed, asking God to take care of Grayson and all of the uncertainty. I lay there holding my young thirty-five-year-old husband as he cried, feeling so helpless and so weightless, as if we were floating in our own little bubble. I can still feel the comforter underneath us, our hands entwined and the wet tears falling down our cheeks. Our new circumstance of such dark uncertainty was such a contrast to the bright light coming through the curtains that bounced off the newly fallen snow outside.

I went out to the living room and gave the terrible news to his parents and my brother. I led Victoria by the hand over to her son where she fell on her knees and began to pray, asking God for guidance and protection. I gave them time alone as I sat on the soft carpeted stairs leading down to the basement and called Grayson's best friend Owen. As I sat there telling him what would ultimately affect all of our lives, I looked down the room at the family room area, envisioning just two weeks ago when Grayson and Owen had watched movies, laughed and shared craft beer. I learned a hard lesson that day of how so much can change in such a short amount of time.

I had to pack up Grayson's belongings so we could head to the hospital. It was January 15th, 2011. I'd just become a cancer wife at age twenty-eight.

~

Your Emotions: It's so important that you take some time for yourself to process what is going on. This was not supposed to happen…but it did. It's okay to feel:

- Angry: This is not fair! Why did this have to happen to us?
- Fear/Scared: What is going to happen? What does this mean for us as a couple? How are we going to pay for all of our bills if my loved one can't work? I am scared I am going to lose them!
- Sadness: I can't believe we are here. I just want to crawl into my bed and hide under the covers.
- Loneliness: I feel so isolated and alone in this. No one I know is going through this.
- Anxiety/Stress: How am I supposed to do this? Can I handle this?
- Denial: This can't be real…can it?
- Guilt/Regret: Was there something I could have done or we could have done so my loved one would have not gotten sick? Was it this or that?
- Hope: I can do this! I love my spouse/significant other and we are going to beat this!
- Positivity will help you tremendously, even if you're faking it for now. Negative thinking will take a toll on your mind and body, but if you can try to use this new knowledge as power, it can help you to try to remain as positive as possible.

  Once you allow yourself to take a few moments to listen to your mind and body and start to process your emotions, you'll be able to move forward in the process to prepare (or at least in my case-attempt to prepare) for what's next.

~

Jack drove us to the hospital as I sat in a daze holding Grayson's left hand, as we were all side by side in the front of the truck. Up to that point in my life, my only experience of cancer was from what I'd seen in movies and television. I usually correlated cancer to the Julia Roberts movie, "Dying Young," that involved a young man who became very ill as he underwent treatment, continually sweating, vomiting and losing control of his body. What I'd seen in general wasn't pretty, and I had no real preconceived notions of what I was going into and would face.

We checked in at the hospital's front desk, and then were swiftly led to a room where Grayson was asked several questions about personal safety at home, emergency contacts, and life. The hours flew by in a blur of tests and scans to gather immediate information on his condition. I was speechless as I sat there in the shiny-vinyl covered wooden chair. I kept telling Grayson I was there and loved him. Fatigue was written all over his face and his exhaustion grew with each poke and prod.

That afternoon was filled with visits from his parents, Jack, Owen and his wife, and all of the medical staff coming in and out of the room. I took a break to go to the cafeteria with Owen and his wife where I detoxed my feelings over a bag of chips and a Coke, while Owen excitedly ate the famed Minnesota tater-tot casserole.

That night I slept at Grayson's bedside on a blue vinyl chair that folded down into a semi-comfortable small bed if I laid in the fetal position. We prayed and had small talk as we tried to get some sleep. As we lay in our respective beds, we held hands and said the Lord's Prayer. From that day on, it would be our nightly before-sleep ritual whether we were together or apart, as we'd recite it over the phone.

As I attempted to sleep, the song, "When You Say Nothing At All," popped into my head. It's a song that I adored from the movie, "Notting Hill," in the end scene with Julia Roberts and Hugh Grant. I jumped up and made my way in the dark to the bathroom, shut the door and looked up the song online on my phone. Once I'd found it, I went up to Grayson, asked him to scooch over, then climbed in and played the song by Alison Krauss as tears dropped down his face. I knew that we'd face this beast head on and no matter who, what, where, when, or why, I'd always be by his side. I learned years later from him that Grayson played that song every night before he went to sleep when he was in the hospital away from me. It was another way to hold us up and together through the storms we faced.

Early the next morning the rounding oncologist came in to formally diagnose Grayson with ALL: Acute Lymphoblastic Leukemia. He said treatment needed to start immediately and it was time to decide if Grayson would receive care there at North Memorial, or at another facility in the Twin Cities. After an hour of research, we decided on the University of Minnesota's Fairview Hospital on the East Bank of the U campus. We were told that he would be admitted the next day, Monday morning, and that next we needed to go to the nearby cryogenics clinic to have some of his sperm frozen, as it was mandatory for young cancer patients to do so- as they could become sterile from chemo and radiation.

~

Diagnosis: Ask as many questions as possible! No question is a dumb question.

- How long do you think the cancer has been present?
- Has it spread into other places in the body?
- Is this treatable?
- How serious is this?
- What are the chances of survival?
- What will the next few hours/days/weeks/months look like?
- My spouse/significant other usually takes medications, do we stop them now?
- If you do not understand something the doctor/medical staff is telling you, ask them to explain it again.
  - o Rephrase your questions in a way that makes the most sense to you-this may help them better understand your concerns.
  - o Don't be afraid to ask for explanations in layman's terms- there are a ton of medical mumbo jumbo words and acronyms to get used to along the way.
  - o It's vital that you get all of your questions answered and you understand what is happening, despite how hard it is to hear.

- Try to write down as much information as you can from now on throughout treatment. It's going to be a lot, and you most likely will only remember a small portion of it when you're trying to balance it all, while coming to terms with the diagnosis. Ask a friend or family member to help take notes if you cannot.

~

We Have the Diagnosis. What's Next?

- You are entitled to get a second opinion and to seek treatment and services wherever your loved one feels most comfortable.
- Your spouse/significant other is the patient now. It's your job now to be the team manager, secretary, cheerleader and point of contact for the medical staff. It's time to put on your Wonder Woman or Superman cape and go get em'!
- Don't feel like you have to think of everything to ask now. Cancer is a long process and things will pop up along the way you'll want to ask more about.

- BREATHE! and know that more information will come in the next days and weeks.

Chapter 4:
Tutti-frutti, Specimen Cups and Hospitals, Oh My!

As if the shock of Grayson's diagnosis wasn't enough, we were also given the odd task of cryogenic sample collection. Jack tried to lighten the mood and make a joke at the awkward experience by saying, "Come on, Rachel, give Grayson a hand!" on the drive over to the clinic. I told him to shut up and laughed in my nervousness at the situation.

The chipper young woman at the front desk gave us forms to sign and a collection cup before leading us to a somewhat darkly-lit room that contained a sink with soap and paper towels, a big brown leather chair and a magazine rack full of porn. Grayson took off his coat and looked at the cup like it was an alien life form. To our bewilderment, songs like "Tutti-Frutti," and "Blue Suede Shoes," were being pumped into the room from a sound system with a volume we could not control. Talk about awkward! He told me he would do the sample on his own and rolled his eyes and grimaced as I sat on the floor against the door holding up a dirty magazine and said, "This is your hall pass buddy, take a good look!"

After a few awkward minutes he told me to leave. I was more than happy to escape to the hallway where I called a friend to fill her in on Grayson's diagnosis. Before we left, we paid the receptionist and set up a payment plan to pay for storing our frozen children, then left that twilight zone to try to relax at home before starting hospital life the next day.

Monday morning I waited in the lobby this time and told Grayson, "Go save our children!" to which he rolled his eyes, smiled and said, "Thanks, Pony!" His nickname for me was "Pony," as he said I reminded him of a My Little Pony when we met. After depositing sperm sample number two, we were ready to check him into the U hospital. I prayed on our way there for God to help keep me calm and level headed. I could not afford to lose it when he needed me to be his rock. Time to suit up and learn my new life as a cancer wife.

~

Emotional Support and Self Care: This is a vital part of the process, second only to the medical treatment itself.

- Choose a family member or friend you can confide in. Having someone you can be your authentic self with through the tears, fears, anger and unknown is key. Your emotions will be on a rollercoaster ride and you cannot put these feelings on the plate of the patient. They are counting on you to be their rock. Try to keep it together in front of them, share those emotions when they come up together, but try to process your own emotions with your own support system.

- Grayson felt terrible that I had to deal with so much and as close as we were, I didn't want him to know about all of my fears, doubts and sadness when he had his own reality and emotions to process and deal with.
- Keep notes of questions you have for the medical staff to ask them privately out of earshot of your spouse/significant other. Go out in the hallway or make a phone call to them when you're not near the patient. This will help ease your fears, doubts and give you knowledge and connection to your loved one's medical world. You're a vital part of this process and deserve to be heard, too.
- Seek spiritual support from your pastor/minister/spiritual leaders or friends.
    - Delegate informing your church about the diagnosis to a friend/family member.
    - Hospitals have chaplains available to meet with when needed.
    - Hospitals have chapels and family waiting areas to meet with your spiritual friends and confidants or just to gather with your supporters when needed.
- Pray. Asking for guidance can be freeing, helpful and can center you.
    - Knowing you have a network of people storming heaven with prayers can be very comforting and you'll feel less alone.
- Rest. You will crash and burn if you do not. Navigating this new world is tough and without enough rest, you cannot be the support you need to be for your person.

- You can do this! Take a few breaths and know that millions of people have been exactly where you are, or will be in the future. You have to do this for your spouse/significant other. I think you will find, like I did, that you have levels of strength you never knew existed.

~

As I sat in the little wooden paneled office in admissions at the U (aka- University of Minnesota) hospital and gave my insurance card to the woman behind the counter and signed on for only God knew what future expenses, I felt like I was stepping onto on escalator that had no exit. I had an idea where we were headed, yet not what any of it would entail. Within thirty minutes Grayson was checked into a temporary room, snuggled among blankets and we were being told by Dr. Lazar, his head MD, that they'd been able to detect that the cancer had only been in his body two weeks or so and that it had infiltrated 91% of his blood stream. As I sat there holding my husband's hand and looking at the stark white curtain near his bed that contrasted with the gloomy gray-painted walls, I took in what the doctor was telling us about the disease that now controlled Grayson's fate. We were told that as far as cancers go, this was considered "the good kind of cancer" as it was more treatable with higher survival rates. Grayson was to start chemo that Thursday, in three short days, after he gave his last cryogenics sample.

Later that afternoon Grayson's parents, Jack and Owen all came to visit. I began to feel calmer with the hourly info updates that provided us with more of a game plan. I felt like the

Titanic had hit the iceberg but instead of it sinking, it was my job as the healthy spouse to get as many resources possible, to crank this baby out of the frozen water, put it back together and steer it as best as I could. By dinner time Grayson was transferred to a single room that would remain his home for the next five weeks. It was warmer and more welcoming than the previous room, with cherry wood trim around the windows and a seated sill, closet and sink. I looked around the room, wondering how I could make it more homelike for Grayson.

When our loved ones had headed home, I rifled around my duffel bag and pulled out pajama pants,   prepping for my overnight stay. That night I learned the routine of setting up my foldable bed that staff had brought in. I topped the three-inch mattress with a sheet, pillow and thin blanket, settling in for his first night there. I later learned about my best friend down the hall, the blanket warmer that held heated treats that somehow made things better when dealing with so much.

Right then in those moments all I could focus on was the fact that we were together and the medical staff had a plan of treatment. The rest was in God's hands, and ultimately all I could do was trust in the process. Were alarm bells going off in my head? Yes. But I had to hit snooze for now and keep moving forward.

I awoke the next day to see a phlebotomist taking Grayson's blood. I quickly learned that these early-morning vampires would be the first ones to come in aside from the rounding nurses and assistants doing vitals (temperature and blood pressure checks) during the night. I stepped out of his room and went to the small family waiting area at the end of the hallway. It contained two small couches, a couple of chairs and a desk with a computer. I sat down and called my boss, informing him of Grayson's diagnosis and that I would need the next week off of work. He was dismayed and concerned at the shocking turn of events and told me to take all the time I needed, that my activities would be covered or cancelled. At the time I worked as an activity coordinator at an assisted living for mentally ill adults, planning in-house events and socially integrating the clientele in the community while doing fun activities. I made a few other calls to close friends, including Grayson's high school buddies that he talked to only a couple times a year, knowing they would want to know the big news about their friend as well.

Later that morning I called our insurance company to go over our plan and coverage details. I'd dreaded making that phone call but as I sat in the glassed-in private room inside another family lounge I'd found, I was pleasantly surprised. We would only be responsible for a $5,000 deductible, then a 30% co-insurance after that, with a maximum out of pocket for the year of $10,000. I was told that ALL was considered an acute critical illness and that if Grayson needed a bone marrow transplant down the road, everything would be covered, including the donor's procedure and travel expenses. Well then, hallelujah! (I tallied the costs of Grayson's treatment after he died and it was roughly $4.4 million, so what we paid was just a drop in the bucket). Thank you, Lord, for some good news!

Over the next few hours I rallied the troops, making more phone calls, sending texts and emails, asking for support and prayers, as we needed as much help as possible to get on the right side of the tug-of-war that was cancer.

Within the first couple days I knew the names of most of the medical staff, when the best foods were served at the cafeteria and how to get discounted parking passes and valet service for when I was too tired to walk to my car or didn't want to face the frigid Minnesota temperatures. The kindness, expertise and knowledge of the medical staff made me feel more secure by the day, especially the veteran nurses who had literally seen it all in their years working with patients in all stages of cancer treatment. I was amazed at my own ability to gladly take the cancer world by the hand, despite the horror of being thrown into this difficult mess. I allowed it to show me the good, bad, and ugly while also feeling at peace that Grayson was in the only place he should be at that time.

It wasn't until months later when we were sitting in the clinic for his outpatient appointments that I'd learn how fortunate we were to have accessible healthcare so close to us, especially oncologists. Many other patients in that same waiting room drove for anywhere from one to three hours, two or three times a week for their medical appointments. We were so blessed and fortunate to live where we did, and to have the choice of top medical facilities. I felt inner warmth to be back on the old stomping grounds of my youth at the University of Minnesota, among the beautiful and charming brick buildings, especially the dorm across the street from the hospital, where Grayson picked me up for our first date so many years ago.

I was able to turn Grayson's hospital room into our own cozy little place. We'd later learn from our favorite nurses that they often referred to Grayson and I as "the love birds in their little apartment" when we were there together. I brought a small table lamp that I put on the windowsill, an 8x10" photo I'd had made of our puppy, Clive, that I taped to his closet door, a quilt from our living room that I put on his bed and a cross with one of his favorite scriptures on it, on a shelf for him to view.

I had a crash course in the lack of privacy for a cancer patient, quickly disarming any societal norms of being modest. My life with Grayson was now on full display for all who came in the room to see. Grayson would become vulnerable on levels a healthy thirty-five-year old would never think about. He was asked dozens of questions by the hour as he attempted to wrap his mind around the new feelings he was having as his body betrayed him more each day. The daily routines he'd known had been thrown a grenade, and he was only offered the solace of a few hours of sleep a day, in the pockets of time he wasn't being checked in on. I learned quickly not to care who came in as I yawned, burped, tooted or was in the middle of a story or joke. We adapted our marriage and life to this new phenomenon that was cancer and held on tight to what had become the bumpiest ride of our lives.

~

Treatment: Cancer treatment depends on the type of cancer, its stage at diagnosis, and the available medical treatments. Your loved one may require inpatient treatment for a period of time in the hospital and/or outpatient treatment in a clinic setting. The American Cancer Society is an excellent resource to research treatments and has helpful decision making tools at: www.cancer.org

Below is a list of questions I would highly recommend asking the doctors and medical staff, based on my experience, and the experiences of other patients and caregivers I've known.

- Do we need to bring any medical history records in addition to what you already have?
- What is the recommended treatment?
o What are the success rates?
- What is the best outcome that we can hope for?
- Are there any complications associated with this treatment protocol?
- Is there anything we can do to prepare for treatment?
- How will the patient most likely feel after the treatments?
- What are the side effects of the chemo drugs/radiation?
- Can I be with them during these treatments?
- Are there any clinical trials available?
o What is the purpose of the trial?
o Why is it believed to be the best option?
o How long will it last?
o What kinds of tests and treatments are parts of it?
o How will you know if it is working?
o Who do I speak with if I have questions along the way?
o Can we quit the trial if it feels like it isn't working, or my loved one doesn't want to participate in it anymore?
o Is there someone we can talk to who has personally been in the trial?
- Will surgery be needed?
- How long do the treatments take?
- Will my loved one be in pain?
- How much experience do you (doctor/medical facility) have in treating this kind of cancer?
- Will they be really nauseated? Are there ways to help with this?
- Will this affect the ability to have kids? Do we need to freeze our eggs/sperm for future children?
- Will my loved one lose their hair?
- Does my loved one need to change the way they are eating or exercising?
- Can my love one work? Will there be a reduced work schedule?

- Ask as many questions as you'd like. If you don't get all of your questions answered when the doctor comes in, request a Physician's Assistant (PA) or another doctor come back later to discuss things more with you. It's their job, and your right to get the answers you need until you feel comfortable and informed.

~

Insurance: Navigating Your Coverage

- Become familiar with these terms and know what they mean!
  - Deductible: The amount you have to pay before insurance picks up any of the medical costs.
  - Co-insurance: The percentage of the cost of an appointment or procedure that you are responsible for after you've met your deductible.
  - Co-pay: The payment that is due when services are rendered. Typically $20, $40, $50, etc.
  - Out of Pocket Maximum: The maximum amount you will have to pay out of your pocket in the form of co-pay, deductible and co-insurance costs all combined until your insurance company pays for all of the medical costs for the remainder of the plan year.
    - Sometimes you may have Individual and Family deductibles: this means that each person has to meet their individual deductible or the family has to meet their combined deductible, whichever comes first. It works the same for out of network coverage as well.
      - Example: You have a: $3,500 deductible with a 30% co-insurance and an out of pocket max of $7000.
      - This means you have to pay 100% of all medical costs until you have spent $3,500, and will pay 30% of the costs of whatever the provider charges for all medical services until you meet the out of pocket maximum of $7,000, then you will be covered at 100% (owe nothing) from then on for the remainder of the plan year.
    - In and Out of Network Services and Deductibles:
      - In Network means providers, clinics, hospitals and treatments are covered within your insurance policy. Always check with your insurance company before going to a provider-to check its network status and any possible exclusions or specifics.
      - Out of Network means providers, clinics, hospitals and treatments are not within your insurance policy and typically it will be much more expensive to receive these services.
        - An out of network deductible is the amount you have to meet for out of network services before insurance will pick up anything.
        - Some insurance policies do not have out of network deductibles- double check to see if you do. If you do not have out of network benefits- you will always pay 100% out of pocket with no option for reimbursement.
        - If you choose to go out of network, you typically are responsible for paying 100% upfront, and filing claims

with your insurance company for every service date rendered. It can be quite confusing, but it is do-able.

- o Exclusions: are there any services that are excluded within cancer treatment?
- o What is covered?
- o Labs
- o X-Rays, CT Scans, MRIs
- o Chemotherapy
- o Radiation
- o Blood infusions
- o Room and Board
  - Is there a maximum on hospital stay days?
  - Is there a maximum on the number of hospitalizations per year?

- o Are clinical trials covered? If so, are there any portions of it that are excluded from coverage?
- o Are travel expenses covered?
- o Clinics: What is the cost of a clinic visit?
- Do we need to have the insurance company pre-approve any or all of the treatments before they occur?
- Are there any other reimbursable expenses? Transportation, etc? (Check with the IRS website as well: https://www.irs.gov/taxtopics/tc502)
- Are outpatient medications generally covered? (I would call before picking up any prescriptions when outpatient and/or double check with the medical staff to see if insurance had been called to make sure insurance is paying to the max for all meds).

- ☐ Take notes on all of the insurance information, as it's very confusing and cumbersome. Feel free to call back and ask the insurance company as many times as necessary until you fully understand your coverage. Cancer is expensive and you want to get it all straight.

~

Making the Hospital Room Cozy:
- Ask your spouse/significant other what they want you to bring from home.
- o Keep in mind there isn't anywhere to lock anything up, so you don't want to bring any valuables or anything you don't want stolen. (There may be times neither of you are in the room; don't leave anything to chance).

- o I took everything out of Grayson's wallet except his driver's license, photos and a small amount of cash. I took home his credit cards and any other personal information.
- Phone charger, pj pants, hoodie, t-shirts, socks, underwear, toothpaste, toothbrush, lotion, deodorant, hairbrush or comb, tissues, paper, pen, etc.
- Photos: Your loved one will need that comfort and familiarity, and it's something to talk to the medical staff about when they come in the room. (Grayson loved talking about our puppy and other photos I'd brought of us and family)
- Entertainment: Books, magazines, card games, Mad Libs, etc. There will be a lot of downtime and you'll need to/want to keep yourself busy at times.
- I had my brother bring us a mini-fridge from Target. It was helpful to store bottles of soda, juice, yogurt, fruit, etc. as the cost of food in the cafeteria can rack up quickly and Grayson didn't always want the food offered from the dining services menu.
- For yourself- if you're going to ever nap or sleep over, make sure you bring a face-mask and ear plugs! They were my air and water. With medical staff coming in all hours of the night, it was hard to be a pleasant cheerleader and supportive spouse when I was crabby and short on sleep. Blocking out the sound and noise every time someone came in was genius!

Think of what you'd want if you were in the hospital, and bring some of you loved one's favorite things from home to surprise them, especially if they are too tired or overwhelmed to think of what they might want you to bring.

~

Get to Know the Medical Staff: When your loved one is in the hands of the medical professionals, you want to make sure you treat them very well for everything they do. It makes all the difference in the world and doesn't hurt to make your spouse/significant other one of their favorite patients. I found that this was key in our journey. I was even told at times that nurses fought over who got to be Grayson's nurse, as he and I were so kind.

- Make an effort to remember the names of the nurses and nursing assistants that work with your spouse/significant other.
- o No matter how tired I was, I'd ask the staff their names until I remembered them, then asked them for help and thanked them by name.
- Ask them how they are when you see them for the first time each day, and say goodbye, have a good day, good night, etc., when you leave.
- Bring treats- cookies, brownies, and baked goods. Even if they are store-bought, it is still a nice gesture. Chocolate, Gummy bears and other sweet candy treats work, too!

Remember these are the people that are taking care of the most important person in your life, every second of the day, and especially when you are not there. They allow you to sleep at night, knowing they are doing their job, helping your person during these hard times.

~

Wednesday was our last day before entering the chemo world. I woke up to a nurse taking Grayson's vitals. After attempting to snuggle back into sleep for ten minutes, I surrendered to the new day and got up.

After a nurse told us Grayson would have a bone marrow biopsy within the hour, I threw on my sweatshirt and shuffled to the bathroom as my husband groaned at the news of having this painful procedure again.

I took the elevator to the cafeteria and grabbed a healthy breakfast of hash browns, two donuts and a Coke. When I returned, we caught up on local events and the frigid weather outside on the morning news on the TV set across the room from his bed. The PA came in to prep Grayson for the biopsy and I stepped it up to be his distracting entertainment.

In that moment I became "Rachel, the Funny Cancer Wife." I hadn't planned on it, and didn't make light of the gravity of the situation, but found this added humor got us through some pretty tough times. As the long thick needle went into his lower back, he closed then opened his eyes, turned his head toward me and watched me sitting on the window sill, eating donuts and guzzling down my liquid caffeine.

"Grayson, you had to be fancy, huh? You had to come here to get more attention, huh? Was I not giving you enough at home?" He let out a sigh and a laugh at the same time, and smiled at me through the pain. The nurse and PA chuckled and told us we were quite a pair. As Grayson winced, I jumped off my perch, knelt at his side and told him to take deep breaths. Within minutes it was done and he lay on his back for the mandated hour with a thick white bandage to seal the puncture wound. He had me check it after a half an hour; I found his sheets and gown soaked in blood. One nurse call and five minutes later he was as good as new.

Bright and early the next day it was time to start chemo. Grayson had to give the last cryogenic sample before treatment could start. The nurses put a sign on the door asking no one to enter and I stood watch behind the white and green curtain blockading the door as he put our last possible kid into a cup. I then wrapped the specimen cup in a plastic bag, set it carefully in an extra hat I had in my purse and left for the clinic. It had to be kept warm, so I bundled it to me as I waited for the valet to bring my car up front. I drove the twenty minutes to the clinic, dropped it off and headed back to Grayson. One of his best friends from high school, Bella, told me later that I could tell our kid one day that it took its first car ride without a seat belt. God bless laughter during these times.

~

Employment: Can Your Spouse Work Anymore or Part-time?

- Contacting Your Spouse/Significant Other's Employer: When the diagnosis is given and the treatment plan is established, the next step is to inform your spouse/significant other's employer. Most likely your loved one will be too overwhelmed to do this, so if possible do this for them. Some employers may require talking to the employee directly, but try to help as much as you can.

- Patient's Inability to Work: If your spouse/significant other cannot work:

o Contact FMLA: the Family Medical Leave Act is a federal legal policy that guarantees employees can take time off of work unpaid due to illnesses, serious illnesses, and caregiving of immediate family without the risk or threat of losing their position within the company, for certain periods of time.

- To be eligible for FMLA, the employee generally has to have been employed by the company for at least a year to qualify.
- PTO: When on FMLA, you first use your accrued PTO–Paid Time Off of your sick and vacation days. When those have all been used, you can use unpaid time off, and your job will still be secured for the agreed-upon period of time off.

o Disability: Contact the HR: Human Resources department to inform of the employee's diagnosis and work status if they cannot return to work during treatment. The Disability Department can help navigate how the benefits work.

- Short-term disability (STD): pays a portion of the employee's income for a short amount of time, depending on the plan, this pay out can generally last between three to twelve months.
- Long-term disability (LTD): pays a portion of the employee's income after short-term disability ends, for the plan period, sometimes for one to two years or more, depending on the company.
  - o Grayson did not have a LTD policy because he was only 35 and didn't think this was necessary. Big Mistake! I encourage everyone I know to make sure they elect this through their employer– it is a crucial move, just in case.
    - Familiarize yourself with how long these disability payments last and what the pay structure is:
      - It can be 80% of the regular pay for 6 weeks, then 60% for 4 weeks, and so on. It varies.
- Updating the Employer: Find out how often the supervisor/HR department will need updates on your spouse/significant other's health treatment/progress.

~

Work Status: If the Patient Can Work During Treatment:
  - o Contact/Meet with the supervisor to go over diagnosis, treatment plan and any physical/mental health accommodations that may be needed as treatments occur.

- Example-if you have a job where you are standing the majority of your shift, can you have a chair or stool, or are there other less strenuous duties/tasks you can do in place of your normal ones while undergoing treatment?
- Most employers these days like to be in the loop about what is going on in their employees' lives, and are willing to make accommodations to best meet the physical/medical/mental health needs of their employees. In addition, the ADA-American Disabilities Act may also apply.
  o Contact FMLA and see if "Intermittent Leave" or a "Reduced Work Schedule" can be applied.
  o This type of leave is on an as-needed basis, or reduces work hours to meet the medical/physical needs of the employee. This can protect your job when you need to have time off for scheduled medical appointments, or unexpected instances when the employee may be too sick to attend work or to perform work duties.

  ☐ It may seem daunting to figure out how all of this works, however managers, human resources, disability and FMLA professionals are qualified and able to help walk you through this process.

~

Caregiver Time Off:
- Inform your supervisor as soon as you can about your new life situation. Again, employers are typically glad to know what is going on and can provide ideas on how to help you regarding possible options or resources.
  o Check with your HR department about caregiver time off. The FMLA program often has allowances for spouses to take care of sick spouses or children. You will need to use your PTO until it runs out, and then take unpaid time off.
  o Inform your supervisor that you may need to leave unexpectedly at times or to take time off without any notice to be with your spouse/significant other. Give as much notice as possible when you know of upcoming appointments or procedures you need to attend. Giving a heads up is always appreciated.

  ☐ Do not be afraid to check in with your supervisor and let them know what is happening. This is a major life change and of course, you will want to be there with your loved one as much as you can.

~

Legalities: Power of Attorney, Advanced Directives and Wills: This is probably the last thing anyone wants to deal with- however it's vital to take steps to put the proper documents in place in case anything happens. I highly recommend doing this even if your loved one has a great prognosis. I believe everyone should have Advanced Directives and Wills put into place, as anything can happen to any of us, and it's better to have your wishes known instead of leaving your loved ones wondering or arguing about what you would have wanted.

- POA: Power of Attorney: This allows the appointed person to act on behalf of the spouse/significant other/patient for any or all legal or financial matters, or if otherwise specified.
  - o I learned the hard way that I needed this when I had to jump through several hoops to take care of things that were only in Grayson's name, like our cable service. I spent twenty-five minutes in line at a Comcast office only to learn I could not make changes without written or verbal permission by Grayson to do so.
  - o You can ask for the hospital notary to come to the hospital room to help fill out and notarize the forms.
  - o Forms: Hospitals can provide these, or you can find them simply by searching the term "Power of Attorney," online with your state.
  - o Do not sign any forms until the notary is present.
    - If you do not have these done at the hospital, you can always go to your local bank and do this there.
- Advanced Directives: This is a document that lists one's wishes on the types of medical treatment one would like when they are no longer able to make decisions for themselves.
  - Are life preserving measures desired?
    - o CPR
    - o Going on a ventilator- life support
      - How long will this last and under what conditions would it continue?
      - If you are on life support and there is nothing that can be done to preserve life, is it ok to withhold nutrition and water?
  - Who can be there during the dying process with the patient?
  - Spiritual preferences desired during the illness, death and dying process
  - Is a memorial, funeral or celebration of life desired?
  - Musical preferences
  - Any other wishes of the patient

- Wills: Living Wills and Wills
- o Living Wills: Similar to Advanced Directives- give instructions to medical staff and family members on what the patient wants in regards to treatment if they become incapacitated or are unable to make decisions themselves.
  - These can be found online by state in a general search or at Legalzoom.com
    - o Wills: Designations of whom the deceased wants their property, items or money to go to after they are gone, along with any instructions or stipulations on how these things are to be utilized.
- National Cancer Legal Services Network http://www.nclsn.org
- https://www.cancerlegalcare.org

☐ Once you have documents in place, you will feel more relaxed and secure in knowing that if, God forbid, something happens, your loved one's wishes have been written down and will be honored.

Chapter 5:
Chemo, Pirate Skulls and Clinical Trials

One of the most common words that goes hand in hand when anyone thinks of the word cancer is chemotherapy. It's the most commonly used treatment for cancer, as it often is very successful in eradicating the diseased cells that are harming the patient's body. We all know it can cause hair to fall out, nausea and for some, vomiting, but for the most part we know it's a necessary evil. What you usually don't think about is how dangerous it is and how something that toxic can be put into someone's blood stream despite the reasons why.

Many of the chemo infusion bags that I saw had skulls and crossbones on them. Some contained neon-yellow liquid that looked like Mountain Dew, and others were so sensitive to light, they were covered in an extra black bag for protection. Whenever Grayson had an infusion –chemo, red or white blood cells, or plasma–two nurses had to be present, which I found reassuring as his life depended on their accuracy and care. One nurse would look at Grayson's armband and ask him his full name and date of birth, then stated the infusion drug name that was listed on the bag, while the other nurse confirmed it all from their computer system.

During the second week of the inpatient stay, Grayson was offered the opportunity to be part of a clinical trial for young adults ages eighteen to thirty-five who were diagnosed with ALL. We chose the U for its world-renowned reputation, expertise and the benefit of it being a teaching hospital. As the lead research nurse Nadia handed me the forty-page clinical trial document, she explained the intricate elements of the study that would last a total of ten years, three and a half of them involving chemotherapy infusions. Grayson would receive higher doses of chemo than traditional regimens that would be very hard on his body. Grayson told us, "If I can help others know what treatments work to hopefully cure this thing one day, then I really want to be a part of this. I'm here anyway and want to help in any way I can."

My mind spun as I looked through the protocol's pages of charts and terminology that I didn't understand yet. When I think of it now, it was essentially like signing him up for boot camp, then dropping him off in a foreign land. I would be there with him to support him as he fought the enemy, but I'd never be able to fully understand the war he fought with his body, alone in the trenches.

I quickly got into the routine of running home after work to let the dog out, then driving to the hospital to spend a couple hours with Grayson before heading home to sleep, and start the cycle all over again the next day. One night I had what I call "The Dreaded Elevator Episode." As I was bundling up to head home, I looked back at Grayson sitting alone in his bed in the cold spartan hospital room, void of a home's true comforts that we all take for granted. I literally could not move. My feet would not move. It felt like they were magnetized to the floor, held in place by a force I could not control. I had an inner dialogue running through my head telling me I couldn't leave him there and go home to our home sweet home, to the house we picked out together, full of our lives' treasures and pets.

How could I leave when he was stuck there all by himself? Waves of uncertainty rocked me to the core and propelled me forward to his bedside where I broke down crying, hugging him and telling him I was so sorry I had to leave him there. We talked for a few minutes then I attempted to leave, but it happened all over again. On my third attempt, I summoned enough strength to make it to the door where I looked back at my husband one last time, told him I loved him and would be back the next day. I looked at the nurses at the station across the hall with a red, puffy, wet face as they gave me sympathetic smiles and told me he'd be well looked after.

I walked as quickly as I could down the hall, then stared at the silver metal elevators waiting for it to arrive on my floor. The doors opened and I just stood there sweating in my winter coat, hat and scarf looking at them but couldn't get myself to go inside. I ran back down the hall past the red, orange and blue matchstick art on the wall, to his room where I cried and hugged Grayson one last time. I said a little prayer and made my way back to the bank of elevators, this time getting on as I said aloud, "I can do this, hell if I know how, but I can do this!"

I walked to the lobby past the fancy plants, the closed gift shop and coffee bar and out into the cold. The valet service was closed at that time of night, so I trekked it the block and a half to the parking garage. I let the whipping winds and frigid temps smack me in the face. This became a regular practice. The cold pelting my skin was the welcomed wake-up trick that I so direly needed after the nightly trauma of leaving Grayson in the hospital. During the day and on most weekends when the valet service was not running, I would use the U's underground "Gopher Tunnels," that connected dorms, buildings and parking garages to be used during the inhumane winter temperatures, but at night during the week I opted to brave the elements outside. By the time I got in my car I had sobered up. I turned on the radio and shifted my mind to what I needed to do at home with my pets, and to prepare for the next day. There really is no place like your own home. It's the ultimate alpha and omega of where we all want to be on our worst days. I wanted to be there all the time, but since my other half was in the hospital, I had to put that desire on hold.

Most of the time on the twenty-minute ride home I'd call my parents, siblings or a close friend to detox. It is a blessing and a curse at times to be the biggest insider, having a front row seat as the spouse/significant other, with the inability to turn off your mind. All I seemed to talk about was the medical mumbo-jumbo. It was hard to remember to talk about fun and happy things as well. Cancer and all it entails is an endless vortex and it's helpful to have distractions from time to time!

Announcement of Illness, Treatment and Support via Social Media:

- Ask your significant other/spouse what they would like. Not everyone will want their new illness broadcast publicly; ensure you have their permission to do so.

- If your loved one is okay with you sharing information, ask what you can share:
    - Are exact specifics okay to discuss- ex: "He/She is having a biopsy today"
    - Or would they rather have you say "He/She is not feeling well today after treatment."
- If you'd like to share information about the diagnosis, it's helpful to include a link to the specific cancer type your loved one has. Links can be found on the American Cancer Society, Leukemia and Lymphoma Society websites, etc.

- ☐ CANCER has to be one of the scariest words known to man, and so many people do not know how to respond to it. Providing info and letting them be a part of your journey can allow them to feel updated and involved, and you can receive support this way as well.

~

What to Do When Loved Ones Want to Visit or Help Out: As soon as you announce the diagnosis and illness, you may receive several requests asking how to help. This can be overwhelming while also comforting to know you're so supported.

- Think of practical things that would help you out, that you may not have the time or energy to do.
- Make a list and let those friends or family members know what you need most and be as specific as possible. I found out that so many of our loved ones wanted to help but didn't know how. When I had specific things to do, people were glad to step up and assist.
- o Transportation: The patient may need rides to appointments if you're working and cannot provide them.
- Chemo/radiation treatments sometimes result in the patient's inability to safely drive to and from appointments. Even if the patient says they are fine, get a chemo buddy to help out and sit there at appointments.
- o When my parents or I couldn't take him to appointments, I had a team of friends that I asked to be with Grayson.
- The American Cancer Society has a program called "Road to Recovery," that provides free rides to medical appointments. https://www.cancer.org/treatment/support-programs-and-services/road-to-recovery.html
- o Pets: Pet care – walking, feeding, litter box, pet sitting. My neighbors who lived behind me were incredibly kind and generous, often taking Greta to their house with their dog, or letting her out when needed and feeding her and the cats. It's so comforting to know you don't have to worry about your pets when you have backup care.
- o Running errands/tasks: Give a list of things you need from Target or the grocery store and let someone help you with it.

31

- o Meals: Often getting a nutritious meal is hard with limited time, especially if you're balancing work, helping/visiting the patient and also if you have children. There are really cool websites out there now that can help organize meals for your family where you can list specific meals desired, any allergies, days of the week you would like food and food delivery time.
- There was nothing like this around when Grayson was sick, and it would have been so cool to have this! Our elderly neighbors John and Betty and Olivia and Grayson would randomly bring over cookies or fresh baked bread and it was the coolest and nicest surprise.
- Meal Sharing websites:
  Lotsa Helping Hands: https://lotsahelpinghands.com,
  Meal Train: https://www.mealtrain.com
  Take Them a Meal: https://takethemameal.com
  Care Calendar: https://www.carecalendar.org
- o Seasonal Help: Depending on the season and weather you may need help with home or lawn care tasks.
  - Ask a neighbor if they can mow the lawn for you or if you can pay them to do so. We had an amazing neighbor, Fred, who was retired from working at an inside job for thirty years and was more than happy to mow our yard during the spring and summer, and was kind enough to plow the snow in our driveway in the winter. Fred and his wife Jan even shoveled us out one time, during a snowstorm when I needed to get to the hospital, and our neighbor Ed helped with the snow as well. We were so blessed for this kindness!
  - Hire a neighborhood kid to mow or shovel if you cannot.
    - o The summer after Grayson died I hired a sixteen-year-old that my church had referred me to, whom I paid $40 twice a month to mow. It worked out great. I shoveled the best I could in the winter, and it worked out fine.

- Your supporters most likely really want to help, but feel helpless in knowing they cannot fix your situation for you. By providing specific tangible tasks, you can receive the assistance you need, and they can feel useful and supportive.

During the third week of Grayson's stay, his supervisor Adam came to visit. They'd worked together several years and although Grayson had been pretty unhappy with his job the last few years and detested all of the extra work he'd been given, he was happy to see a familiar face. Adam brought him some books and magazines to keep him entertained, along with a very nice card and gift card from all of his coworkers. I watched Adam as he grappled with what to say to Grayson, as anyone would have in his shoes, as this was not something any of us had dealt with before. Grayson carried it all with grace and kindness, attempting to crack

32

jokes and make conversation during the awkward silences. Grayson told me earlier that day that literally two weeks before his diagnosis, a coworker had actually said, "Everett, you look really pale and weak, what do you have, leukemia?" then laughed. Oh. My. Goodness. I wondered how they felt after learning of his diagnosis.

~

Online Social Support: Establishing a virtual social support base to update family, friends, loved ones, co-workers and anyone who cares about you and your spouse/significant other is a great thing/important thing to do.

Reasons to do so:

- One central place to share information.
- You can either update it yourself from first person, or assign a close friend or family member to do it. (I did ours and at times Grayson shared his own posts).
- You can ignore all of the texts and emails you may be getting from many people, opting just to do an online blog post that everyone reads. It gets you off the hook from feeling like you have to contact everyone when you're too busy and too tired to respond.

CaringBridge: If you've never heard of CaringBridge, you are in for a treat. It's a website where the patient themselves, loved ones or family members can post medical updates, hospital information and photos to share with family, friends and supporters. It quickly became a pinnacle part of our journey where I began to update our support system via a shared link that required a login and password, so the entire world couldn't know about our lives, but those in our army would.

CaringBridge: Jan. 26, 2011: Today Grayson is doing and looking great, in my opinion as well as the medical staff. Zoe, my oldest friend from childhood, is here for a few days, which combined with Rachel = many entertaining antics, jokes and constant laughs for Grayson. So far we've had lunch, done crosswords, and played 'Fact or Crap,' testing our trivia knowledge. Yesterday I chopped off 6 inches of my hair in honor of Grayson's impending hair loss to support him! We thank God for friends and family! Love Grayson and Rachel

Zoe came to visit the week after Grayson was diagnosed; the trip had been planned pre-illness. I met her in first grade and she was my kindred. We are very extroverted, weird, nutty, authentic and connected. It was an absolute Godsend that she was there during that time, as I was craving familial support, but my parents and siblings were all in different states. Zoe came with me as I cut my locks to support Grayson and watched me fix the not-so-stellar cut at home, shaping it into a cute pixie cut. We went on mini-adventures to the Mall of America to the Sanrio Hello Kitty store, Panda Express and just walked around talking about how odd and unknown my life had become so quickly. We lit candles, held hands and prayed through tears at the Basilica of St. Mary, wondering what would come next. My red-headed spitfire best friend, who had been my maid of honor when I'd married Grayson many years ago, brought so much laughter and joy to us when we needed it most.

CaringBridge: Jan. 29, 2011: Grayson is doing great. He continues to have his wit and dry sense of humor that make all those around him laugh. He has had 3 treatments so far and is progressing well. Love Rachel and Grayson

~

Self-Image and Hair Loss:

During week three, Grayson's hair began to fall out. The beast that is cancer doesn't allow hair to fall out gracefully, but then again, it isn't a ballet, either. There can be beauty in the journey depending on your attitude, but cancer is a beast no less. Luckily, Grayson and I both had a great sense of humor, which made his hair loss from chemotherapy not as sad as it could have been. When his began to fall out in clumps, he got the idea to do a Saturday Night Live-esque version of cutting it off in stages and dancing as I took pictures. Grayson started out the process by shaving just the sides, creating a Mohawk, then leaving bits and pieces, reminding me of the characters in the game "Guess Who?" When he got to the last chunk of hair, he frowned to himself in the mirror and said "Here we go!" then shaved the rest. I sucked in a deep breath, feeling my stomach hit my feet. My husband now looked like a cancer patient. He was hairless, losing weight and mostly confined to a bed while hooked up to wires and IV poles. Breathe in, breathe out. This was the new us, whether I liked it or not.

The experience of losing one's hair can be very difficult, as we most often identify ourselves to others to somewhat of a degree, by our outward appearance. It's the first thing someone sees when they look at us, as they have no idea of our inner character, or who we really are. We express ourselves by how we dress and style ourselves, and cancer can very quickly strip away that ability. Many men opt to sport being bald, some wear hats and others are already bald or balding. For most women this can be a traumatic experience as it most definitely immediately changes things, especially if you've spent years growing out longer hair. Luckily there are more and more options created each year to provide women undergoing cancer treatment with wigs, hats and scarves to choose from online.

Keep in mind, no matter how you think you look, or what someone might choose to think about you based on those looks, you are a warrior on a path that no one can know unless they have been there themselves!

During this time my dad and I saw a little boy in the cafeteria one day who was singing while he held onto a tray in one hand, an IV pole in the other and navigated his way to a table. This bald child no more than ten years old, was in pjs, and had wires going from a shirt pocket above his heart, connected to a battery pack, but he sang and pushed along to his destination acting just like any other kid. My dad and I smiled at each other and discussed how if that kid could find joy in the storm of it all and choose positivity, then so could we. He gave us faith and hope in Grayson being okay too, just by witnessing his spirit. Even all these years later, my dad and I reflect on that little kid who showed us what happiness in the storm could look like.

There are many websites that offer help with self-image and hair loss during the cancer process including: www.headcovers.com
American Cancer Society: https://www.tlcdirect.org/Wigs-for-Cancer-and-Chemotherapy-Patients-TLC-Wig-Collection-American-Cancer-Society-TLC-Direct
Livestrong: https://www.livestrong.org/we-can-help/emotional-and-physical-effects-of-treatment/body-image
https://www.cancer.gov/about-cancer/coping/self-image

~

Tattoos, Endless Driving and Exciting News
CaringBridge: Feb 1, 2011: Today is day 22 since the start of this journey & day 16 of Grayson being at the U. We continually pray daily for strength, thanking God that Grayson is in this setting with experts and kind, understanding hearts. On Sunday I got a tattoo to honor Grayson so I could not only carry him in my heart, but also on my wrist. ~ Love Rachel and Grayson

As Grayson got farther into his treatment, he began to have super crappy complications of more intensive night sweats, insomnia, and stomach cramping, despite the pre-meds given before the infusions. My sweet husband had begun to become frustrated with his body that was betraying him more each day. He could no longer sleep without the help of meds, and even when he was able to sleep, he was often wakened for blood draws, infusions and vital checks. He quickly learned that food didn't taste as good as it had before chemo started, to his frustration. He had a menu to choose from for three daily meals – whatever his taste buds would permit at the time, but after a couple weeks of getting his butt kicked by chemo, that became a chore. His energy was zapped and the desire to eat was nil.

At this point, I was used to balancing my work schedule of 8-4, 10-6 or 12-8 depending on the activities that I was doing, pet care and going to the hospital. Due to this major life change, I had to quit my part time nanny job that was one night a week and weekends, as well as resign from the LGBTQ Aging board I was on at the time. I only slept six to seven hours a night, and was running on pure adrenaline every day out of the super power strength that I could feel coursing through my veins. I had no choice but to keep chugging on. When I think back on it, I have no idea how I did it all. All I knew was that the love of my life was in the hospital facing the biggest challenge of his life, and our life together, and that I wanted to be there for him as much as I could. As scary as it sounds, I could basically drive back and forth to the hospital from our house on auto-pilot. You know when you drive somewhere and when you're partway through the drive and you realize you've been zoning out and question how you've been safely driving and gotten to that point so far? It was like that, constant zombie tiredness, yet running on love and a mission to take care of it all, to be by Grayson's side.

One day when I was leaving the hospital room to go home for the night, I gave Grayson a hug. As I started to walk away from his bed he said, "Don't leave me. Please don't ever leave me!" with tears falling down his face. I dropped my purse, ran to the bed, and hugged him while wiping away his tears, and reassured him that would never happen, that I loved him, he was my world and I couldn't imagine my life without him.

I have no idea how in the universe, world or God's green earth, cancer patients do it. Over time I saw how extremely painful, scary, frustrating and alarming it was for Grayson to be at the daily mercy of this seventh circle of hell that was cancer. The loneliness that enveloped him was something he didn't often express to me, but I knew it was present, like the elephant in the room. I'd call him every morning on my way to work, in the afternoon, and to say goodnight. We'd recite the Lord's Prayer together when I got home from the hospital. Living for weeks, literally within only the four walls of a hospital room, surrounded by machines, medical smells and medical staff was quite a sight to behold, and anyone's version of a nightmare. I continued to try to figure out how I could bring joy to his face each day when so many things continued to be taken away from him.

It was after that night that I decided to get "Grayson" tattooed on the inside of my left wrist, in a cursive script with a small purple star. When Grayson and I were dating and I worked at a garden, I purchased a commemorative brick there that was printed with "Rachel Loves Grayson, You Are My Star," forever stamping my feelings for him. I would write him poems over the years and would always do a little star on the page with line-like sparks coming out of the star. I got the tattoo done at Steady Ink Tattoo, where I'd had rebellion eyebrow and nose piercings at ages eighteen and twenty-two. I was excited and apprehensive at the same time; this was my first tattoo. The buzzing of the machine pen made me jump in anticipation of the pain, when I walked into the shop. Ready or not, it was happening. I was hell-bent on doing this to honor Grayson. After having my desired script traced, put on paper, then onto my wrist for approval, the inking began. As each letter was etched into my skin, I felt pride in doing this for my husband. I paid, got my after-care sheet and walked around the block to the hospital to show Grayson. He was so blown away, that he told anyone and everyone that came into his room for the next week, his smile oozing with pride.

Several frustrating things happened during these first five weeks. His mom, Victoria, had given us a new Teflon cookware set for Christmas, even though Grayson specifically asked for stainless steel. I went to Macy's at the mall to exchange it, only to be told I could not do so until the next day during the planned sale. As I stood there at the counter, sweaty in my winter coat and gear, I freaked out on the cashier. I told her, "I cannot come back tomorrow! I have no free time, my husband has cancer and is in the hospital and I work full time and I can't come back tomorrow!!!" The poor lady looked at me with wide eyes, picked up the phone, called her manager, then did the exchange. It's crazy how a task like exchanging something at a department store, can make you lose your mind when you're balancing what I was at the time.

Another time I was at Target in a food aisle and overheard a lady on her phone complaining about a lingering cold. I had to bite my tongue not to go all Mr. T on her. I wanted to yell, "Shut up! You don't know how good you have it! My husband is lying in the hospital, fighting for his life and you're here complaining about freaking cough syrup?" I know everyone has their own life battles and problems, but when you're in a fishbowl like mine was at the time, you tend to be super sensitive. I had a younger coworker who was worried about whether her boyfriend was going to get her a certain desired gift for Valentine's Day. I almost went off on her as well- as my fuse was short. It's amazing how our bodies and minds go into defensive mode, and our life struggles are magnified on the Jumbotron of our minds. At any point in life it's really hard when you want to be in too many places at once, but with Grayson in the hospital, I felt like a victim on a firing line. My life and what I knew had been taken from me (hopefully only temporarily). While it was happening, my fuse was burning faster than I could run.

Each weekday I called Grayson mid-morning to get the morning report after the doctors had done their rounds. I had down pat what levels his white blood cells, platelets and hemoglobin should optimally be. I knew the chemo drugs he was taking and their possible side effects. I visited as many nights as I could, sanitizing in the hallway, then giving him a hug and kiss before I'd run upstairs to grab dinner before we caught up on each other's day. Most nights I had black bean burgers, fries and soda. It was not the healthiest, but it got me through, and I ate salads for lunch at work. I ended up gaining weight because of my poor diet, but took it all in stride. I was doing the best I could to balance everything.

Grayson was so goody-two-shoes kind, which makes me giggle to think back on. While undergoing chemotherapy, I was not permitted to use the bathroom in his room, as it was possible for me to come into contact with the toxic chemicals that he peed out. The nurses had to suit up each time they measured his urine output, and after seeing how much of a production it was to put on a gown, masks and gloves, Grayson began to write the amounts he'd peed on the white board in his room to save the nurses from having to get dressed up, to their surprise and delight. He was just so very kind and considerate all the time. I witnessed him making staff laugh many times when he'd ask, "Can I trouble you for something?," when he'd need something, being so kind as if he was putting them out by asking them to do their job.

We tried to be as normal as possible by playing cards, doing Mad Libs, watching movies, having sleepovers, and occasionally having a friend or two visit if Grayson felt up to it. My sisters sent him fun shirts with the Kool-Aid Man, Smurfs, Superman and the Muppets on them that became conversation starters with the staff who entered his room. Felicity and Diana kept him stocked in pajama pants, Goldfish crackers and sweet treats, which he enjoyed.

CaringBridge: Feb. 8, 2011: Thank you again for all of your stories, notes & well wishes! Grayson is doing great. He is taking a couple of walks every day and doing exercises. We thank God for his strength. He seems like himself with his witty sense of humor and amazing smile. He was taken off his IV pole, which I named Trudy (I would tell him "Trudy follows you around everywhere you go!") giving him more independence! GO TEAM GRAYSON! Love Rachel and Grayson

CaringBridge: Feb. 10, 2011: Hello All! Grayson is continuing to do well! We love all of the support, kindness and stories! We thank God for all of you! R & G

I knew when Grayson came home he wouldn't be able to navigate our house as he had been able to pre-illness, which meant he wouldn't be able to do the stairs to get to our entertainment and TV watching area in the family room in the basement. I decided to replace the mismatched sofas with covers on them upstairs, along with purchasing a television and stand. I wanted to make a new cozy haven for him as he'd be spending all of his free time outside of clinic visits at home. I ran from store to store in the winter weather in a bundled-up, sweaty mess and was satisfied with my purchases in the end.

CaringBridge: Feb. 17, 2011: Today is day 29 of Grayson's 29-day Induction Phase of Chemotherapy! Please pray while we wait for the results of his biopsies that will tell us whether he can go home in a week, or if he has to be inpatient for an additional 3 weeks. He is doing great and is truckin' on! Love Rachel and Grayson

CaringBridge: Feb. 20, 2011: Amazing, Amazing, Amazing news! Grayson's tests came back and after 35 days in the hospital and his hard work: HE IS IN REMISSION!!! And COMING HOME ON MONDAY!!! We thank God so much for all of our blessings! He starts outpatient chemo on Thursday. Please pray and/or think about us as we venture into this new uncharted territory & help us celebrate our blessing! Love Rachel and Grayson

~

Health Status Updates from the Medical Team:
- If you are unable to attend appointments or to be at the hospital when the MDs do their rounds, you can call the nurses' station for an update. It's your right as the spouse/significant other to get the most up-to-date information. Your loved one may be able to recall everything the MDs told them, but with so much information being told on a daily, sometimes hourly basis, and depending on how they are feeling, they may forget pertinent info you will want to know. You can ask them:
  o What is the most recent update?
  o Are there any new side effects I should be aware of?
  o Do you think that treatment is going as planned?
  o Is there anything we/I can do to help out the patient that is not currently happening?

  By asking these questions you will have more peace of mind and feel secure in knowing you aren't missing any pieces to the puzzle if you cannot be there.

Chapter 6:
Coming Home and Our New Life

W e were originally told that Grayson would be good to go and ready to come home the following Monday, but on Wednesday Grayson's doctor called, telling me my husband would be discharged on Friday instead. My sister Felicity had graciously paid for a cleaning service to come sanitize and prep for Grayson's arrival, helping clean the whole house and get rid of pet hair from our two cats and dog. As soon as I heard of his early discharge, I could not stop shouting, "I'm not ready!"

Green Darlene, a cleaning company owned and operated by a husband and wife team that created a green and cancer-friendly cleaning service after the wife's own cancer experience, was scheduled to come and clean that Friday. I called them and this lovely couple who would later become family friends agreed to come Friday morning to meet our needs. Despite my relief, I still couldn't stop yelling, "I'm not ready!" to my parents, siblings, and friends and on Facebook, as I asked for prayers. I had to put together the new TV stand, set up the living room and make the rest of our house safe for my husband. I rearranged our bedroom so he would be closest to the bedroom door. The couches wouldn't be delivered for another week, but that wasn't a huge deal to me in the big picture. Grayson was out of his mind excited to see our cats and dog, while I was freaking out like a chicken with my head cut off to get everything ready, work full time and going back and forth to the hospital. I went to the store to buy produce and healthy meats for his meals to fill the small standing freezer I'd purchased the week before.

Before Grayson was allowed to come home I had to take an hour-long crash course in cleaning his PICC line (peripherally inserted central catheter), to my dismay. This central line that was implanted in his arm was used each time he needed blood draws and infusions, eliminating the need for a new IV each clinic visit. I trained on a dummy lying on a table. I learned how to clean the two small catheters that hung off the line, as well as how to rip the entire line out of his body via his arm if it became infected. It was all a bit scary at first to be responsible for something so vital, but I got used to it in time.

Friday morning I worked a half day, and then went to pick up Grayson, feeling a mix of excitement and fear. The discharge process involved another crash course in medical care, as I received nearly twenty pages of printed instructions on his new med schedule, symptoms and side effects to look for in the coming days, weeks and months. It all made my head spin, but I worked on deep breathing to remain calm.

While waiting for his meds at the pharmacy, I saw a tall, thin, exhausted bald man who looked a lot like Grayson at the time. When asked about a caregiver by the pharmacist, he said he was alone. In that moment I felt so terrible for this stranger, and reflected on how lonely and difficult it must be to be on that journey without a key person for support. I carried the large shopping bag of pills back to Grayson's room, thanking God for the life Grayson and I had together. Grayson was wheeled downstairs by staff to his waiting beloved steel gray Subaru WRX. He gingerly got into the front seat and sighed in relief with an ear to ear grin. I drove very carefully in the falling snow in his car that I nicknamed "Clint Eastwood" due to its grizzly and manly gear shifts, feeling like I had a newborn baby beside me.

We arrived to the welcoming committee of Rufus, Puddin' and Clive that met us at the front door with squeaks, meows and tail-wagging. As Grayson relaxed on a sofa, I began to try to make sense of his complicated medicine regimen. He had to take multiple pills daily at 8 a.m., 10:30 a.m., 2 p.m., 6 p.m. and bedtime. He was tired and mentally taxed from treatment, so it was up to me to figure it all out for him.

That night I silently freaked out at bedtime, thinking he would somehow fall out of bed and break all of his bones. Pre-illness Grayson was a lean 180 lbs., and now he was down to 145 lbs., which was so teeny on his 6'2 frame. He seemed like a fragile doll. I wished I had a padded ring around the bed and everywhere he went just in case he fell. I had put up grab bars on the shower walls and purchased a shower chair for when he was too weak to stand.

That first week after he was home, I ran to Walgreens no less than six times and spent hundreds of dollars to get the medical equipment we found was necessary to check his vitals and emerging health needs. I had to purchase several large days-of-the-week pill boxes, a blood pressure gauge, a new scale, a digital thermometer, lavender baby lotion and creams for his sensitive skin, gauze and netting to wrap around his PICC line like an arm band, baby tooth brushes for his sensitive teeth and gums, Pedialyte for dehydration and countless other small items.

~

Preparing Your Home for Your Cancer Patient/Loved One:

- Discharge Prep: Ask the medical staff what your spouse/significant other will need at home, and what the next treatment steps will be as soon as you get the discharge timeline. It's better to know what you might need to run around and get ahead of time, and what the upcoming schedule will most likely look like, then to be unprepared later on.
- I highly recommend these items and staples based on what Grayson needed/desired:
  o Blood pressure monitor
  o Digital thermometer
  o Lavender lotion -for sleeping and relaxation
  o Ginger ale- for nausea or upset stomach
  o Lemon Ginger tea- for nausea or upset stomach
  o Saltines or similar crackers- for easy calories with loss of appetite or upset stomach
  o Boost or Ensure protein shakes for easy calories

o   Ginger chews or hard peppermint candies -for nausea or upset stomach

o   Plenty of hand soap for every sink

o   Hand sanitizer for at home when they are too tired to sanitize at the sink after petting animals, before eating, etc., and also to have on hand when on the go.

o   Sanitizing wipes-to keep counters, common surfaces and door handles clean

o   Shower chair- (I bought Grayson a $25 one at Walgreens that helped him tremendously)

o   Shower Safety grab bars- Walmart/Home Depot. Make sure the suction cup is secure. It will need to be refastened every few days which is an easy task

o   Journal -for the patient to record symptoms, schedule, whatever they want to write down. (Grayson recorded the names of family or friends he talked to over the phone or visited, to add to his daily schedule. He also wrote down the gifts he received so he could write thank you cards.)

o   Slippers or fuzzy cozy socks- to keep your loved ones feet warm; they will often be cold.

o   Bathrobe- to keep them warm as they will often be cold and too tired to dress in layers or may fall asleep on the couch and become cold, needing that extra warmth.

—   Getting all of these things cost more than I expected, but it was worth it to have the items that he needed for comfort, and we needed for peace of mind.

~

CaringBridge: Feb. 24, 2011: Grayson is home and doing well. He's happy to be in our bed, not eating hospital food & with our pets! In the next few days he will have inpatient and outpatient chemo. Please continue to keep us in your thoughts during this tough transitional & busy time. Love Rachel and Grayson

Despite the turmoil that cancer created in our lives, one of the biggest blessings was the time Grayson and I were able to spend with my mom and dad. They'd hatched a plan back when Grayson was still in the hospital, committing to being Grayson's long-term caregivers after I shared with them the intense schedule of clinic appointments per the clinical protocol. I never thought in my wildest dreams that I'd be twenty-eight and feel comfortable having my parents live with me, however I never thought I'd be in the situation I'd found myself in, either! All those years I'd wanted to break free as a teen had been replaced with a young woman who needed her mom and dad to help keep her afloat, and make sure someone was there to care for her very ill husband, monitoring him for fall prevention or to drive him to the emergency room if he had a temperature of 100.1 or above. I am so grateful to my parents to this day, unable to fully articulate how much they rescued me and provided me with the love and support I needed during those years.

Grayson had known my parents for nine years at this point, but we all learned more about each other on more intimate levels by living together in our three-bedroom rambler home.

Marie and Ryan moved into our guest bedroom a week after Grayson came home from the hospital, which provided me with sense of peace I didn't know I'd been missing. Grayson had clinic appointments five days a week for three months, then three times a week for three months, then two times a week for two months, then one time a week for two and a half years, then every other week for six months and so on. There was no way I would have been able to manage that without the help of my kind and generous parents.

Grayson quickly became accustomed to waking up to the smell of breakfast meats cooking and having the option of eggs, pancakes or French toast from my dad, his chef. This was the dad that all of my friends adored; my house was the one they wanted to stay at for sleepovers when I was little, as a big breakfast was customary the next morning. When he stayed with us, he would walk around the house and sing Elvis, Johnny Cash, gospel or hymns as he did chores, cleaned, dishes and laundry. Grayson loved having the company and cheer around him after he'd been so isolated and alone for all of those weeks when he was hospitalized.

My mom is a power-punched, 5'2", kooky little lady with a heart of gold who talks your ear off until the wee hours of the night. I get my creativeness and chattiness from her and unending desires to help others from both of my parents. It was my mom's mission to make sure that Grayson did not want for a cup of tea or beverage and that he was always covered up with a blanket, just in case. She'd forget her own beverage in the microwave, reheating it several times, resulting in an endless beeping that made us want to scale the walls, but she'd always make sure you had what you needed. I quickly became fine with my parents folding my underwear when doing laundry and knowing where everything was in my house. I was too tired to care after working a full day and taking care of the pets and supporting Grayson. My parents and I alternated between setting the table and cooking dinner each night. I was so grateful to have all the help that I did.

In contrast to the warmth of Marie and Ryan, Grayson's parents Victoria and Bernard were a whole other tale. I'm including everything that occurred during this time because I've always been an open book and I want to remain true to what this journey entailed.

I was exposed to maltreatment from his mother during almost the entire eleven and a half years I was with Grayson. Victoria made it clear with rude comments and statements that she didn't approve of my physical appearance, my dyed hair, facial piercings, later tattoos, what I wore or my dietary choices. She was never able to keep her thoughts to herself. I knew I was the hippie vegetarian that stole her baby from her, but the blatant disregard for my feelings and disrespect I received was not warranted or appreciated.

In the second week that Grayson had been home after his hospital stay, she sat down at the dining room table with my parents and her son, while I sat in the living room reading. Victoria was a former professor and artist diva who wore fancy pantsuits with jewelry and expensive perfume no matter the occasion. She would wear black pants to our house, then complain when pet hair got on them and demand a lint roller. On that day in our home, she took out her bright red planner to go over Grayson's clinic schedule, reminding us she was very busy with all of the committees she was on, as well as her church and social obligations she needed to attend. When she said she wasn't able to take Grayson to many appointments, my parents stated that they were going to take shifts taking him to the clinic. Victoria thumped her fist on the table and said, "But he is my son!" My dad said, "He is our son too," as he grabbed Grayson's shoulder. This is a prideful moment I hold close to my heart, as my parents provided Grayson with the mental, emotional and physical support he lacked from his own mother and step-dad during his cancer journey.

Despite the treatment I received from Grayson's mom, he did have extended family members who were pretty great. He had a very cool Aunt Anna, an ally of mine who lived in Louisiana. Her adult sons Jason and Dean, also in Louisiana, were so fun to hang out with during the holidays, as they had the same dry wit that Grayson and I had. They were my kindred and I appreciated them very much.

Grayson's sister, Natasha, three years younger than him, lives in Louisiana; she had been less warm than the other crew. When I sent her an email telling her how her brother was doing, she sent me back a long reply, basically stating that he may have long stretches of not feeling well, but he would get better and feel fine in time. She was more focused on telling me how she was working long hours with a lack of support and how lucky Grayson and I were to have what we had.

I thought my bleeping brain was going to explode. Statements like that coming from his mother or sister shouldn't have surprised me, but they always did. The audacity to be non-empathetic just didn't flow through my veins. Bernard, his step-dad, could be very sweet at times but could blow up and flip on a dime as well. I never felt very comfortable around Grayson's family outside of his aunt and cousins, in my eleven and a half years with my husband.

Grayson was the kindest man and deserved the best. I knew in my heart during the whole cancer journey that each person deals with illness differently, but taking things out on me was never acceptable. It was tragic and sad that Victoria had lost her husband, and Natasha had lost her dad at such a young age, but going through this with Grayson wasn't a trivial thing or a time to be unkind. Challenges and struggles with these women continued to bubble to the surface this whole time and all I could do was give it to God and seek the support of my family and friends.

CaringBridge by Grayson: Feb. 27, 2011: My first post! Thank you to everyone who has been thinking about us and praying for Rachel and I over the course of the last month and a half. I feel very blessed to be in remission. I really appreciate all the uplifting and inspiring comments, jokes, and funny stories. I also love the cards I've been receiving. They mean the world to me, and I treasure each one. Things are going well here at our house and I'm getting terrific in-home support from Rachel, and my two wonderful in-laws, Ryan and Marie, not to mention my mom Victoria and step-dad Bernard. I'd also like to especially thank my brother-in-law Jack and his family for all their help and continued support. I'll be starting my next round of chemotherapy on Monday and thankfully it will be outpatient, so I will not have to

43

stay in the hospital. Please continue to post, and pray for us as we go into this next week of uncharted territory. I am very positive and confident about the treatment I am receiving, and I know with God's hand and all of your support, I will get through this. God Bless, Grayson

~

Finances and Figuring Out How to Support Yourselves During the Cancer Process: Step one of the cancer process is seeking out the best available medical treatments. You need to worry about life and money, but survival is what is on the docket first, so you put those logistics on the back burner for the first few days.

Once the medical plan is in place, you may need to look at your finances to see if things will change based on your spouse/significant other's ability to work. I was fortunate to have a great job, six months of Grayson's disability payments and Grayson's late father had left a trust fund that his mother gave us monthly support from to pay for the mortgage. I'm not sure I would have taken the help from his mom if I'd known how many strings were attached; however, it was very helpful not having to worry about money as much while balancing everything else. The beast that is cancer does not discriminate who it attacks and most people like me, are not financially prepared for this kind of catastrophic illness and the financial burden it causes.

If you do need to look at your finances, I want to recommend filling out the below chart to analyze your monthly bills, see what you could cut out or down on, and add in the medical costs of deductibles, uninsured expenses, medications, medical items at home, transportation and gasoline- all that will most likely accrue over time. Many service providers are more approachable than you'd think, and have the ability to help lower costs if you take the time to call to inform them of your spouse/significant other's illness.

- Credit cards: See if you can negotiate a lower interest rate.
- Internet: Ask for a lower monthly payment/discount.
- Utilities: My natural gas provider offers an option to spread out the total annual cost of services by having a monthly payment based on the mean of all of the combined months, resulting in me not having to pay more in the winter or summer when the furnace runs more for heat or air conditioning.
- Student Loans: Try to negotiate a lower monthly payment or see if you can defer your monthly payments. Deferment allows you to stop making the monthly payment amount due in the negotiated or vendor's offering, in increments of 3, 6, 9 or 12 months. During deferment the principal does not have to be paid, but interest is still accrued.
- Medical Bills: The billing departments at clinics and hospitals are often willing to help you set up payment plans to meet your financial needs. Depending on what you can afford to pay per month, as long as you can pay something on your bill, it can even be in amounts as low as $50 or $75, the provider will be happy.

  It is important you live within your means, not above them!

44

Monthly Expenses:		
Mortgage/Rent:		
Electricity:		
Natural Gas:		
Trash/Recycling:		
City Quarterly Fees (homeowners)		
Association Dues: (Townhome or Condo owners)		
Cell Phone:		
Internet:		
Car Payment:		
Car Insurance:		
Student Loans:		
Entertainment: Hulu/Netflix/Amazon Prime or Cable:		
Childcare:		
Homeowner's Insurance:		
Credit Cards:		
Groceries:		
Medical Bills: Co-pays, Deductibles, Co-insurance		
Prescriptions:		

Transportation: Bus/Train/Parking Passes:		
Snacks/Meals at Medical Facilities:		
Gasoline:		
Misc:		
Misc:		
TOTAL EXPENSES:		
INCOME:	Pre-Illness:	Income after Diagnosis:
What areas could you cut out or decrease?:		

I spent nearly twenty hours looking online for available funding sources to help us offset the unexpected expenses we continued to accrue. Below is a list of resources I highly recommend checking out:

Additional Funding Sources:

- SSDI: Social Security Disability Insurance/SSI: Supplemental Security Income www.disability-benefits-help.org
  - o To qualify for this, the type of cancer has to be considered "acute" and within the guidelines stated on the Disability Benefits'-organization webpage. There is a page with an A-Z index of what are considered "Compassionate Allowances Conditions" that you can check to see if your diagnosis is listed as qualifying for benefits.
  - o To qualify you will need to take the short and simple quiz on the homepage, along with submitting proof of income, tax records, medical reports and a history timeline of medications and treatments.
  - o You can apply for this online or in person at a local Social Security office. (Due to having an acute cancer diagnosis- ALL-Acute Lymphoblastic Leukemia, Grayson was able to apply and we were fortunate to receive a monthly payment that started about eight months after his diagnosis.)

o   Another great resource to navigate the SSDI/SSI process is the website https://thedrlc.org/cancer/
- VA: Veteran Affairs: if you or your spouse/significant other have been in the armed services check with the VA to see what you may qualify for at www.va.gov

Cancer Aid Organizations:
- Cancer Financial Assistance Coalition: https://cancerfac.org   Financial help listed with qualifying diagnoses, assistance type needed and zip code.
- Cancer Care: https://www.cancercare.org Limited funding by need, income and/or availability. Funding can vary over time, ranging from helping with co-pays to transportation, child care, etc., based on cancer types/diagnoses.
- CancerHorizons: https://www.cancerhorizons.com   Prescriptions, rent/mortgage, utilities, travel and other assorted living expenses. Caregiver financial resources and assistance, list of pediatric resources as well.
- The American Cancer Society: www.cancer.org Help to understand the costs of cancer and treatment, and a place where you can find local resources under the tab "Treatment and Support."
- Cancer Finances.Org: Food, childcare, general living expenses, home cleaning, treatment comfort and cosmetic needs, health insurance premiums and deductibles, home-care and caregiving, prescription drugs, travel and transportation. Funding varies by qualifying diagnosis types.
- The Leukemia and Lymphoma Society: www.lls.org Funding that varies in amount and type based on blood cancer type and diagnoses. Co-payment assistance, Patient Aid Program, travel assistance, transportation, prescription drugs.
- The Lymphoma Research Foundation: www.lymphoma.org Helps with uninsured expenses and those struggling to pay for treatment and bills that have lymphoma diagnoses.
- SusanG.Komen   https://ww5.komen.org/FinancialAssistanceAndInsurance/   Local and national resources for financial and personal wellness.
- Sisters Network Inc.: https://www.sistersnetworkinc.org   Financial assistance to African-American women diagnosed with breast cancer with utilities, rent/mortgage and medical accessories.
- Healthwell Foundation: https://www.healthwellfoundation.org/ Financial assistance for medical and life expenses for certain kinds of cancers or illnesses.
- Sarcoma Alliance: https://sarcomaalliance.org/ Provides up to $500 for a second opinion with a specialist.
- My Good Days.Org: https://www.mygooddays.org Provides co-pay help if insurance pays at least for 50% of the medical costs.

- The Bone Marrow Foundation: www.bonemarrow.org   Assists with the expensive costs of a bone marrow transplant including pre-transplant matching and testing, medications, medical equipment, home and child care services, transportation, housing and expenses related to the transplant procedure.
- The National Organization for Rare Disorders (NORD):   https://rarediseases.org Assists with medications, insurance costs, diagnostic testing and travel to clinical trials or meeting with disease specialists.
- PAN Foundation: www.panfoundation.org Helps older adults with medical costs for qualifying cancers and other medical diagnoses.
- Patient Services Inc.:   https://www.patientservicesinc.org Insurance co-payments, premiums, transportation, Medicare Part D co-insurance.
- Fifth Season Financial:
  https://www.fifthseasonfinancial.com   Helps those with late stage and terminal illnesses.
- Livestrong.org: www.livestrong.org/we-can-help has a handy page where you can look by assistance type needed, and are walked through any possible financial, legal, medical needs you might have.
- https://www.vitaloptions.org The Selma Schimmel Grant helps patients and families going through cancer and other serious illnesses.
- Brain Tumor.Org: https://braintumor.org has a long list of funding and emotional support for patients.
- Pinkfund.org helps with costs associated with breast cancer undergoing current treatment.
- Bmcf.net Brenda Mehling Cancer Fund:
  https://www.cassiehinesshoescancer.org/resources/financial/financial-assistance/the-brenda-mehling-cancer-fund-bmcf/ assists patients ages 18-40 up to $500 as they undergo treatment with living expenses and medical costs.
- Stupid   Cancer: https://stupidcancer.org/get-help/financial-assistance/   List   of financial resources.
- There are also many websites out there to help child cancer survivors pay for college!

Prescription Assistance:
- https://www.needymeds.org
- https://patientassistantprograms.org
- Bristol-Myers Squibb: Patient Assistance Program: www.bmspaf.org
- https://www.genentech-access.com/patient.html#patient-assistance-tool-page   For meds made by this Rx manufacturer.
- https://www.gskforyou.com Aid to pay for certain oncology medications.
- https://medicineassistancetool.org Matches patients with med assistance programs.
- https://www.pfizerrxpathways.com Assistance program search and match

- https://www.rxassist.org Helps find ways to reduce Rx costs.

Fundraising: There is no shame in asking a friend or family member to create a fundraiser on the behalf of your spouse/significant other. I had a couple of these when Grayson was sick, and they helped us tremendously to pay for meals, gasoline, parking, transportation, medical costs and other life expenses.

- https://www.gofundme.com is the most popular and utilized website for fundraising out there these days.
- If people want to give you money or gifts, ask for practical things like gift cards for gasoline, groceries, Target, etc.

- These are ultimate blessings and so needed when you least expect it.

Chapter 7:
Team Grayson

My brother Jack developed the idea of "Team Grayson" a couple weeks into my husband's illness by outfitting Grayson and I, our parents, siblings and their spouses and children with maroon fleece jackets and hats with gold lettering, the colors of the University of Minnesota. It was heartwarming and inspiring to see close family members wear their gear in his honor through the photos sent from all over the country. It was amazing and made me feel less alone.

I also began a "Team Grayson" Facebook group around this time, where many of the posts in this book originate from in the upcoming posts and beyond, when labeled "Facebook." This group brought me so much comfort, especially on the really tough days.

CaringBridge: Mar. 3, 2011: Grayson is doing well. His lengthy and complicated clinical trial is kicking his butt but we are giving it to God. This protocol allows closer observation and attention to meet the end goal of a total cure. Please keep us in your prayers and thoughts, Love Rachel and Grayson.

CaringBridge: Mar. 8, 2011: Hello TEAM GRAYSON! Grayson is continuing to do well. He has outpatient chemo many days this week, which is long, tiring and at trying at times. Please send good thoughts and prayers his way! Thanks, Love Rachel and Grayson

Facebook: Mar. 9, 2011: I am annoyed at several things and need to let them go! Sarah McLachlan concert, taking clients tonight!

That night I took my assisted living clients to see Sarah McLachlan at the fancy State Theatre in Minneapolis. It felt wonderful to escape for a few hours through the beautiful voice and lyrics of one of my favorite singers. It fed my soul, but also made me wish Grayson was with me, as the last time I'd seen Sarah, he'd been in the seat beside me.

CaringBridge: Mar. 15, 2011: Grayson is doing well. He amazes me every day via his positive attitude and the way he faces it all with grace. I feel humbled and lucky to be around this strong and courageous man. This week he has 2 days at the clinic versus the past two week's schedule of four times a week. Please continue to keep us in your thoughts and prayers, Love Rachel and Grayson

Facebook: Mar. 16, 2011: Grayson- you are a warrior!

- o Thank you, my warrior Princess. It's hard to be down when you are around. Grayson

Facebook: Mar. 18, 2011: Early and shortish work day, we had Buca de Beppo to go for lunch, digging into rich pasta, garlic mashed potatoes, lemon green beans and garlic bread. In addition, we've had 1.5 days alone together. Woot!

In mid-March I bought "Team Grayson" green silicone bracelets that I sent to family and friends all over the country. These two hundred bracelets were reflected back to us in photos of our supporters proudly wearing them smiling, flexing muscles, being angry at cancer and also cheerful in their belief and support of Grayson beating it. Grayson was thrilled to no end and felt so honored and loved. He kept a bracelet supply in the bright yellow messenger bag I had made for him that had a cartoon picture of a cowboy on a donkey on it, that said, "I Am a Cancer Buttkicker," that he took to the clinic.

Facebook: Mar. 21, 2011: Supporting my amazing husband Grayson as he goes through Leukemia. GO TEAM GRAYSON!

- • Go Team Grayson!!! Thinking of you both daily.
- • For Rizzle!
- • This is so great! Glad to join Team Grayson!
- • Our prayers are with you two.
- • GO GRAYSON GO!!!....Thoughts & prayers sending your way
- • Grayson, you have a tremendous amount of strength and courage. Team Grayson is going to kick some booty!
- • Grayson and Rachel, I am thinking of you both and praying for you! Inspired by you!
- • Grayson and Rachel, you guys are awesome! You are a fantastic team, hugs to both of you!

CaringBridge: Mar. 21, 2011: Today is day 21 of 56 days in Phase 2. Please keep Grayson in your thoughts today. Last week he had an allergic reaction to one of his chemo drugs (he is doing fine!), which meant the medical team needed to find an alternative drug. The replacement is a giant shot-yikes! Please pray for strength and comfort for him. I'd like to thank my parents for helping us and Victoria for staying last week when my parents took a break. Thank you to our supporters- we truly could not do this without you. God has certainly blessed us with all of you! This time has been a shmorgishborg of feelings, emotions and major life changes; however Grayson and I are finding strength, pride, joy and happiness each day!

- • We are very excited to get to see you soon. I am so glad everything is going well. You are a very strong woman, but I knew that the moment you walked into our lives and then had to entertain my children. We love you and send all our love and prayers your way.

CaringBridge: Mar. 24, 2011: Hello! First off, Grayson is doing great! Yesterday he had the new chemotherapy shot that his body is accepting so far. On Monday his medical team discovered a blood clot in his arm so they took out his PICC line. He is being monitored closely and taking blood thinners via a belly shot 2x a day. Grayson is a definitely a super trooper. He has clinic tomorrow with new drugs then will go in 4x a week for the next two weeks. **I want to take a second to talk about my gratefulness for all of the love and support from all of you. I was just telling a co-worker about all of the continual kindness we keep receiving and was brought to tears. God is truly blessing us every second of every day. Yesterday after yet another big snow storm, I shoveled the wet and heavy snow in our driveway, only to have the city snowplow throw eight inches of the rocky and hard stuff at the end of the driveway. Our neighbor Fred across the street came and plowed it out, and when I went to thank him, he told me he'd been praying for Grayson and that he'd take care of our yard for the entire year!!!! An hour later another neighbor came by with a loaf of hot pumpkin bread. Friends have recently donated online to our fundraiser to help offset our medical bills. We know friends and family are thinking about us daily and praying. My co-workers are sporting Team Grayson bracelets I see peeking out of their sleeves during staff meetings. All of these things fill my heart with so much love and appreciation. This is the hardest thing I hope I will ever have to go through, and I wake up each day happy, joyful and take ultimate pride in taking care of this amazing man! I am so fortunate, lucky and blessed! Thank you all so much! Sincerely, Rachel and Grayson

CaringBridge: Mar. 25, 2011: Grayson is doing great. I had the morning off so I was able to take him to clinic. All the ladies love him there!

Taking Grayson to the clinic proved difficult for me as I am not a patient person by nature. Working with small children for decades, then adults with mental illnesses had made me immensely patient, I think more than most people, but the boredom I experienced at the chemo appointments drove me bananas. In the hospital I had books to read, games to play, shows to watch, and could go for walks. At the clinic in contrast, waiting five minutes to be checked in, then twenty to be called back for labs and vitals, then another twenty to thirty until being called to the infusion floor, then an hour to three for chemo just took the wind out of my sails. I think it was the combination of the florescent lights and gray and white walls that made me so sleepy and irritable most days. I struggled to stay awake and alert within the little partitioned curtain area he was assigned to, and found it made me crabby and antsy. I always felt like I had that twitching sensation I got at times when I was attempting to stay awake reading or watching TV at night, but my body was signaling me to give up and surrender to sleep. It made me feel like a total jerk, bad wife and definitely a bad clinic caregiver and supporter. I hid it well for the most part and held his hand or got him snacks if he needed them as the chemical toxins pulsed through his veins. Occasionally I'd fall asleep in the chairs, but usually just read magazines to try to stay awake while Grayson listened to music on his headphones as he lay back with his eyes closed.

Facebook: Mar. 25, 2011: I am extremely tired every day, but I love my life, I love my job, I love my friends, love my co-workers, love my family and LOVE each and every day with Grayson! ☐

  • Hang in there Rachel so many prayers are being said for strength & love for you & Grayson.

  o Rachel: thanks everyone! I am so lucky and privileged to have Grayson!

CaringBridge: Mar. 28, 2011: Hello all! This week Grayson has to go into the clinic every day Monday-Thurs for chemo. Please keep him in your thoughts. He is amazingly patient and continues to take it all with grace and courage. GO TEAM GRAYSON!

CaringBridge: Apr 2, 2011: Again want to THANK all of you for your continual thoughts, love and support! We could not do this without you. This week has been long and tiring, but Grayson and I are now relaxing on the couch with family watching the NCAA playoffs. He continues to prevail and take each day with grace. GO TEAM GRAYSON!

~

Baseball, Grandma Irene and Easter Sunday

CaringBridge: Apr. 8, 2011: This has been a long clinic week for Grayson, but he is taking it like a pro. He had outpatient chemo Mon-Thurs and today is getting a blood transfusion to boost his energy level. We are happy to have an upcoming relaxing weekend together. Today I am going to the MN Twins opener with my dad. Next week Grayson has treatment on Mon, Wed, and Friday. Please keep him in your thoughts and prayers as always. Thanks so much! Rachel

That day I went to the new Twins stadium at Target Field with my dad to see the first Twins' baseball game of the year. I wore the green Twins jacket that I'd gotten Grayson, so I could bring him to the game with me. My dad got emotional during the National Anthem, hat in hand watching the gigantic American flag cover the field with six jets flying over our heads, as he himself and other family members had been in the armed forces. As a tear dropped down my seventy-one-year-old dad's face, I leaned up on my tippy toes and kissed his cheek and told him I loved him.

CaringBridge: Apr. 11, 2011: TEAM GRAYSONERS: If you have a bracelet- please take a pic of yourself wearing it and post! If you need a bracelet- email me and I will send you one! I finally got to grow the beard out a little, too. Rachel calls me her "little bald cutie"...lol. I am so blessed to have an enormous amount of support, and top notch medical care. I believe the prayers are making all the difference! ~Grayson.

CaringBridge: Apr. 13, 2011: MN, MN! We never know what to do with you! The last few days we have had nice weather, this past weekend reaching 76 degrees, but this weekend we are expecting a lot of snow. Oh well, what to do? Grayson is doing well after an eight hour day at the clinic Monday, and will hopefully have a shorter day today and Friday. He finishes this phase of the clinical trial on Easter Sunday, and then we wait to see how his body responds before Phase 3 starts. All of these clinic appointments get very tiring, please keep him in your thoughts and prayers for patience and strength! Love Rachel and Grayson

It was during this time that my friend Irene became ill and died. She was a little curmudgeon who was a part of the seniors group I facilitated during my grad school internship. I was her surrogate granddaughter, the only young person in her life, and had taken care of her and helped her out when needed. She succumbed to death due to a lifetime of smoking and many falls at age seventy-six. I spent weeks sitting in the hospital at her bedside. Weeks later my friend Ashley had a heart attack at the gym, leaving behind a six month old daughter and husband. I felt so saddened by both losses and felt blessed that Grayson's health seemed to be going in the right direction at the same time.

CaringBridge: Apr. 20, 2011: This is Grayson's last week in Phase 2. He goes in on Monday, Wednesday and Friday for outpatient chemo- then will start Phase 3 next Monday. Please post in his guestbook to keep his spirits up during this long week! Thanks!   Rachel

Grayson was getting into a pleasant rhythm with his appointments, yet was still discouraged to be at home most of the time, not working or being productive. I told him to treat this life like a full time job despite how tired or reluctant he might be to leave the house yet again for another appointment. It was his war and he had to soldier on through, no matter what. He found a friend in his physician's assistant Tessa, whom he saw on a regular basis outside of his check-ins with Dr. Lazar. Tessa was very cute with glasses, tons of freckles, had gotten married on the exact same day as us, was a joy to be around, and had two small children she'd fill him in on. Grayson had an innocent crush on her and I didn't mind one bit. She had a great sense of humor and was a good ally in all of this.

CaringBridge: Apr. 24, 2011: Happy Easter! I want to thank all of you for your love and support on this important day. We are so very blessed to have all of you. Tomorrow Grayson starts Phase 3, which will be rigorous in its initial few weeks. Please keep him in your thoughts and prayers! Love Rachel and Grayson

We spent this Easter in St. Cloud at Victoria and Bernard's house. As my mom and I were getting ready, Grayson walked into the dining room looking sharp in khaki pants cinched with a brown belt, a white and blue checked shirt and what I call a "Newsies" cap. I could feel myself tighten and sucked in a breath as I took in my husband's extremely thin frame. I snapped back into focus as my mom grabbed my arm and shot me a stern look to keep me from exclaiming aloud how skinny Grayson looked. I hadn't seen him in dress clothes since the Christmas before, and we hadn't gone anywhere together besides medical appointments due to his compromised immune system. We opted to skip the germ-a-palooza of church and headed straight to his parent's house.

Over the years I'd shared with my mom tidbits of holidays at my in-laws in their fancy museum-like home. I'd never felt comfortable in the cold living room with the giant grand piano, white couches I wasn't allowed to put my feet on, grandfather clock, Faberge egg and lifeless art on the walls. Often there were fancy towels hung in the bathroom that we were instructed not to use, like the time we were shown the new $100 bath ones.

Holiday meals were spent around the intricately carved dining room table where we'd sit for hours eating off of china as Victoria and Bernard talked about people we didn't know. It was this same table that I'd received dirty looks for accidentally scraping the chair leg on the table leg when scooching in closer. My mom was aware of the manipulation and verbal abuse I received from my mother-in-law over the years, and I was glad to have my own mama there as back up support for this holiday.

Bernard and Victoria bickered a couple times across the table as the three of us sat there in our own awkward silence. Halfway into the meal Victoria did her usual song and dance of boasting about her former students to Grayson, telling him about their recent accomplishments, jobs, new expensive homes or children. I had no idea why she seemed to take so much pleasure in comparing her former students to her own son and his wife, implying that our life wasn't fulfilling or good enough. The worst I'd ever heard was when my sister Felicity told me that as my grad school cohort crossed the stage at my graduation years before, Victoria leaned over to Grayson and said "You know if you ever went to school again, you could have a ceremony like this, but it doesn't seem like that will ever happen." After all these years I still cannot believe she said that to her own kid, let alone to anyone. I felt grateful then and now -that I've always had a kind and supportive family. Even if we didn't/don't always get along, I always knew they had/have my back in the end.

For years Victoria would make rude comments and say demeaning things to me out of Grayson's earshot, which I'd tell him about on the long car ride home. That inevitably meant we'd then argue, as he thought I may have been blowing things out of proportion. He always wanted to give her the benefit of the doubt, as she was his only living biological parent, which I completely understood. It wasn't until years later when Victoria would cut me down in front of Grayson that he fully understood what I'd been telling him for so long.

Two years before cancer rocked our world, I confronted Victoria when I couldn't handle the abuse anymore, calling her and giving her a piece of my mind. She attempted to deny any maltreatment and stated that no one had ever told her anything like that before. I'd heard from many people that she was feared by students and even some peers, which lead me to believe no one would dare cross her. Despite it being a nerve-wracking experience I was thrilled that I'd told her I deserved to be treated with respect in general, and as Grayson's wife. The call did not end well and the next time I saw her she acted like it never happened, treating me as she always had, alternating between snippets of kindness and smiles with snide comments and making me feel like I was a tolerated houseguest that she wished was anyone else. I really do think she wanted to like me and to have me be a part of her herd of fluffy white sheep that frolicked in the field together, but instead she saw me as the black sheep that her son saw as a diamond in the rough. I tried really hard for years but sixty to seventy percent of the time when we were together, I was just so uncomfortable. I was never appreciated for being the quirky, fun, smart and kind girl God made~

Support Groups/ Outside New Emotional Support: Finding social support for your spouse/significant other is vital. There are hundreds of support groups out there for all different types of cancer. Past and present patients and survivors can provide priceless insight, support and validation to your loved ones in ways you never can. They have been through it, are going through it and can relate and provide invaluable advice and comfort to help guide you and your loved one along the way.

Grayson joined the Leukemia and Lymphoma Society's Young Adult support group that provided weekly online chat groups with members across the country. Each Monday night he would log on at 7p.m. and have a forum to talk to other blood cancer patients on topics like work, sex, relationships and friends, finding kindred connections that he couldn't and wouldn't find elsewhere. It was exciting to see his eyes light up when he'd later fill me in on a joke or story that someone told or how he'd connected well with someone and was now Facebook friends, allowing them to freely talk whenever desired.

Grayson and I began attending the local Leukemia and Lymphoma Society's (LLS) monthly support group at North Memorial Hospital near our home. It was odd to both of us to walk into the hospital where Grayson was diagnosed with cancer, after facing what he just had at the U. We entered with slight excitement mixed with nerves. We found the meeting room and joined fourteen other participants who each had their own journeys and stories to tell. We looked forward to what they had to say and what we could learn from them. I had been thrown into the cancer world with a force of Thor's hammer, and since then I'd been comfortable around other cancer survivors, their loved ones and supporters in ways I may not have been prior to my husband's diagnosis.

Cancer was an odd club to be a member of; its membership was paid for in blood, sweat, tears, money and exhaustion. Grayson was the youngest patient among the mid-forties to mid-sixties group. As each participant went around the circle sharing their name, diagnosis, illness status, and whatever else they wanted to share, I found myself thinking that Grayson had it easy in so many ways. Several of these people had faced several kinds of cancer, had had multiple bone marrow transplants, and were living with dire complications. As each person shared, the other participants would nod in agreement in non-judgmental, unconditional understanding. It was humbling to hear other perspectives and tales of the paths they'd each been on. This was the type of safe place that Grayson had been craving so badly and needed.

~

Online Resources for Patient and Caregiver Support:

- One on One Support: https://imermanangels.org Mentoring Program of Support
- Emotional/Mental Health: https://www.cancer.org/treatment/treatments-and-side-effects/physical-side-effects/emotional-mood-changes.html
- How to Cope With Cancer: https://www.ctoam.com/services/monitoring-and-support/support/emotional-support/for-cancer-patients/
- Cancer Care.org
  https://www.cancercare.org/publications/262-the_value_of_oncology_social_workers this link connects to counseling resources as well as an option to find online, telephone or in person on the East Coast support groups.
- Springboard Beyond Cancer:
  https://survivorship.cancer.gov Self-empowerment management
- American Cancer Society:
  https://www.cancer.org/treatment/support-programs-and-services/resource-search.html You can put in your zip code and "Support Groups," to get a page of results of groups in your area.
- Leukemia and Lymphoma Society: https://www.lls.org/support/support-groups Groups for patients and families
- Stupid Cancer: https://stupidcancer.org Support for patients 15-39.
- Livestrong: https://www.livestrong.org/we-can-help/just-diagnosed/your-emotions-after-cancer-diagnosis

Chapter 8:
A Sleeping Dog, Trainers and a Guinea Pig

CaringBridge: Apr. 28, 2011: I've had a relentless terrible string of bad days and last night accidentally stepped on my sleeping dog and was bitten on one of my calves and a hand. Pain, urgent care & antibiotics + a traumatized dog.

CaringBridge: May 2, 2011: Grayson is doing well. This is the second week of Phase 3. He has clinic appts., 4 days this week, prayers please. As I said in my last post I accidentally stepped on our sleeping dog that was tucked partway under the couch that woke up startled and sunk his teeth into my leg. I had to go to urgent care to get checked out and was put on antibiotics. When trying to wrestle a sock away this weekend, he bit Grayson on the hand which meant Grayson had to go to the ER to get checked out. We have a dog trainer coming to try to help us out for 6 weeks. Many people have told us to give up. This is our baby we've had since he was 8 weeks old, he is nearly two. Please send us your thoughts and prayers that we can keep him. Love R & G

CaringBridge: May 2, 2011: As many of you know my parents have been here in shifts living with us, taking care of Grayson. Last week my mom walked in when I was watching a few minutes of American Idol, saw Steven Tyler and said, "Who's that really unattractive woman on the left? She has not aged well!" Love it! R.

CaringBridge: May 6, 2011: Last few days with my mom here. We've had my parents rotating shifts with us for the past 12 weeks. We are so blessed! TEAM GRAYSON!

CaringBridge: May 8, 2011: I just saw a great play about Nat King Cole called "I Wish You Love" at the Penumbra Theater with my mom. This was very cool and I learned a lot! Thank you Dad, for the tickets!

CaringBridge: May 9, 2011: Hello all! Grayson is doing well. This week he finally gets a break from having chemo several days a week. We continue to gather strength and patience through our faith and all of your support. It amazes me how fast time has flown by and how relaxed we feel at times despite the craziness we are living through, thanks to the help of my parents. We feel so grateful to have them here with us. Thank you for the support and prayers. Please keep sending messages for my Grayson as they keep his spirits up! Love R & G. P.S. The dog training is going well so far!

CaringBridge: May 10, 2011: I am watching The Voice with Grayson and my mom. She just said about Cee-Lo Green "I'm sorry but he looks like he just escaped from somewhere with all that red on and clown shoes!" Ahhh love it!

My mom, Grayson and I had become addicted to watching The Voice when it premiered for the first time ever. It started in March and we watched it every Monday and Tuesday since. It was scheduled to end the second week of May but it had been extended a third day into that week. Mom was supposed to go to my brother Jack's on a Wednesday but when the show was extended she called Jack and fibbed, telling him she needed to stay with Grayson an extra day. It was hilarious.

CaringBridge: May 12, 2011: Crazy stressful day, but soon I will have from 2:30pm today until 5 pm Saturday to spend with Grayson. My mom leaves today which is hard, but Grayson and I get our house to ourselves for the first time since early January

Facebook: May 26, 2011: Today is a very long intense clinic day with Grayson. Good prayers and thoughts please! So glad my amazing job allows me time to be with him!

~

Our little Pembroke Welsh Corgi, Clive, turned out to be more than we bargained for during Grayson's illness. He didn't adjust well to Grayson being gone for five weeks, nor to the different parents, friends and medical staff that had been in and out of our home. After being bit quite severely myself, then getting called out of a cancer conference by Grayson because our dog bit him, I had a big decision to make. We had to get professional animal support or give our beloved Clive away. We decided to pony-up and pay the $450 for a behavioral training company to come to our home to teach us how to work with Clive. We had failed at training attempts in the past, a year before having the hair-brained idea to put pennies in a Coke can, tape the top shut and shake it at him when he did something wrong. Can you tell we were pros?

The behaviorist didn't seem to help much no matter how hard we tried. During the third week of the six-week program, our cute little chunky man bit me when I was trying to stop him from eating seeds out of a lawn spreader in the garage. It was time to make the tough call.

I stood in the darkened afternoon shadows of our kitchen and looked out the window as I called shelter after shelter seeking one that could take our dog. No one could guarantee he wouldn't be put down because so many organizations were filled to maximum capacity. I tracked down the breeder in rural Minnesota we'd gotten him from, and was relieved to hear she was willing to rehab him on their farm. I sat down on the office floor with Clive asleep between my legs as I told Grayson who sat above me at the computer, that I'd found him a home and that the next day we'd have to say good-bye. My husband cried and asked me if I was sure. I was scared of this twenty-five pound dog, wondering if I moved, would he sink his teeth into my flesh like he had weeks ago? I could get another dog, but I couldn't get another Grayson.

CaringBridge: May 27, 2011: Please keep Grayson and I in your thoughts and prayers. We had to give our dog, our baby, Clive away. We drove to the farm where we got him and dropped him off with the twenty or so other little chunky cute Corgis, knowing he would have open land to run on, and would be rehabbed, trained and one day hopefully would have a new family. We cannot afford the risk to our family and Grayson's health. This is surreal and is going to leave a big gap in our lives. We will miss him dearly. Grayson is doing well health wise. His treatment is going well and he needs your prayers for strength and perseverance. We feel blessed to have you all. Sincerely, Rachel and Grayson

- I'm sorry.
o Thanks, we are devastated but have to keep perspective on Grayson's health & safety.
- I understand. You have to do what you have to do though. Keep your heads up
- Oh guys, that sucks, I'm so sorry to hear that. I know you did the best you could. Hugs
- Sad, I'm so sorry to hear that.
- I'm sorry to hear about Clive

~

Oh my goodness. What a funny, funny girl I am. With Clive gone I somehow thought I needed to replace him with another pet. Two days after Clive left our home I went to PetCo, picked out a caramel-and-white-colored guinea pig and purchased a cage, water bottle, bedding and toys. Spontaneity and impulsiveness had been a fault of mine at times, just like the time Grayson and I went to PetSmart when I was twenty, after I'd been sipping off of his beer at dinner one night and insisted I needed to adopt the large white doe-eyed cat that needed a home. At the time he told me, "You cannot have that cat Rachie!" to my chagrin. I had to be told at times, "Rachel, look both ways before you cross the street!" if I was in a hurry or "You probably shouldn't have ice cream or candy for breakfast again!" Sometimes I needed reining in and this would have been one of those times. I thought this guinea pig would be a great distraction for us, which turned out to be true as we loved to hold her as she squeaked and wiggled in our arms as we held her little warm body in a towel because she peed all the time.

Facebook: May 30, 2011: We are grieving the loss of giving away Clive, but I just surprised Grayson with a baby guinea pig we named Iris. She is so tiny and will be Grayson's new little girl!

We fell in love with Iris quickly. Her tiny squeaks sent the cats toward her whether she was in her cage or we were holding her. In the whirlwind of purchasing her I didn't factor in the fact that Rufus, my wily hunter of a cat, might want to eat her. I'd put her cage on a coffee table in our dining room and when she would squeak, Rufus slowly approached the cage, literally licked his lips and touched his paw to his mouth. He'd bat the cage and try to figure out how to get in. This was an actual game of cat and mouse. Three days after I purchased Iris I had to take her back to the pet store in shame, as I'd learned that guinea pigs are in the rodent family that could potentially spread infectious diseases to my cancer patient that could result in dangerous or fatal results. That was the beginning and end of Iris the guinea pig in our lives.

CaringBridge: June 6, 2011: Hello, Hello! Sorry it's been awhile. Grayson is doing well. He is finally getting a break from multiple visits per week at the clinic! He only goes in 1x a week and is about to finish Phase 3, and we are waiting for more info on Phase 4. Grayson is adjusting well to being at home more, and we're quickly finding out that the days after the actual treatment are worse than the infusion days. He's enjoying playing the new Wii tennis game I got him as well as reading the Star Tribune newspaper cover to cover each day. We cannot believe it is June already! He is 4.5 months into this 3.5 yr protocol, and we thank you all for your continued support and want to ask you to please hang in there with us! R & G

CaringBridge: June 10, 2011: Please pray and think good thoughts for Grayson and I. Our cat Puddin', our beloved ball of black fur and squeakiness, is quite ill after he jumped out of my arms and fell backwards onto our coffee table, hitting his head on the hard surface. As we watch him unable to focus his eyes and walk sideways due to vertigo it seems, we fear we may face another loss soon. We took him to the emergency vet and two hours, two tests and $450 later were told the next few days would determine his longevity.

CaringBridge: June 15, 2011: I thank the Lord a million times over for all of the blessing and puzzle pieces falling into place during this tough, unpredictable and trying journey...and that our cat Puddin' turned out to be okay!

CaringBridge: June 18, 2011: Grayson is in remission! His bone marrow biopsy just came back Friday and there are no traces of Leukemia! He's been given a week between phases and starts up Phase 4 on Monday the 27th. THANKS BE TO GOD AND ALL OF OUR SUPPORTERS!!!

~

More Chemo, Chicago and Another Loss=Stress Is Trying to Bite Us!

Facebook: June 18, 2011: I am enjoying Grayson telling my mom what a nunchuck is. Lol.

CaringBridge: June 27, 2011: Today Grayson starts Phase 4 of treatment. I am writing this to ask all of our supporters and followers to keep us in your hearts, minds and prayers. In the last Phase, 3, Grayson only had to go into the clinic 1-2 days a week. He will now have to go in more times per week as the phase progresses. We've been told the intensity will ramp up and will most likely be draining on us both emotionally and physically. We're trying to prepare ourselves for the possible side effects and changes that could happen. My husband continues to amaze me daily with his courage and spirit! Love R & G.

CaringBridge: July 9, 2011: Grayson is doing well. He just finished week 2 of Phase 4. He is currently relaxing in St. Cloud with his parents while I am away in Chicago for a mental health conference. I miss him greatly but am happy to have time away to explore Chicago with my friend Julie, and am quite enjoying the respite it's providing. Grayson is fatigued, but doing well as we head into the weeks filled with more clinic visits. We've been extremely fortunate to have all of you in our lives and on our team! Love Rachel and Grayson

Chicago was just what I needed at this point. I felt like I'd been running around lost in a corn maze for the past few months. Julie, my friend and co-worker twenty-two years my senior, and I road-tripped there while listening to classic rock and sharing our life stories. I'd reserved our hotel online that appeared nice and was on the outskirts of Chicago, only to find that it was subpar, was sandwiched between a church and a Hooters and the "continental breakfast" consisted of a silver pizza tray stacked with Hostess Ding-Dongs into a pyramid shape. The room was hot and sticky, the floor was a tad damp, and I injured my leg on a spring that was popping up out of the mattress.

The NAMI- National Alliance on Mental Illness conference was amazing, though. It was there that I was able to fall into the crowd of two-thousand attendees in a posh hotel to learn best practices to work more effectively with my mentally ill clientele, to understand them better. I'd been working with individuals with schizophrenia, bi-polar, anxiety and depression for several years by then and it was very rewarding to hear first-hand experiences and life stories of individuals who had these mental illnesses themselves. Throughout the three day conference of lectures, breakout sessions and the expo, I met so many incredible people that added so much richness to my professional and personal life. I learned how to advocate for this population more fluently and felt so blessed that my employer paid for the conference.

On our downtime we explored the wonders of Navy Pier, perusing booths of colorful wares. I saw nuns in habits eating ice cream, drank Sangria and danced at a music festival we stumbled upon in Grant Park, and had several outdoor meals at amazing restaurants. We spent one morning at the Shedd Aquarium walking around in joy and awe at the exotic frogs, fish, birds and every kind of aquatic creature, and that afternoon went to the birth place of Ernest Hemingway in Oak Park. I've been an "Erniephile" since I discovered his literary works at my hometown library at age seventeen, as well as biographies about his interesting and tragic life. We attended a tour of the house, then ditched it, opting to take photos and look around the house at a faster pace in the sweltering heat. This trip allowed me to recharge my batteries, ready to come home to Grayson feeling refreshed and prepared to take on the next phase of his treatment and our crazy, busy life.

In mid-July I went to an aging conference with my mom in Duluth, two hours north of the Cities. I was geeked to attend this three-day event that would provide me an arena to expand my knowledge base and spend time with my mom in this wonderful lakeside city. We had many great meals; drove on Bob Dylan Way; toured the historic Glensheen Mansion, the site of a long ago family murder; and walked along Lake Superior.

One evening my sister Diana called as we were relaxing in the hotel, to inform us she'd eloped that day in St. Croix in the Virgin Islands. I sat on the bed shocked and felt excited for Diana while also being annoyed and upset that there wasn't a wedding for me to attend. Selfishly I was thinking how like Ryan Adam's song I'd hear years later, it was about time to "Gimme Something Good." Life had been so hard and this would have been a happy event to attend and separate me from all of the illness, losses and life upheaval that 2011 had brought so far. I cried for a couple minutes, wiped my tears away and thanked God for Diana and Oscar, her new husband, and the other blessings that I had received that year and those hopefully to come.

Life at times brings us surprises that we didn't know we needed, wanted or would appreciate. That summer our surprise came in the form of a little Golden Retriever-Cocker Spaniel mix that Grayson's sister Natasha gifted to us when she'd heard we had to give away Clive. Our pup was chucked out of a truck in Natasha's Louisiana driveway along with five other little puppies at the tender age of two months. Greta, as we called her, was such a joy and brought us endless hours of laughter, entertainment and distraction from the cold, cruel world of cancer.

Grayson had wanted to name her "Louie," and I voted for "Greta" as in the actress Greta Garbo, as she has always seemed like a graceful, collected lady in old movies, especially if she'd been cool enough for Madonna to recite her name in the song "Vogue." The dog did not in fact come to Grayson when he called her by his pick, but happily trotted over to me when I called her Greta. Natasha decided to gift us the dog as she knew her brother would be disabled, homebound and could use a buddy, so she graciously rehabbed, trained and drove Greta all the way up to Minnesota with her boyfriend Ken.

We received this precious fourteen pound little lady on a hot summer day when I had a terrible cold. I alternated between petting her fuzzy light tan fur, and blowing my ever-dripping nose. Greta looked like a little lamb and her "Papa" Grayson was so proud of our new little family member. I was so thankful to Natasha for the gift we didn't know we wanted or needed. We'd later learn how scared Greta was of men, especially those in hats; she must have been abused at such a young age, all of which made her such a good guard dog and the trust process between her and I, so rewarding. She's been my constant companion all these years after Grayson has been gone, and I still thank God for her daily. (She's lying at my feet now as I write this, age nine and just as much of blessing as she was from day one.)

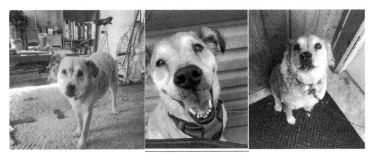

My Greta

That same summer my maternal grandmother died after living ten years with dementia, six of them with Alzheimer's. I flew into Detroit, was picked up by my dad and learned the schedule of events for the next few days as we drove to my hometown. When we arrived home I was greeted by Jack, his wife Maddie, my three nieces, and Felicity, Diana and her husband Oscar. We hung out in the living room while my mom rushed around organizing for the next day. I later sat on my parents' bed and watched my mom try on dresses for the funeral. I reflected on the year I'd had, and how I prayed to God that Grayson wouldn't die until we were in our nineties, just as my grandma had.

The day of the funeral I rode with my parents and Felicity to Battle Creek, the same city that my parents met in while both working at the Kellogg's Cereal Company, back in 1965. When we arrived at the church we helped set up the post-service reception and greeted family and friends, as my grandma lay in an open casket outside the sanctuary doors.

My expertise on Catholicism was very limited at that point, and I'd gone into the service with an open mind as I walked into the sanctuary, holding onto my crying mother's arm with my father on her other side. Mom was crying heavily and I had no idea what that felt like or how to help, so I just held her hand. We sat in silence listening to the service, until my mom put her hand on my arm and warned me to not squeal or yell as I typically do and cannot control when I'm surprised. The priest began to wield what I can only describe as a medieval-looking, smoking, wrecking ball thing that he swung around in the air. We then sang "On Angel's Wings," before filing out of the sanctuary and attending the luncheon where I was asked dozens of questions about Grayson and our new cancer life by extended family members.

Later at the cemetery I kneeled on the ground with my five and seven-year-old nieces in the hot sun and watched the casket get lowered into the ground as I wiped dripping sweat off of my brow, arms and out of my knee pits. It was surreal and odd. There goes another loss in 2011. On the way home we went to Meijer's, where I bought sangria that I later handed to my mom and instructed her to drink when I saw she was in a stressed-out daze. She accepted it despite having only drank maybe a dozen times in her life. My parents, siblings and I shared stories of my grandma that evening. The next day I hung out with Zoe for a few hours, then got on a plane and returned to the cancer caregiving zone.

Caring Bridge: July 27, 2011: Hello, Sorry it's been so long. We've had a whirlwind of weeks of rigorous 4x week treatments. Running back and forth to the clinic combined with my work schedule is really stressing me out and stretching me quite thin. We are blessed at his prognosis and know each time he goes in -it's one more step towards the end zone. We still have a long climb and are taking each day as it comes. Just in this past month we have had friends die, an ill cat, my grandma die, and were gifted a puppy. I was sick for the first time since his diagnosis which resulted in us having to quarantine in separate bedrooms. We continue to keep the faith every day, appreciate each other and our blessings, and try to stay as positive and strong as possible. Please continue the supportive posts, as we love and need them so much! Love R & G

Facebook: July 31, 2011: from my friend Immaculate: Rachel you are a diamond. Stronger than anybody I have ever met in my life. Go Team Grayson!!

- Grayson: Thank you, Immaculate! The Lord has really been my strength throughout all of this. And Rachel. You are the sweetest, pretty-lady.

Chapter 9:
Convertibles, Weed Whackers and Hospital Beds

That spring, in honor of my parent's forty-fifth wedding anniversary, my dad bought my mom her dream car, a red convertible Mustang. She drove it to Minnesota that summer from their home in Georgia where they lived in the winter, to take Grayson for joy-rides. They would get in that thing and go for drives and temporarily forget the world of cancer. I went for a ride only one time with the top down, as I ended up with a wadded nest of hair despite wearing a scarf over my head. I sat in the back seat with the wind whipping me in the face, as my mom rocked out to Rod Stewart's greatest hits. It was so cute to see my mom in her scarf and sunglasses, and Grayson in the passenger seat in his shades and Minnesota Twins ball cap with such big smiles and his face- so lit up and full of life. I liked that these long drives were just theirs, road trips where they bonded while immersing themselves in nature out on the open road, in contrast to the weeks and months they'd spent/spend in the clinic.

Grayson became really frustrated over the course of his illness with his inability to do what he deemed "guy stuff" like mowing the lawn, shoveling, raking leaves or other outdoor tasks he enjoyed. Besides doing the WiiFit, and physical and occupational therapy, he was limited to low impact activities. His immune system was compromised and too much exertion could lead to fevers and other complications.

On one particular weekend when my parents had both gone back to Michigan to spend time together between switching caregiver shifts, Grayson and I looked forward to spending a couple days alone. I had to go into work for a few hours that Saturday night to take my residents to an annual church festival, and explicitly told Grayson not to go outside to do yard work, which he'd been talking about wanting to do all day. He dropped me off at work so he could put gas in the car and get out for a little bit. On this hot, sticky evening I danced it up for hours to a live band, under a tent with my coworker friend Julie and the residents, ate fair food and had a great time. Around 9 p.m. I received a panicked phone call from Grayson saying he had gone outside to use the weed whacker for fifteen minutes until exhaustion hit, and then he crashed on the couch. He had a 101 temperature and needed me to take him to the hospital. Julie had just left and I had no car. Grayson was too ill to drive. I called Julie to come back and tried to remain calm in front of my clients until my ride arrived. By 10 p.m., two Tylenol and a twenty-minute drive later, Grayson and I were in the ER. I spent the night on the low mattress next to him, holding his hand and talking him through his bouts of frustration and sadness at being back in the cancer wing again.

The next morning when our favorite nurse Saja saw me walking down the hall, she ran toward me and went in for a hug while exclaiming, "Hello! Oh, my gosh! You're here and you're still together!" It was so surprising and bizarre to hear. I replied "Of course we are together! What do you mean?!" Saja told me that fifty percent or more of the patients she'd seen over the years had their significant others leave them, or their marriages did not make it through the cancer process. I could not imagine leaving Grayson, and even if I did run away in frustration one day, I would only make it an exit or two away before I'd come running right back. What I'd been told just then was so sobering and encouraged me to reflect on all of the blessings and positives I had to hold onto, when the waves of cancer tried to rock me out of the boat.

CaringBridge: Aug. 7, 2011: Hello all, Grayson is back in the hospital due to a fever and neutropenia (having a very weak immune system). He spiked a fever Friday night, we were in the ER from 11pm-2:30 a.m. and we finally were able to get some sleep in his new hospital room by 3:30 a.m. That Saturday morning the oncologists made the decision to keep him inpatient for a few days on antibiotics, as he needs to remain in this germ free bubble until his white blood cells increase. Please pray for his wellness and for our strength. After going to dinner the next day with a friend in town, I came home to find our puppy with her foot trapped in her cage, resulting in a trip to the emergency vet. I've now been in both the human and animal ER in twenty-four hours. Some days I feel like I am only running on fumes and only able to keep going by the sheer grace of God. Despite it all, I feel lucky to take care of this amazing man. He is so strong, kind and brave. I am proud of him and love him to bits. Love R & G

Grayson was so discouraged by his current circumstances that I decided to dip into his savings to buy him an iPad. I knew it would provide endless hours of entertainment when he was stuck in his hospital bed. When I gave it to him, he immediately said, "Pony! We could have saved that for a trip or something you wanted to do!" I replied, "Grayson, you have a full time job of fighting cancer and deserve this!" He spent the next days and weeks happily discovering new apps, looking at reviews and creating music playlists. It was a welcome distraction to him and a comfort for me to know he'd be able to keep himself busy.

Facebook: Grayson: Aug. 10, 2011: Thank you all for the prayers and good thoughts. I was able to break out of the hospital and be home by Monday afternoon. My fever had gone down and my white cell counts were up to acceptable levels, so my doctor deemed my immune system strong enough for me to leave. I was expecting to be there for another day, at least. That was a real blessing to be able to go home earlier than I thought! Anyway, I'll be taking it easy this week, and Rachel and I go to see my primary oncologist on Thursday to get the full report before I start up with more chemo next week. I'll keep you posted! ~Grayson

- Sending you happy thoughts!
- You both are always in my thoughts and prayers! Great to hear that you were able to go home early! Keep up the faith and strength! You are incredible!

CaringBridge: Aug. 16, 2011: Hello all! Grayson's chemo schedule had been pushed back a couple weeks due to the recent hospitalization, and the fact that treatment has been so hard on his body during this phase. This week he still has to go in to have his vitals checked, but we remain upbeat and hopeful as he is still in complete remission. I continue to be overwhelmed and depressed, but I am getting better. I opened a membership at the YMCA and am working out a lot, attending spousal support groups and connecting with my girlfriends when I can. Please keep us in your thoughts, minds and prayers.

Facebook: Aug. 19, 2011: On Saturday I am walking in the American Cancer Society's annual event to honor my amazing husband Grayson on our 7th Wedding Anniversary, 8/20/2004. I Love You Grayson!

- Grayson: Thank you, Rachie. I am extremely proud of you for everything you do for me and those others who are in need of support. Happy Anniversary. I love you

~

Cowboy Boots, More Chemo and Lit-up Balloons

Facebook: Aug. 24, 2011: Miranda Lambert!

In the past couple years I had become a modern country fan, which I had never expected. I always thought, "Yuck! Country! Dogs, broken hearts and broken trucks!" It turned out that a lot of the modern country on the radio was what would heal my soul through its focus on love, family and wanting a simple life. I could identify with that and had really gotten into Tim McGraw, Miranda Lambert, Keith Urban, Lady Antebellum and Darius Rucker, artists I was lucky enough to see in concert for free when taking my residents to the shows.

Miranda Lambert's lyrics of raw beauty and struggle cut me to the bone in "Heart Like Mine," and "House that Built Me." When I saw tickets go on sale I knew that I wanted to go to the show, even if I had to go alone. I'd been doing so much for Grayson that year and wanted to treat myself. I drove to Mankato, eighty-five miles from my home to attend the concert wearing a tank top and jeans. Seeing my clothes when I went to leave, my mom said "Are you sure you a want to wear that? You don't want any men to hit on you in that sexy top." I rolled my eyes, told her I wasn't eighteen, hugged and kissed Grayson as he silently laughed with his shoulders shaking. I listened to our local country station K102 all the way there, singing along.

Once there I purchased a tee, got a soda and found my seat. I wasn't too familiar with Jake Owens the opener, but sang along to the one song, "Barefoot Blue Jean Night," I'd heard a few times on the radio. When Miranda came out, I sang my little heart out, enjoying the show. I texted Grayson a few photos, telling him I was having a good time and that I loved him. I raised my arm in the air and danced along to "White Liar," "Gunpowder and Lead," and chair danced when Miranda's bandmates for her side project, The Pistol Annies, joined her on stage for a few songs. After the show I drove to a motel, had a vending machine snack, called Grayson and slept like a log. It was a great night and a smart choice to do that for myself.

~

Caregiver Self-Care:

It's important to take time to do things for yourself when your spouse/significant other is ill. At the time it may seem selfish or neglectful when your person is going through the hell of cancer, however it is vital to indulge and get out on your own or with friends to do something you enjoy. When you're in the role I was in, your mind is constantly focused on the needs of the patient. I will say it again- take time off for yourself! Your person depends on your sanity and care, and you need to reboot in order to be able to take care of everything.

- Go for coffee or tea with a friend/friends.
o Have them come to the hospital if need be and meet you-if you need to be close by.
- Have a meal with someone out or even at the hospital cafeteria. (My friend Vera did this with me a few times and it was so refreshing.)
- Go for walks. Whether it's around the outside of the hospital campus or in your neighborhood, even 10 minutes- can add energy and focus to your day. I also used to walk up and down the flights of stairs at the hospital.
- Read, draw, paint, knit, do crosswords or Sudoku. Work your mind and fingers to keep busy and immerse yourself in a hobby.
- Take naps! When the patient sleeps, try to as well!
- Go to a movie or concert with a friend. You're not leaving your person behind, you're regenerating your soul!
- Binge your favorite TV shows or watch movies that you love- it's comforting and effortless.
- Do whatever you used to do for fun even if you have to adapt it.

CaringBridge: Aug. 28, 2011: Tomorrow starts the last week of Phase 4!!! Grayson has clinic this M, W, Th, F, tests on Sept 7th, and starts Phase 5 (the final one) on the 12th. After that he will only have to go to the clinic every 28 days for chemo, and every other week for blood draws, then will have chemo in a pill form daily for the next 3 years. Last week we celebrated our 7th wedding anniversary by taking a two hour road trip. Grayson continues to inspire me with his attitude, strength and positivity. Somedays I don't know where either of us gets the energy or strength, but of course it is from each other and God! Please post! We need the inspiration! Love Rachel and Grayson

CaringBridge: Sept. 10, 2011: Great news! Grayson got his Phase 4 test results back from the most recent bone marrow biopsy and is still in remission! We thank God for his health and blessings. On Monday he starts Phase 5, which will last for 3 years- he will have clinic chemo, then not again 'til mid-October. It's been a tough transition for him to get used to being disabled, unemployed and homebound. It's a difficult world and reality for cancer patients.

Please send Grayson good thoughts, prayers and cards to encourage and inspire him. He is doing well but needs extra support; this transition can be just as psychologically and emotionally hard as being in the hospital. Love Rachel and Grayson.

CaringBridge: Sept. 17, 2011: Hello all! Grayson is doing great. Monday chemo didn't happen as his white blood cell counts and neutrophils were too low, so he was sent home to rest and recharge his batteries for now. Please keep up those prayers. Thanks to my mom who lived with us the past 4 weeks and left this past Wednesday. When I was depressed and overwhelmed she was able to relieve some of my stress by taking Grayson to his appointments, doing laundry and making meals. We are extremely lucky to have so many earth angels on Team Grayson! Love R & G

CaringBridge: Oct. 1, 2011: Team Grayson Supporters! Sorry it's been so long. A week ago Grayson started Phase 5. We are so grateful to be in this last phase after this rollercoaster of a year. The at-home pill chemo is much more convenient of course, but still has the same crappy side effects. He's had a rough few days after taking steroids too. Last Sunday we participated in the Leukemia and Lymphoma Society's "Light the Night," which was humbling, sobering and life changing for us. We were able to see how fortunate we are for Grayson's remission status on the forward path to wellness. Love Rachel and Grayson.

Light the Night is an experience that I will never forget. It is one that to this day, can suck me right back to sitting in my seat at Target Field in the Minnesota Twins stadium, holding Grayson's hand as I looked out at the sea of balloons all around me. Light the Night is the Leukemia and Lymphoma Society's annual fundraiser that unites patients, survivors, families, friends and supporters together for one night to light balloons corresponding to one's status as current patient, survivor or to honor those who have passed. It is beautiful and heartbreaking all at the same time.

Grayson and I met up with our dear friend Sandy as we were in the plaza area decorating the banner we would carry later as we walked around the stadium. Grayson wore his Minnesota Twins ball cap and went to socialize with his friends from his LLS group, as they all excitedly chatted and gave each other hugs. Sandy and I put "Team Grayson," on our banner and chatted away while we made flowers and designs around the edges. Our group captain let us know that it was time to get inside the stadium, where, once inside, we purchased nachos, hotdogs, sodas and Grayson's beloved kettle corn before we found spaces to sit amongst our group. The program began with a greeting from the event's MC, Keith Marler, one of our local morning news meteorologists. He discussed the importance of LLS, and welcomed a child and adult survivor on the stage as the year's honored attendees. Next an LLS staff member went over the organization's mission and shared exciting statistics of increasing survival rates of blood cancer patients, as well as the new developments of chemo drugs and treatments.

I looked around at the beautiful sight of hundreds of balloons in red, white and gold held by people of all shapes, sizes, ages, genders and ethnicities as they flipped the switch on the light inside the balloons. Within seconds, Grayson and I were sitting in a wonderland of red, white and gold. As we sat in the stands awaiting our turn to walk around, we watched the smiling faces of hundreds of families come across the Jumbotron screen as they proudly waved while holding their balloons. Children and adults alike were giddy and excited to be on the same turf that our famous baseball players set foot on. When it was our turn, we gladly lined up like cattle in a queue, and made our way up the stairs to the main level where we began walking through the concrete structure, before making it out onto the field. Sandy and I took turns holding our banner with Grayson so we could take photos with our beloved blood cancer super hero. Grayson beamed the whole time, so cute and as lit up as the balloon he was holding.

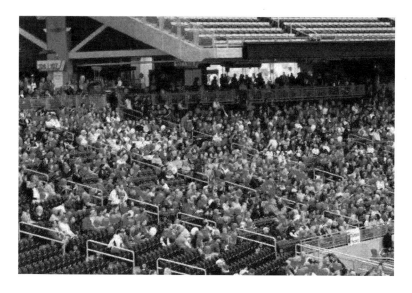

I got goosebumps when it was our turn to walk onto the field as I leaned up on my tippy toes to give Grayson a quick kiss and tell him I loved him, as we headed in with our support group friends. We kept watch on the Jumbotron and soon enough we saw ourselves on the big screen! "You are an athlete running a long distance event,!" I told Grayson. "Thanks Rachie!" he said. Sandy, Grayson and I were in awe and so thrilled to be there. When we had finished walking around the stadium we met his group outside and talked for a little bit then gave hugs to everyone, thanked Sandy for coming and walked to our car. On the way home Grayson was walking on air as he continued to smile nonstop and talk about that night's experience. It was great to see him in his element and with his peers, when so much had been taken away from him in the last year.

Chapter 10:
Road trip, Hospital, Halloween and Chemo

Facebook: Oct. 7, 2011: Cannot wait for my sister Diana to come visit Grayson and I!!! Am so excited!!!

Diana, who is two years older than I, was my favorite childhood toy. We didn't always get along, but we had a great time creating adventures, songs, dances and games throughout the years. Diana lived in New York City and hadn't visited our home in several years, so we were thrilled she was coming for a visit to see her buddy Grayson.

I took Friday off from work so we could all hang out and catch up, and that evening we had Mexican takeout from our nearby favorite, El Loro. We told stories, talked and watched movies over our fajitas and burritos. The next morning we woke early to drive to an apple orchard thirty miles away, where we spent the day in the sun picking apples, drinking cider, going on a hayride and taking silly photos. It was so heartwarming to see the smile on Grayson's face as he did normal and fun everyday things outside of the medical world. I'd seen him vulnerable in ways I never thought I would, and there he was proudly holding bags of apples he'd picked with a cheesy grin on his face as I took his picture with Diana. That night we made dinner, apple crisp and played games.

The next morning we loaded the car and headed north to Duluth. Grayson drove, Diana was shotgun, and I happily sat in the back alternating between reading magazines, chatting and looking out the windows. The fall colors were so beautiful and refreshing to view as we got closer to our destination. Our first stop once we reached Duluth was the Rocky Mountain Chocolate Factory, followed by Starbucks for Grayson and Diana, then we perused the local bookstores and art galleries. We walked along the shore of Lake Superior and felt the cool breeze on our faces as I thanked God for our time together that day and never giving up on Grayson and I.

When my travel mates went to get coffee again that afternoon, I sat on a nearby bench and reflected on how odd my life had been that year, and how blessed I was to be there with two of my favorite people in the world. We were away from the chemo bags, white clinic and hospital walls and all of the other junk that went along with cancer, in exchange for this waterfront view. We feasted on wild rice burgers and seasoned waffle fries while we drank local ale at Fitger's Brewhouse and Grille, talking about our favorite parts of the day. The beer was a rare treat for Grayson, the former beer connoisseur; as he wasn't allowed to have alcohol while in treatment. I felt a surreal sense of peace and normalcy that I hadn't felt in a very long time that day, which would turn out to be one of the highlights of our year.

CaringBridge: Oct. 17, 2011: Due to having a high fever and chills, Grayson was admitted to the U again today. His white blood cell count was zero and his immune system was severely suppressed. He's been quarantined in a private room and is taking antibiotics and white blood cell boosting meds. His head MD, Dr. Lazar, said that the combination of the high doses of chemo in Phase 4, along with 16 days of chemo pills have taken a toll on Grayson's body. Please pray for him as we are trying to remain as positive as possible. I will keep you updated as always. I'm sitting in my pjs in the lounge outside his room by the loud computer, with a bad headache as I prepare for this unplanned hospital stay. The man I love is being watched like a hawk and on the road to recovery! Love Rachel

- I'm sending prayers for both of you. Take comfort in how many people love you deeply and how you touch the lives of each of us. There are great days ahead. Keep strong, love each other, and keep looking for that elusive corner you'll someday be able to turn.

Facebook: Oct. 19, 2011: I'm exhausted to the bone. I love you Grayson! Get better so we can get you out of that hospital!

CaringBridge: Oct. 28, 2011: Sorry to not update sooner. It's been a busy week. Grayson came home Saturday the 22nd. He's doing well, his immunity and white blood cells have greatly increased from the meds he received while inpatient. His levels continue to fluctuate so he cannot have contact with many people for now, and his chemo is being withheld for another week as his body recovers. He is very thankful to be home, as is our puppy who missed her papa. Thank you for all of your prayers, wishes and thoughts, keep them coming! Love Rachel and Grayson.

Over those weeks we binge-watched Arrested Development and Seinfeld on DVD. Back in 2011, there wasn't an option for instant online streaming like there is today, but we made it work as we snuggled on the couch and laughed along with the silly humor, attempting to have a semblance of normalcy during the marathon that was cancer.

Grayson's 36th Birthday: Oct. 31, 2011: Grayson's wishes for his birthday that year were to have lunch at Buca de Beppo with his best friend Owen, Julie and I, and to dress up in a costume at home. I found a beer bottle costume online that he was ecstatic to wear that day. The giant green bottle with a silver cap on top, that was my husband, did little dances around the dining and living rooms, including pretending to open himself up with a bottle opener. He was so cute and funny, and this giant Heineken-looking bottle was very interesting to our little Greta, who was dressed up herself as a bumble bee, antenna and all.

Victoria came over for a couple hours that morning, bringing a large sheet cake with a ghost and a haunted house on it. She opened the cakebox lid, wanting me to take a photo of her and Grayson standing in front of it. I warned her twice that she may just want to hold the cake or take a photo of just the two of them without the cake with the box closed, as Rufus our cat had a thing for jumping on the table when we had sweet treats out. Of course, Victoria ignored my advice, and within seconds of getting in her desired photo position, I heard a slurp, slurp, slurp noise. I jetted around Grayson and his mom to see my beloved wily tabby cat licking a divot into the middle of the cake, as he slurped up the sweet frosting with his little sandpaper pink tongue. Victoria lost it, yelling and shooing away Rufus as he froze, took one last look at the cake, then jumped off the table and ran to hide. Later at Buca we had a wonderful lunch of pasta, veggies, bread and another rare beer for Grayson, as we celebrated his victory of living another year, making it through the beast that was cancer.

CaringBridge: Nov. 10, 2011: Hello all! Grayson is in the swing of things again, receiving outpatient clinic chemo and pill form at home. He's having an extremely difficult time with the awful protocol of taking steroids in a rotation of 2 weeks on, 2 weeks off then starting all over again. He is consistently uncomfortable and fatigued. I myself, am suffering from extreme exhaustion from balancing work, home life, Grayson's illness and trying to carve out some time for self-care. This year has flat out sucked, but I wouldn't have it any other way than to be by Grayson's side. R.

~

Thankfulness and Snowflakes

Facebook: Nov. 19, 2011: This year has been overwhelming, the past few months have been very hard, recently harder, however, **** The Snow * ** blankets everything and creates a gentle wonderland that makes me extremely happy and thankful for each day.

Thanksgiving that year was spent at Grayson's aunt and uncle's house in St. Cloud. I came prepared with my own food to make sure I'd have enough to eat, as the holiday fare was often laden with dairy and meat, despite our pleas to have dairy-less veggies because both of us were lactose intolerant. I ate my green beans with almonds, amazing vegan apple sage and faux meat stuffing, pumpkin cookies and attempted to remain quiet during the political discussions I didn't agree with.

Years prior I had had lovely things happen, like the time I spent hours in the basement bathroom after eating rutabagas that had milk in them, unbeknownst to me. I sat there on the pot while hearing laughter and snippets of conversations upstairs during dessert time while I was pooping nonstop and wishing a magic carpet could transport me home. This year I drank a Coke with the Chex-mix I made. I quietly watched football and zoned out before the big meal.

Later that afternoon when I was alone in the family room, I watched in horror as Bernard went to change the channel from the Ellen Show that had come on, stating that "She is too dyke-y for me," before chuckling and exiting the room. This shouldn't have surprised me coming from the man who once stated, while driving down Lyndale Avenue in Minneapolis, "Look at that colored boy walking across the street who needs to pull up his pants!" Grayson had to hold my arm in the car that day as I nearly flung myself out of my seat to protest. On this holiday I sat there in silence wondering what would happen next. Happy Thanksgiving Ya'll!

CaringBridge: Nov. 30, 2011: Lord Above, I cannot believe how long it has been since I've written an entry! Time is flying by! Grayson is doing well. Although we've gotten him through the most intensive parts of treatment, he's still having a really hard time with strength and energy post chemo. While he is in full remission and we rejoice in that, we still have a long winding path to follow, and feel a bit discouraged as we thought he'd feel stronger by now. Grayson's ability to still be sweet, kind, home all day with pets, and a spectacular cancer warrior- amaze me daily! I have caregiver burnout, and my own health issues have begun to surface again, to the point that Grayson has to care for me some days. Despite all that, we're excited to have time to spend enjoying some of the Twin Cities Christmas events that we have never done before in our 10 years together, due to our opposite work schedules. Please continue to keep us in your thoughts and prayers. We need them! Love Rachel and Grayson

~

OT and New Ways to Adjust to Life

That fall and winter Grayson worked really hard on Occupational Therapy. He had to work on adapting his ADLs: Activities of Daily Living Skills (bathing, dressing, resting, eating) and IDLs: Independent Daily Living Skills: (cooking, cleaning, exercising, laundry, household tasks) to learn new ways to do the daily tasks he'd been able to do on auto-pilot his entire life pre-cancer.

Grayson was no longer the healthy, vibrant man he once had been, who could do housework, run to the store or work a full time job. He worked with an occupational therapist on ways to structure his day so that he'd do tasks that required more energy earlier in the day, leaving the less strenuous ones for the afternoon. He came home with worksheets on ways to learn to stand, sit, lie down and lift with this new body of his, as well as how to create "activity stations" like putting a stool in front of the sink to do dishes when he was too tired to stand (we did not have a dishwasher), or an extra lamp in the office to add more light for when his eyes became fatigued.

I learned a lot about my own husband as he would show and explain his goals to me with great confidence in having a game plan of things he could at least try to control, for the first time in a long time. It made me extremely sad for him, though, the times I'd come home from work and find him so frustrated that he would be yelling or crying, angry that he hadn't had enough energy to do the dishes or laundry. He'd often tell me how he felt like a failure and had no control over his body or world. I'd bite my lip and try not to cry along with him, reminding him that his job was to get well and that housework could always come later. I'd calmly tell him how much of a warrior he was to be fighting as hard as he was, and a very kind one at that, to top it all off. We worked on fine-tuning his goals to break them down into more tangible tasks, which allowed him to take pride in what he could and did accomplish, resulting in smiles and excitement when I'd come home from work. It's important to remind your loved one that things won't always be this way, that this is temporary and in time they most likely will be able to do more things just as they could before the illness.

Facebook: Dec. 13, 2011: Ryan Adams concert tonight with Wyatt!!!

I was out-of-my-skin excited to see Ryan Adams live. I'd been a fan of his since 2005, falling in love with his voice and lyrics after hearing "Come Pick Me Up," on a mixed tape from a friend. I met Wyatt at the State Theatre in downtown Minneapolis for dinner at the Rock Bottom Brewery where we discussed our favorite songs and what we hoped Ryan would play that night. We had great seats off to the left and fifteen rows back. Every song I hoped I'd hear, he played, creating a Zen-like break from the craziness of cancer wife life for two hours. It was a great night that was well deserved.

Christmas 2011: Grayson and I spent Christmas alone that year while my parents were in Georgia, my siblings were at their respective homes, and Grayson's parents were in Louisiana with family. We felt fortunate to be together with our pets in the comfort of our own home, in front of our decorated tree, thanks to God's grace. So much had been up in the air since the start of the year and we were able to testify to the power of love, faith, resiliency and perseverance.

On Christmas Eve we had planned to go to the evening service at our church down the block. Once I was ready, I calmly sat on the bed and watched Grayson get dressed as I'd done so many times before. He was upset, huffing and puffing because none of his pants fit due to weighing 190 lbs., ten more than his normal weight from the steroids he'd been taking. Grayson was trying to jam his little belly paunch into his khaki pants while swearing and grunting as we prepared to go praise the Lord's birth. He told me he couldn't go and to go without him. I begged him to come with me as it was a special time of year and service. As he struggled to zip his pants I said, "Now you know what it is like to be a girl and not have your clothes fit when you gain weight. Welcome to my world, dude!" It was not the most helpful thing to say, but I tell it like it is, and it was too late to bite my tongue. He squeezed into the pants, pulled on a sweater and we walked the three minutes to church in the beautiful snow and cold night air.

We stood for only five minutes before he needed to sit. Within another ten, he lightly grabbed my arm and leaned over to tell me he didn't feel well. He was sweaty and looked miserable, so I immediately grabbed our things and got us out of there. The walk home was slow and quiet as he apologized over and over. I told him it was fine, and that his comfort and health came first. We snuggled on the couch and watched Christmas movies until we were tired and went to bed.

The next morning we woke to fresh snow, opened presents and had breakfast. We played Nat King Cole, Harry Connick, Jr. and Bing Crosby, then had Skype calls with family. We thanked God for all of our blessings and took an afternoon nap.

Therapy: Just before the end of 2011 I gave in and began researching mental health therapists to start seeing, as I had a lot swimming around in my mind that I needed to process. I had a wonderful support system in my family, friends and co-workers, but needed professional help to discuss my fears, doubts and struggles. After looking online for a while I ended up meeting with Jamie, a therapist in her forties who had experience in serious illnesses, marriage and balancing life. I had no idea what to expect. This was my first time seeing a counselor, and I was pleasantly surprised with my experience from the first appointment. There was a Chipotle near her office and I'd often unload about my life as I ate my burrito bowl and sipped my soda, as she helped me come up with ways to reframe my thinking to help me cope with all that was going on in my world.

Most days I just wanted to hide under our bed and be magically transported to a foreign land where cancer didn't exist. I'd live there, Grayson would meet me there and all this medical madness would be gone. But since that wasn't a possibility, I instead used the gusto and moxie the Lord had given me, squeezing out every last bit to support, honor and walk alongside the man I loved. There was so much that I didn't tell Grayson, like my fears of him dying and none of this working, how hard it was to balance it all, and how sick and tired I was of medical facilities and pills and everything that went with cancer, that I was able to talk about with Jamie. I found my hours with her freeing and reveled in the solace I felt each time I'd walk back to my car in the parking lot after each appointment.

~

Caregiver Therapy and Support:
Reasons it's important to get professional help:
- It's helpful to have a third party person, someone outside of your world, who can be your sounding board to vent and cry to, and can help you learn coping techniques.
- Share everything you feel. All those fears, frustration and things going on in your mind and body need to be processed. Don't hold onto those emotions, let them free.
  o Holding in emotions is like holding in poop. Emotional and mental distress can cause physical symptoms like stomach aches, headaches, sleeplessness or sleeping too much. You don't want to keep these emotions in, unprocessed; later you may feel fear and resentment.
- The rollercoaster ride that is cancer will have its ups and downs, and just like a car, you will need maintenance from time to time. Tune up your mind and soul with the help of a counselor/therapist.
- Take your spouse/significant other to a session or two with you. My therapist requested that I do this, and it helped to get a clearer picture of my relationship with my spouse by doing so, and it also helped Grayson feel more included as well.

- Tele-health is now an option that many insurance companies offer. You can have your therapy sessions via FaceTime, Skype or Zoom, allowing you to make the appointment time work from home, work, or even the hospital if need be.
- EAP: Employee Assistance Program. Check with your manager or HR dept. to see if they offer this prepaid program, separate from your health insurance that offers a set of counseling sessions at no cost to the employee and household members.
- 7 Cups of Tea: https://www.7cups.com Offers a free 24/7 chat, self-help guides, or a paid subscription to therapy on their website.
- Behavioral health/mental health benefits: Call your medical insurance company to see if you have counseling coverage.

Caregiver Support Groups
o   https://cancare.org Caregiver one on one support
o   https://www.cancer.org/treatment/caregivers.html
o   https://www.cancercare.org/tagged/caregiving
o   https://www.cancersupportcommunity.org/living-cancer-topics/caregivers
o   https://www.livestrong.org/we-can-help/caregiver-support
o   https://www.helpforcancercaregivers.org/content/caregiver- burnout

Chapter 11:

This New Year Has Gotta Be Better!

The year before, 2010, had ended with the, "You're about to have a major life change," fortune cookie that had led to the rollercoaster that was 2011. We'd had an epic year of changes, losses and gains, and as ugly as cancer was, we were given the gift of spending more time together, which made our marriage stronger than ever. The New Year had to be better than the year before, it just had to be. I thought to myself, "2012, come and get me! I've been through hell but hear me delight in God's sovereignty. No matter what I face, I can do it with God on my side!"

The second week of January I went to Boston for a mini four-day vacation, thanks to my sister Felicity. I was able to spend time with Felicity and Diana, who took the train from NYC to Providence, RI, where we gleefully picked her up to join us for the weekend. I saw my sisters only once a year, twice if I was lucky, and lived for these times. We opted to stay inside most of the time due to the frigid winter temps, making cookies and painting while listening to Prince, and ventured out one afternoon to walk around the famed Quincy Market. I had a horrible cold most of the time I was there that kicked my butt, but was still able to have a good time nonetheless. It was a wonderful reprieve.

Facebook: Jan. 13, 2012: Yesterday I took residents to Super Target, the same one I was at exactly a year ago to the date when Grayson texted me saying he needed a blood transfusion, that started the whole cancer process. Strange huh?

- Funny how we remember things like that.
- Does this mean no more Target?
o   No, I looooove Target

Jan. 15, 2012: One Year Anniversary! To commemorate the fact that we'd made it a full year, I decided to get a tattoo as a testament of the tenets that had been keeping me going: strength, faith and courage. It certainly had taken a lot of strength to get through this rollercoaster, my faith in the Lord had kept me grounded every second of every day, and it had taken a lot of courage to keep it together for us both. I went back to Steady Ink Tattoo, this time with Grayson, who attempted to distract me from the pain by making funny faces and telling stories. I had lowercase "strength, faith, courage," inked in that order on the inside of my right wrist with a small flower on either side. We paid the artist and headed next door to Sally's for dinner to celebrate over their fabulous curly fries drenched in honey mustard and veggie burgers. We wandered down memory lane over the last year -at a quiet table in the back, reflecting on how uncertain we'd been and although we didn't know what the future held, we knew we'd already walked hand in hand through the fire and could get through anything. We'd made it through hospitalizations, endless clinic visits, nights in the ER, fevers, late nights, early mornings, shed hundreds of tears, and said hundreds of prayers. We sat there smiling at each other, so in love and felt like we were kids on a first date.

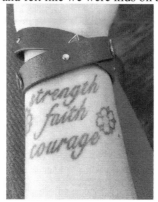

My new tattoo with my LLS bracelet.

CaringBridge/Facebook: Jan. 15, 2012: Sorry it has been such a long time since our last entry. We have had some joint ups and downs but nonetheless are good. We had a relaxing Christmas and New Year's Eve. I've felt so fatigued the last month that it's resulted in depression. I've started seeing a therapist and am reading self-help books. I thank God for my family, and continue to need the support of my family and friends, as we still have a long road ahead. Grayson is feeling well on the first anniversary of his diagnosis. He still amazes me daily with his lovely spirit, kindness and resilience, and being pretty cute doesn't hurt either. I think the word 'remission' usually leads people to think that everything is honky-dory and back to normal, but we still need so much encouragement, prayers and support please. We know everyone is busy, but need our village to keep up the cheering! With much love and joyous hopes for 2012, Rachel and Grayson.

- I love y'all.
- Sorry to hear it's been tough. I wish you and your family the best. Your wife rocks with her fancy new ink in honor of your strength
o Grayson: Thanks! That means a lot to me. I think we are doing well and staying strong. I am incredibly proud of Rachel for all that she has had to endure, and I could happily get one to show my support for her too in a couple of years when my treatments are complete

Grayson was also feeling depressed at this time, and increased the dose of Zoloft he'd taken since diagnosis. On the way home from work the Monday following the new tattoo, I called his sister and left a voicemail telling her he was depressed, and asking her to check in with him.

Instead, two hours later as I was getting dinner out of the oven, Grayson's mom called, berating him about why I "defiled my body." Apparently instead of calling Grayson as I'd asked her to, Grayson's sister Natasha took it upon herself to call Victoria and tell her about the photo I posted of my new tattoo on Facebook. Grayson began yelling, "I don't care what you think, Mom. It's none of your business what one of us puts on our bodies. That tattoo is really meaningful to Rachel and I. You don't have to get it, and don't have to understand it, but it's important to us." The biscuits that came out of the oven that we ate after that phone call, tasted especially good, as we ate them, rolled our eyes, and continued on with our night.

CaringBridge: Jan. 30, 2012: Rachel Love Love Love Love Loves Grayson! He is so much stronger than he'll ever know. We are having ups and downs with this journey due to chemo, etc., but he is a warrior!

~

TNT, and Not the Explosive Kind

In January of 2012 I embarked on what would be one of the most valuable and rewarding experiences of my life. The Leukemia and Lymphoma Society runs an amazing program-TNT: Team in Training- that partners fitness and fundraising to benefit patients, survivors and loved ones, by raising money through endurance events. Participants choose to do a half marathon, marathon, triathlon or bike race without having to have any prior athletic ability. That definitely was me! Aside from Saturday morning basketball in elementary school, and the freshman year girls' basketball team, my exercise was limited to yoga, Pilates, recently machines at the YMCA, and walking my dog. TNT is a very well-orchestrated program with a kickoff event, coaching, mentoring, and Wednesday evening and Saturday morning practices. I was nervous yet excited and soon found myself enveloped in support as I walked miles upon miles to honor Grayson.

Diana happened to be visiting the weekend of the shoe clinic where TNT participants had the opportunity to have their feet measured and fit to their specific comfort needs at a local running store. She helped me pick out the pair of pink, black and white Nikes that I still occasionally wear to this day and treasure. That evening Diana and Grayson helped me create and edit the "ask" letter that I would send to family and friends, requesting donations to go toward the mandatory goal of $1,500 I'd committed to raising. Participants chose their type of event and race location while also factoring in the set dollar amount they'd need to raise. Along the four to five month training program and process, I was delighted to receive cool TNT prizes like gloves, water bottles, a duffel bag and pins. I put my heart and soul into that letter and hoped for the best.

I knew that the training would kick my butt, but what I hadn't anticipated was the amount of emotional support and the connections I would make along the way. I became good friends with my mentor, Angela, seventeen years my senior, as we shared our life stories, tastes in music, books and movies over the endless miles where we talked and walked all over various trails and roads in the Twin Cities. I was fortunate to meet many other great friends like Ella, my cheerleader on frigid Wednesday nights. She pushed me as I alternated between running and walking sprints as she talked of losing her good gal pal the year before to blood cancer. I became friends and had great allies in my coaches that pushed me to keep going and doing exercises I didn't like or want to do, when everything inside me screamed to stop and eat a candy bar or chips with a Coke instead.

Each practice started with a "Mission Moment" where participants take turns sharing who they are honoring and the story of why they are walking or running. It often becomes emotional for a minute or two for some. After that we'd do a team cheer before we'd head out to train. I had more positive news at the time as Grayson was in remission, but often heard up-to-the-moment news of someone losing their battle, a new diagnosis or the anniversary of a loved one's death. This gave us all the more reason to pound the pavement as we worked toward punching cancer in the face and raising money for new treatments and cures.

~

Excerpts from my Team in Training fundraising page:

Feb. 6, 2012: Teams are made up of individuals. Without them, there is no team. I have a mission to help find cures and more effective treatments for blood cancers while honoring my husband Grayson. I'll be participating in the Minneapolis Half-Marathon this June in hopes of raising money to fight leukemias, lymphomas, Hodgkin's diseases and myelomas. I'm also improving my quality of life through exercise, as it's important to practice self-care as a caregiver spouse. I look forward to this experience and hope you'll join me as I walk on this journey that will be long, but nothing compared to what those that are fighting blood cancers experience. Rachel

Feb. 12, 2012: Team Grayson: Winning One Day at a Time. This past year has been a wild ride beside my wonderful husband Grayson, as he's battled Acute Lymphoblastic Leukemia. 2011 was the hardest year of my life and also one of the best. Cancer has such an ugly connotation for good reason, but amongst the rubble of our constant struggles, Grayson and I have grown stronger individually and together. I will never be able to fully explain how difficult this has all been, but with your constant prayers, support and God's grace, it's been more doable. Please support me as I walk these 13.1 miles in honor of Grayson, who has walked millions of miles in the past year of his journey. We have 2.5 more years of chemo to go. Go Team Grayson! Love, Rachel.

Facebook: Feb. 14, 2012: Valentine's Day is overrated, albeit I like all the red and pink. It's so commercial and leaves out all those who aren't in relationships, etc.

- I used to agree, but now I see it as a day to celebrate love in general. I wish my kiddo, my parents, my friends, etc. ALL a Happy Valentine's Day! Any day you get to celebrate love is a good day in my book.
- Grayson: Don't be mad Rach. I still love you - even if you set fire to the holiday chocolate isle and card section at Walgreens.

- I agree about celebrating love.
- And you never know, Valentine's Day might be the best reason to tell someone who doesn't even know you that you like them... Maybe that cute librarian, or that nice lady who works at the truck-stop.
  - Rachel: I am the girly-Hello Kitty, pink and purple loving, girly girl but still hate most of it. I lurvvvvve Grayson tho!

Facebook: Feb. 20, 2012: I'm watching old Michael Jackson videos with my sister Diana like we did when we were little. Yes, I did dance a little.

Diana came for another visit, which was always wonderful and welcomed. We spent a majority of the time inside due to the subzero temperatures, making food and watching movies, had one clinic chemo appointment, and had a blast just being together with our beloved Grayson.

CaringBridge: Feb. 20, 2012: One Year Remission!! Grayson and I are thrilled to be celebrating this huge milestone tomorrow! We continue to take one day at a time through our trials and triumphs. He is doing well despite the home chemo kicking his butt with pain, discomfort and fatigue, as he takes it all like a champ. He's getting stronger inside and out by the day. We thank God for our blessings. Love R & G.

Team in Training: Feb. 29, 2012: The Beginning= Strength and Focus: TNT is kicking my butt (in a good way!) in forms other kinds of exercise never have. I've been walking in all kinds of weather 4-5 x a week, for at least 30 mins. Last Saturday I walked 4 miles in 15 degree weather with a zero degree wind chill. I'm finding this training challenging and difficult, while also enjoyable as I connect with others who authentically understand my story and circumstances, in ways my own family and friends do not. It's rewarding to be part of something bigger that helps me spiritually, and provides such amazing emotional support. I'm working on toughening up my feet that are not used to this much wear and tear. I took quite the spill on a huge sheet of ice the other day, and hope to be back at it in a day. I walked 14 miles total last week, including walking to and from work one day in frigid winds. Please hang in there with me as I navigate this new challenge. Love, Rachel

CaringBridge: Mar. 5, 2012: Grayson is doing great! He still has some really tough days ahead but looks amazing and is surpassing anything I would have thought possible a year ago. We're blessed for all of your support. Grayson helped me prep and send 200 letters all across the country for my TNT fundraiser. Peace, Love, Blessings and Walking! Love Grayson and Rachel

Team in Training: Mar. 6, 2012: March Madness: It's been a very odd winter here. I love the snow but don't mind the clear sidewalks. I walked 2 miles to work, ran ½ mile errands then

85

walked home all in 16 degree temps. Brr! I was able to shave 5 mins off since the last time, to my delight. Per my coach, I need to start strength and core training, adding in riding our Schwinn Airdyne bike that has arm rowers, 10-15 minutes after each walk. Saturday Grayson and I walked Greta for 1.5 miles, and boy was it cold! I want to graciously thank all of you who have donated so far! I feel very loved, supported and more inspired to do this every time I receive another donation. Each time I say to Grayson "We got another donation" not "I did" because I want to include and honor him in this big life challenge I have taken on for the next 13 weeks. More to come....keep on steppin'! R.

~

My Health Struggles: Endo is Endless

In the fall of 2010 I was diagnosed with endometriosis via a laparoscopic surgery to clear adhesions from my reproductive organs. In 2004, shortly after we married, I had an ovarian cyst rupture that was misdiagnosed as an infection by the genius staff at the urgent care center I went to at the time. Since then, I had not had any issues in the past six years. Nowadays there are commercials, magazine inserts, and PSAs on endometriosis awareness and treatment, but back when this was all happening, I was pretty much on my own, when I could have used help most.

In the summer of 2010 I was driving home from work and had such sudden severe pain that rippled through my pelvic area, I thought I was going to combust. The eight-minute drive home, during which I shrieked in terror, felt like the longest of my life. I was only able to get home by the grace of God, dragging myself into the house and to the bathroom. I checked my underwear to make sure nothing was coming out of my body, which it was not. I remember looking into the mirror gripping onto the counter and seeing myself fall over in horrific intolerable pain, like nothing I'd ever felt before.

I made it to my bed and collapsed in darkness as I couldn't make it to the lamp, and rode out the pain in the dark. I didn't have time to take any over-the-counter meds, and was there alone. My legs shook and a thunderstorm of pain and electric shock ran through my body. After fifteen minutes the pain subsided a bit and I looked down, expecting a baby to be there after the amount of pain I'd just experienced. I righted myself, then hobbled to find my phone and called the doctor, only to be transferred to urgent care as it was after 5 p.m.

An hour later I dragged myself to my doctor's office where I signed in, then sat awkwardly in a vinyl chair for twenty minutes until my name was called. I called Grayson and attempted to fill him in on my recent horror show amongst the loud industrial machines running in the background at his work. He told me he was sorry and wished he could help, as I looked up to see Father Time walk in the room. This doctor, who looked too old to practice, asked me, "Have you had a baby yet?' as he went to grab forceps for a pelvic exam. When I said "no" he loudly told the nurse, "Get smaller ones for her!" I rolled my eyes and took a deep breath. He told me that it must be an infection, gave me an antibiotic and referred me to my general physician.

The next week I saw my nurse practitioner who always had her act together, and she referred me to a gynecological specialist. The gyno surgeon stated, based on my symptoms and ultrasound results, he would need to do an exploratory surgery in order to make a diagnosis. I felt relieved and scared at the same time. Two weeks later in my groggy post-surgery daze, I was told that I had endometriosis, could return to work within a day or two, and needed to follow up with the gyno surgeon in three weeks.

Victoria came to stay with me as I wasn't able to maneuver around that well with all of the pain I was experiencing. It kept me home a week, not the two days I was told it would take to heal. The icing on the cake was when the power went out while Victoria was there. Then, after she'd gone home, the temperatures outside got so cold I could not stay home in the dark with no heat. So Grayson dropped me off at a motel near his employer while he worked. I was seething in pain at the time and bitter and upset. I writhed in pain and ate my Cheetos with root beer while I watched cable TV between painkiller doses and icing my incisions.

When I found out the severity of what endometriosis entailed at the follow-up appointment with the specialist, I panicked. I wondered if I'd ever be able to have a baby, doubled with the scary reality of the pain and reproductive issues I'd most likely have for decades to come. I went back to my nurse practitioner and was put on an anti-depressant to help me manage the sadness felt after my diagnosis. When Grayson was diagnosed only months later, I was so glad I was already on the medication to help me get through the terrors of cancer I'd soon face.

Pain began to rear its ugly head again while I was training for TNT, but I chose to shove it aside and do the best I could while taking Tylenol and ibuprofen to make it through those painful days.

Team in Training: Mar. 8, 2012: Last night I trained at Lake Nokomis for our weekly Wednesday practice, which was tough! Between the pre-walk Rockette kicks, jumping side to side, balancing exercises and the threshold intervals, I am toast! I did the best I could while breathing in the freezing air and making sounds like a Muppet as I struggled. Yesterday I watched Grayson have an impromptu bone marrow biopsy. It was awful and painful and if he can do that, I can do this through the bruises and my clumsiness! I do this all for you Grayson! Rachel

CaringBridge: Mar. 12, 2012: I am realizing more by the day how important my TNT training is. I have sore feet and aching muscles but it's nothing compared to what cancer patients deal with. I'm such a chicken with blood draws despite having a husband who is poked so much he says at times he feels like Swiss cheese. Leukemia is one of the leading causes of childhood death, and when I feel like I can barely go on, I suck it up and move my biscuit to honor those babies and my husband. This week I clocked in 21 miles! Onward I go. Thank you, Rachel.

Team in Training: Mar. 19, 2012: This past Saturday I walked 7 miles in the unusually humid yet beautiful March weather. Each practice I feel closer to the TNT mission. Those I train with willingly give up their nights and weekends to raise funds and gain awareness for people like my husband. I continue to walk, walk, walk then nap and soak my aching feet. I love doing this and thank all of you for your support! Love Rachel

During this time Grayson began to consider seeking professional help to process the dark thoughts he said would creep into his mind from time to time. As close as Grayson and I were in this journey, I had no idea what was going through his head, aside from what he'd share with me or I could read from his body language. Cancer is a beast that rips out the heart and lungs of the wolf, or the tornado that picks up the house and throws it back down a mile from its original resting place. Something that catastrophic changes your life forever; it is something that only a therapist who specializes in treating oncology patients can relate to. After making pro and con lists of reasons to see a therapist, the pros won out, thank God, and Grayson began to see a psychologist in a building adjacent to his clinic appointments. I was excited that he had the support of a professional who gave him helpful advice, tips and ideas on how to work through his emotions and ways to cope on the long journey ahead.

Facebook: Mar. 23, 2012: Team Grayson Update: Per his clinical protocol, Grayson is back on the steroid train, to our dislike. This week has been difficult and very painful for him. I'm using the strength I've gained from the six miles of running and walking down hills to compensate for Grayson's weakness, attempting to fuel him with smiles, jokes and love, all the while trying to ice my sore knees. Cancer is so ugly and beautiful at the same time. A year ago Grayson depended on the care of others and now is able to drive himself to appointments and the 75 miles to his parents. This man is why I walk and train. Thank you to those fighting cancer, and to the LLS. I walk for you.

Chapter 12:
Stupid Cancer, Easter and IV Poles

In my quest to find resources to support Grayson, I stumbled across Stupid Cancer, an organization geared specifically towards individuals ages 15-39 who have been diagnosed with any form of cancer, which was perfect for my husband. Through its online website, Stupid Cancer offers a plethora of resources, a podcast, blogs, forums, merchandise and a place for young cancer patients and survivors to belong. This non-profit organization was founded by Matthew Zachary, a brain cancer survivor, offering an authentic experience and platform for the young cancer world. Grayson and I attended their annual conference in Las Vegas in April that year for an experience we'd never forget.

The month before the conference, I nominated Grayson for the "Get Busy Living," award that honors young survivors who are taking life by the reins and living positively. I sent out links to our supporters and Grayson ended up being one of the top ten finalists. Grayson was healthy, had a head full of hair, was still going to the clinic regularly for chemo and taking tons of pills, but was able to travel for this welcomed vacation and escape. I found a deal online for the Bellagio and off we went to explore Sin City for the first time!

We spent five days there in the arid desert, spending the first three at the conference and the other two on day trips. The conference was held at the Palm Casino Resort where we explored their engaging expo, collected conference materials and swag, and learned of new organizations. We connected with other participants, some we'd end up being friends with for life. We met Yelena, who had fought blood cancer like Grayson and was also in remission. The following days were filled with invaluable sessions about health, nutrition, sex, mental health and just living and surviving in the world of cancer.

Each morning we enjoyed Nutella crepes from the patisserie in the hotel and treated ourselves to room service one day. We explored the glitz, glamour and cheesiness of the strip, including attending a Bally's burlesque show that Grayson badly wanted to see. I giggled and raised my eyebrows through the Titanic-themed show and paid for a photo I'd never display in my house of Grayson and I with one of the flamingo girls.

We watched the famous Bellagio fountains, walked through the Paris Hotel and International row, and gambled at the hotel casino. I made a small amount of money, then lost it. Grayson became frustrated with one of the slot machines on one occasion, chalking it up to needing to smoke. He'd been a smoker in his early twenties for a couple of years, and as he bummed a lighter then went looking for smokes, he kept saying, "I need a f&%$ing cigarette!" As I sat there drinking the free bottomless soda I tried not to yell at the top of my lungs, "You know you're at a CANCER conference and you're smoking right?!?!?!" as I rolled my eyes. It was another aberration on this rollercoaster of ours and I gave him a free pass. The irony of it still makes me giggle to this day. The last evening of the conference we got dressed up for the dance night looking like a "normal" healthy dapper couple, but I unfortunately had to leave early due to a migraine.

The next day we shuttled to the Hoover Dam to hear of its impressive construction and history. I had to have my photo taken doing karate kicks in front of the bridge where I'd seen fight scenes in James Bond and Transformer movies. On our last day we took a 5 a.m. bus ride to Los Angeles for a day trip I'd found. We were so close to the California that I came to know as a teen when my sister Felicity had lived there, that Grayson had never known. In the span of one day we were able to go to Mann's Chinese Theater, the Walk of Fame, Mel's Diner, Rodeo Drive, Beverly Hills and to the Santa Monica Boardwalk. He took photos of me from the boardwalk above from his safe and warmer perch as I drew "Rachel Loves Grayson" in the sand and played in the cold ocean. It was a great day and a wonderful trip full of lifelong memories and experiences that I hold so dear to my heart.

CaringBridge: Apr. 4, 2012: We had an amazing time at the Stupid Cancer conference in Las Vegas. It was great to see my husband just beam from having such peer support. Will Reiser who wrote and directed the movie "50/50" based on his life was there, and the theme song of the conference was "We Are Young," by the band Fun, that will forever be connected to this event. I feel blessed we were able to have this vacation and time together. Grayson has a procedure today. Pray please ☐ R.

Facebook: Apr. 7, 2012: Grayson entry: Thank you to everyone who voted for me for the 2012 Stupid Cancer "Get Busy Living" award! I am grateful to you all for your support, not only for believing in me recently, but for the outpouring of positivity and kindness you've passed on for over the last year. Rachel and I had a wonderful time and I brought back resources to share with others here who might be empowered to make positive impacts in their healthcare community. Treatment and survivorship for young adults is the one area of the cancer sphere that has not improved over the years, unlike those programs for children and older adults. This is one group that is looking to see that changed for the better. Love, Grayson.

For my thirtieth birthday I got "The Luckiest" tattooed on the inside of my left foot with an orange butterfly on one side and a purple one on the other. This Ben Fold's tune had been my song with Grayson from the first week we met, and the first dance at our wedding. Grayson felt crabby and tired that day, so I went alone to have it done. God had given Grayson and I this extra time together and I wanted to permanently mark my love for him in another way to keep close to me forever.

CaringBridge: Apr. 20, 2012: A New Day: I have 6 weeks until my marathon day. I hope to increase to walking 20+ miles a week which includes my solo 3-4x a week and group practices 2x a week. I feel lucky to have the opportunity to do this!

~

Side Effects Are Not Fun.........

Facebook: Apr. 25, 2012: Grayson is getting an MRI right now for muscle and bone pain that he's been experiencing for many weeks in his entire body and especially in his legs. We need prayers and good vibes! I love & adore you Grayson!

- Good thoughts are coming your way, you guys.
- Love BOTH of you...stay strong.
- Prayers for Grayson.
- I am sending love, hope & prayers!
- Thinking of you.
- Rachel: Tough news today. More info later. Side effects of being in remission are hard. Prayers for strength please.
- Prayers have been sent.
- Sending healing thoughts your way.

CaringBridge: Apr. 30, 2012: Today we received another pretty big blow. After a series of tests and scans, it was determined that Grayson has Osteonecrosis or death of the bone in both of his hips as a result from all of the steroids he took in Phase 1. The red blood cells that are supposed to be present to surround the hip bone and socket are not there, so his bones have been rotted away, causing so much pain. Today we are going to see a specialist to learn more. Nowhere in the forty pages of the clinical trial did we read this could happen. Sigh. Despite this terrible news, we are glad to know the cause of his pain. Please pray as we wait to learn more, Love R & G.

~

The wheels on the bus continued to go round for Grayson but holes began to form in the tires as the journey went on. As if the nausea, weight gain, anxiety, depression, frustration, anger and fatigue weren't enough, we now had added osteonecrosis to the shopping cart as well as neuropathy. Grayson experienced neuropathy, or tingling and numbness, and at times dull or stabbing pain in his fingertips, hands, arms, legs and feet. He had trouble feeling pressure, picking things up and often dropped objects. He also had less ability to feel cold or hot extremes in his extremities. He often told me he felt like he was all thumbs at times, unable to button, tie or zip clothing or shoes. Many times I'd help with tying his shoes

His feet became so inflamed and large one time, he couldn't put on socks and had to wear compression stockings. It reminded me of Rosanne trying to stuff herself into her jeans that just would not fit in that old 80's episode. I felt so bad for him and there was nothing I could do. He had Frankenstein feet that caused them to be so heavy by the end of the day he'd drag them behind him; his body almost seemed to lead him first. At his request we went to play tennis one day at a park near our home, as he'd loved playing in high school. We took opposite sides of the court and began to play. I will never forget the sight of him attempting to run to get the ball, as his feet loudly dragged behind him. It was horrifying and slightly comical to see at the same time. This superhero didn't let it get him down, though! He yelled at me, "Come on, Pony, go get the ball, don't be afraid to whack it over the net at me!" and darned if he didn't try his best despite his disabling condition. We didn't play too long as he got tired quickly, but man, was I proud of him and to be his wife. The Rock had nuthin' on Grayson!

Grayson and I optimistically went into the osteo clinic thinking we would feel empowered with information and treatment options when we left. Oh, how naïve we were. We waited in the ancient exam room beside a hanging skeleton with Nadia, the clinical trial's lead research nurse.

The specialist confirmed that the steroids had destroyed both of his hips; the left being particularly bad. If you hold up your left hand in the letter "C" and then fist your right hand into that letter- that is how your hip bone fits into the socket. Now imagine a crack in the bone that will increase in size until it completely cracks and falls out of the socket. That is what my husband was facing. I rubbed Grayson's hand with my fingers trying to be as reassuring and calm as I could be. I knew my eyes were saucers and tried to cast them downward out of his sight. Lord above, was this another wrench in the toolbox we had.

The doctor turned to Nadia and blurted out, "What is his life expectancy?" I about peed my pants right then and there. I could not believe he just asked that. That he said that aloud. He told us that hips had to be replaced every ten to fifteen years for the rest of Grayson's life, and once replaced, he would need to rest. It wasn't realistic at that point as he was so young and had to be mobile for his lengthy clinical trial. So basically this stellar chap told us Grayson would be dragging that bad boy of his hip along for the ride, suffering in pain until we heard otherwise.

I had an appointment scheduled with Jamie, my therapist that afternoon that I wasn't going to make in person, so I called her and did therapy over the phone. I stood in the darkly lit hallway among the white cement walls and unloaded the information I'd just learned. From then on Grayson took Vicodin on a daily basis to deal with the pain of his collapsing hip.

Team in Training Post: May 31, 2012: This is it!!! Race Day in 3 days! I am very nervous, excited and proud for race day to come. This has been a hard process, Grayson has faced a lot of hardships recently and I have had a lot of health issues myself. Endometriosis has made training hard, but I will kick butt on Sunday regardless. I'm so inspired by the infants, kids, teens, adults and elders who are fighting blood cancers. I've met many wonderful people along the way. I want to thank my husband Grayson: I Love You So Much and Walk for You!

~

My Feet Kept Walking on for Grayson

The day before the marathon I felt such nervous anticipation mixed with pride and fear. My months of training had brought me to that point with God's grace, along with resilience and perseverance that kept me going when my muscles screamed at me to stop, sleep in or just miss the 7:30 a.m. Saturday practices.

Grayson and I picked up my race gear before heading to the Team in Training "Inspiration Dinner," where we walked through the throng of TNT coaches and volunteers decked out in TNT gear, wearing silly giant neon pink, yellow and green glasses, leis and beads while shaking cowbells, blowing kazoos and jumping up and down for the participants. I filled my plate with Caesar salad, tortellini in white sauce and garlic bread, but passed up the red pastas because of my tomato allergy. I took my Lactaid pill for the dairy and happily ate as we listened to Greg, a fellow cancer warrior, tell his inspirational story of survivorship and success so many years ago. I was so proud to see my Grayson's face flash across the large screen at the front of the room, as he was listed as my honoree for the event. Grayson felt such comfort and inspiration in hearing Greg's story, that he went up to him after dinner and thanked him for sharing.

On the road home I felt a calmness I hadn't anticipated. I was prepared and ready. Minutes within entering our house, I felt an unpleasant rumble in my stomach. Yup, you guessed it. I was on the toilet for the next hour and a half expelling dinner as I panicked, only twelve hours before my first half-marathon was to start. It was my own personal nightmare. I put my head in my hands and looked out the bathroom window at the trees outside and sighed. I was able to get in bed by 10 p.m., chugged water, took Tylenol PM, prayed and fell asleep.

At 5:30 a.m. the next morning I woke, dressed and ate brown sugar instant oatmeal mixed with peanut butter. I shellacked myself in SPF 70, put Chapstick on my eyebrows so that the sunscreen would not run into my eyes, a trick I learned from my teammates, and got my belt pack together. The pack was filled with my water bottle, energy chews, iPod and tissues. I tied my shoes super tight, put on my Darius Rucker ball cap and my TNT neon green emergency contact tag on my shoe with Grayson and Felicity's numbers inside. Grayson drove me to the Minneapolis Depot where my team gathered. I stretched and did the warmup practices I learned during my training.

By that point, I was so filled with nerves I thought I might puke. I felt like I had to pee even though my bladder was empty. Doubts that filled my mind quickly cleared as my team did a group cheer and got ready for take-off. We got in line where our paces were marked, me going farther back as I was a walker, not a runner. I couldn't believe that it was really the time I'd been waiting for. I reached my belt and felt its contents, checked my shoes and my sanity. I was good to go. A voice came across the PA system, the gun went off, I pushed play on my iPod and off I went.

In the first few minutes several hundred people passed me and soon enough the first mile marker was in my sights. I looked around at the beautiful trees along my trail, then heard the devil psyching me out, saying, "No way you can do this!" I had to push it out of my mind. I knew I could do it, God had me covered and darned if I wasn't going to do that to honor my husband who'd been going through his own version of hell. This doubt would hit me in all my future races and I'd learn how to go on, blocking it out. I guzzled down the water passed out at each stop and waved at the TNT supporters who yelled encouragement along the way as they held up signs.

At mile eight I made a friend, another TNT participant thirty or so years older than me, whom I happily chatted with for the next four and a half miles as we huffed and puffed up and down the hills. I hit the metaphorical wall by mile ten, chewed up my Gatorade energy bites, chugged more water, thought of Grayson and soldiered on.

By mile eleven and a half as my muscles screamed, I pictured my guy getting bone marrow biopsies and began to walk faster. One mile later I could feel a rush of adrenaline as I knew the end was in sight. I cranked up my last tune, pumped my arms and made it to the finish line as sweat dripped down my body in places I never knew I sweat. I collected my medal. Two hundred feet later I saw Grayson holding a sign with "Go Rachel!" and a giant heart on it. He was wearing a red polo shirt, blue jeans, his Twins ball cap and a fuller face from treatment, with a smile so big I thought his face would crack. I hugged him tightly, getting him all sweaty as he said, "Pony, you did it! I'm so proud of you!" That was a healing balm to the aching body and feet I would have for days afterwards.

I joined my teammates at the TNT tent and was hugged and high-fived by my coaches as I received my 13.1 pin. My friend Sandy came to congratulate me and sit with us as I rested in the grass before hiking it the half mile up the hill past the hundreds of spectators to Grayson who'd brought the car to me. When I got home I showered then iced my body with the coldest shower setting to help my torn muscle fibers heal, then laid my feet on the pillows Grayson had stacked for me, and passed out. The next day I hobbled around in pain I had never felt before, but with a smile on my lips at what I'd accomplished due to all of my training, support, love and faith in God.

~

Career Changes

By this point in my life as a cancer wife, I'd decided I needed more of a professional challenge. When I'd interviewed at the assisted living four years previously, I honest to God thought it was a position to work with senior citizens, not mentally ill adults. It was only during the interview that I learned the clientele had serious and persistent mental illnesses. I had zero experience in this arena, and had no idea I'd love the population I worked with so much, or find it so rewarding- that I'd end up working in this field long term. That summer I applied for a job as an ILS: Independent Living Skills Worker and was hired on the spot, receiving the highest hourly rate I ever had before, along with great health insurance benefits. I needed to have health coverage as soon as possible, as Grayson was in treatment, so my new employer allowed that day, July 1- to be my start date for the coverage, as well as coverage for a $30,000 life insurance policy for each of us. I went home walking on air, excited for my new life change.

I spent the next two weeks job shadowing a woman who I'd be taking over for when she went to Iraq as a nurse. I had a caseload of twelve individuals who had county waivers to pay for the ILS services to help them meet their independent living skills goals. My job was to help them create and work on attainable goals such as banking, grocery shopping, paying bills and balancing a checkbook, accessing healthcare, setting up appointments, transportation, housing searches, or getting out of the house and socializing/doing something fun. I was their advocate and cheerleader and at times teacher, as they worked towards these goals, as well as someone who would defend their medical and mental health conditions and diagnoses to healthcare providers that had not provided adequate care or treatment in the past.

I helped a hoarder clean her three-bedroom apartment, unearthing boxes filled with rotting, bug-infested potatoes in order to avoid eviction, and a woman with such anxiety that she called me five to ten times a day, could never sit long enough to let her painted nails dry or wait the twenty minutes for the hair dye to set before sitting against her couch, which left several red and brown head shaped spots on the fabric. I had good rapport with a bossy and blunt, yet soft-hearted older lady with two little dogs, that I showed up to help one day and was told she was in jail for hitting a neighbor over the head with a frying pan when they'd argued as she was frying chicken. I was able to help my clients work on their goals, no matter the situation. Even the guy who lived with his hot-tempered ex-girlfriend in a urine-drenched house with twenty-plus cats and a snorting pit bull, that let the felines eat an entire rotisserie chicken off the dining room table, not giving us a place to work on papers when I'd visit. I would do my job, Lysol myself before I got in my car and went to the next person that needed my help. It was quite a trip, but I enjoyed my job and found it rewarding as I drove all over the Twin Cities to my clients.

~

June 16, 2012: Two weeks to the day after my first marathon, I participated in the Lady Speedstick Half-Marathon. I walked the 13.1 miles this time with my friends Sandy and my TNT mentor Angela as we laughed, joked, shared stories and encouraged each other as we huffed up and down the race trails in Bloomington. It was a joy to be with friends and know this time that I had actually completed a half-marathon before and could do it again. At the end I received a really cool medal in the shape of Minnesota on a rainbow-colored lanyard. Two half-marathons in the books- Cancer, you can't keep this wife down!

Chapter 13:
Silent Retreats and Bare Feets

One of the most important things you can do as the spouse/significant other of a cancer patient is self-care. I gave myself pockets of time when I could find them, going to dinner with a friend, a concert or visiting my sisters, even times having Owen, Grayson's best friend come over to stay with my husband so I could go out for a break. I found it hard to shut down my cancer wife brain, and one day got the idea to unplug and be quiet, to shut out the chaos and noise around me.

Grayson encouraged me to take quiet time away, as the month before he'd gone to Florida with his parents for a long weekend, when his mother had a conference. He was able to relax and visit Sea World and Cape Canaveral. I signed up for two retreats- one at the Minnesota Zen Center in July and the other at the Franciscan Retreats and Spirituality Center in August.

The first retreat ran Thursday night through Saturday evening. The Minnesota Zen Center is a white three-story Art Deco-looking building that's snuggled amongst the expensive homes and mansions along Lake Calhoun Parkway in Minneapolis. Ten minutes to 6 p.m. I walked up the light cream-colored stone walkway past the perfectly manicured lawn and knocked on the front door. A kind-looking man wearing all black opened the door, smiled and mouthed "Welcome," to me while handing me that day's info sheet. The greeter cleared his throat and said to me and to the seven other participants standing in the foyer, "In five minutes we will begin the silent retreat. There will be no talking for the remainder of your time here. If you plan on sleeping here please see me for your arrangements." I was given a sleeping space on the third floor in one of their classrooms, and was told that I may have a roommate show up late that night.

I walked up the gray carpeted stairs with my green sleeping bag and overnight duffle to the room on the top left. All of the doors and windows were painted a bright white that gave this attic area a homey feel. I opened up the door to my "motel room" for the next couple days. Oh my. It looked like a pre-school Sunday school room with thin blue carpet, low to the ground built-in bookshelves, a chalkboard easel, a poster of a figure doing yoga in front of a tree, a window seat bench that looked out onto a backyard and one ceiling light. I laid out my sleeping bag and realized I'd have to make my clothing into a pillow since this retreat apparently didn't subsidize pillows. I didn't mind the low-key accommodations but knew I probably wouldn't get much sleep on the hard floor. I looked at the schedule, then texted Grayson that I'd made it there safely.

I went downstairs and was directed via the smiling greeter by his arm movements to the dining room. I found a seat at the dark wooden table in the narrow tan room with matching hardwood floors. Within minutes the table was filled with attendees as we sat in silence. Many people closed their eyes and appeared to be praying or meditating, which I took as a cue to pray. The woman at the head of the table handed out a stack of black bowls, napkins and spoons to pass around the table. The host came out of the kitchen carrying a large wooden bowl with a ladle. We each took turns dishing out black bean, rice and kale soup into our bowls. I had given them a heads up that I was allergic to tomatoes, but was wary the meal might contain traces of it. I tasted onion and celery, and choked down the celery to my chagrin. I silently thanked God that I packed emergency cereal bars that were in my bag upstairs.

After dinner we were instructed to get up, carry our bowls to the kitchen, then follow the host to the main room. There were ¾-inch tall black mats on the floor with an 8 inch by 8 inch circle shaped pillow atop it. Each mat was set up like a station with five feet between each mat, all facing the wall where we'd meditate for the next hour. I did a couple stretches then arranged myself on the little pillow, took a deep breath and closed my eyes. This was it: time to relax, unwind and let the silence take me away. Zen was going to be my companion for the next two days and we'd become best friends. I immediately had two or three songs swirl in my head, causing me to twist my lips into a grimace, willing my mind to shut off. I'd done a lot of yoga over the years but never this much straight meditation.

I tried to think of one of Moby's instrumental calmer songs and waited for my brain to clear. The only sound in the room was someone's occasional sniff or throat clearing. I thought, "It's so quiet. Oh my gosh. No one that knows me well would believe I'd be quiet for a whole weekend, but here I am. Quit talking Rachel. I'm not talking. You're talking in your mind, so you're talking." This went back and forth for a couple minutes then I reached a state of calm that I hadn't felt in a long time.

I imagined sitting on the sand at the edge of the ocean. The beach was empty, except for me. I could hear the rolling of the tide and was working on smelling the salty sea air. A smile came to my lips as I entered a happy place and in no time I heard the sound of a gong. I opened my eyes and saw a couple people leaving the room, others still seated and stretching. I raised my arms above my head, into a deep stretch, got up and headed to my luxurious abode.

I closed the door, ate a strawberry NutriGrain bar, chugged some water then went to the bathroom to brush my teeth. I pulled on some pajama shorts, and lay atop my sleeping bag, holding up my book to block the ceiling light while I read. I called it a night at 9:30 p.m.; the first session started at 6 a.m. the next day. I lay inside my sleeping bag and on my pillow made out of t-shirts and waited for sleep to come. I looked around the quiet room that was lit only by the light of the moon and the street lights, then got up and looked outside. I reflected on what had brought me there, and how I was proud to have taken the time for myself. I didn't initially rest well as I kept one eye trained on the half-inch gap under the door, not wanting to be surprised if my latecomer roommate were to come in after I fell asleep.

I awoke to the sound of my phone alarm at 5:40 a.m. I grabbed my clothes and toiletries and went to the bathroom that looked like it belonged in a cabin, lit only by the bulb above the sink. I pulled back the shower curtain and was horrified to find a claw foot tub that had seen much better days. There was no way I was going to lie in that thing. Right before I got in the tub, I looked around for towels. Of course there weren't any, just the brown folded paper towels in the metal box underneath the sink mirror. Yup, like the kind you find at the gas station. Lovely. Why didn't they say on the website that linens were not provided? I got into the tub, crouched down on my haunches and turned on the water. It was barely more than a dribble. My hair certainly wouldn't be washed for a few days, then. I did a quick wash of all the essential parts the best I could, then rinsed off with cupped amounts of water before drying off with the rough paper towels. I checked my phone, said aloud, "Good Lord, this is just like camping!" and padded down the stairs, hoping the rest of the time would go smoother.

I took my place on my mat as the others arrived and reflected on the fact that I'd hadn't had to be responsible for anyone on two or four legs but myself, for the past fourteen hours. For the next sixty minutes I was able to take myself to a place of calm and quiet.

Soon enough, the gong chimed to signal breakfast. I was delighted to see oatmeal and berries that I devoured within minutes. The next two hours were spent meditating as daylight cast a welcomed warmth into the windows. I let Tori Amos's "Jackie's Strength," flow through my mind as I worked on leaving and flying to another place.

I was tapped on the shoulder a little bit later to signal my turn for my thirty-minute meeting with a monk. I was lead to an upstairs office lined with bookshelves and lit only by daylight. A monk sat on the floor by the window behind a gong, a burning candle and a succulent plant. He introduced himself and asked me what had brought me there and if I had any health issues. I filled him in, and in return he said, "My, that is a lot to have gone through and to be going through." He also told me that if I meditated for ten minutes a day, my health would greatly improve. When my time was up, I thanked him and returned to my mat.

I am not sure when it happened exactly, but I remember feeling so sleepy. Apparently I'd been so relaxed meditating, that I fell asleep. Mind you, not like someone may in a car, on a plane or couch. I'd slid sideways and woke up with a start with my head half on the mat, half on the floor. I was super embarrassed at first, then shook it off as I saw the others had their eyes closed and most likely hadn't noticed. I repositioned myself on the mat. What do you know?, the same thing happened again. Face on floor.

I collected myself when the gong sounded, shaking off my odd meditative nap and headed to the dining room. We feasted on tortillas, seasoned peppers, onions and greens which I happily ate before heading to the kitchen for my assigned chore duty. I scrubbed pots and pans and loaded the industrial dishwasher in the darkly lit kitchen with my passive aggressive teammate.

Kitchen time was followed by a walk outside in what I can only describe as what I called "the prayer pose dippity dopitty stoppity." We all lined up in a single file to walk barefoot on the gray labyrinth stones in the backyard for a slow pattern on the count of one: walk, two:

walk, three: bow down to the earth and the person's back in front of you for three counts, then repeat. I kept going too fast, almost bumping into the person in front of me. When I tried to slow down, I was too slow to an exaggerated fault and almost bumped into the person behind me. This wasn't enjoyable to my exhausted body and mind. I dreamed of napping under the big inviting tree nearby as I continued to walk in the circle.

After fifteen minutes of this we were each assigned our afternoon chore from the sheet posted on the back steps. I saw my name and didn't think "Garden Work," looked too bad. I soon learned I was to pull weeds! It wasn't a horrible task but I guess I was expecting a more spa-like Zen time and swirling those balancing balls that came in a silk box case like the ones I got in Chinatown in San Francisco when I was twelve, instead of pulling weeds from cement. I had a ton of weeds to pull at home in my sidewalk, and didn't even have time to do that.

Apparently the host must have thought I looked as exhausted as I felt, because he asked me if we could talk. We sat on one of the white metal benches in the yard as he said, "I've noticed how you seem really tired and not like you're enjoying yourself or really centering in, in your time here...." I quickly filled him in, nut-shelling the madness that had been my life for the last eighteen months. He was a little flabbergasted and didn't quite know what to say. He told me he was glad I was there and suggested I take a nap for a little while to rest up. I agreed and was fine getting out of more garden duty.

I took a mediocre nap, no longer than fifty minutes, waking up to silence instead of the yard work I'd heard prior to falling asleep. I looked out the window to an empty yard, so I crept down the stairs to find everyone in their happy places on their mats in the front room. I took this as a sign that it might just be time for me to go. Nope, not downstairs returning to join them- but to get the freak out of Dodge.

I crept back up the stairs to gather my things. I first considered how I could chuck my belongings out the window and climb down off the roof, however that didn't sound too smart as I wasn't a ninja. I was too exhausted for a trip to the emergency room, so I opted to sneak out the front door. I went one step at a time, stopping to see if anyone heard until I reached the landing, located my sandals on the mat among all the shoes, then bolted out the front door, silently giggling and running to my car as if wolves were chasing me. I hopped in my car, turned on the AC and the radio, then peeled out of my parking spot. I felt like I was cheating on my quiet time but knew I couldn't stay awake during the next day and a half of meditating. I thought "God bless those monks and attendees, now where do I get some food?" I decided to hit up Whole Foods for something delicious from their hot bar, as they often had amazing veggie entrees and salads that I liked. I pulled into the parking lot and looked around and behind me as if the silent retreat staff or Zen masters were going to come get me.

My parents started taking Diana and I to a church when I was ten that had staff that would come find you if you skipped Sunday School, which we tended to do in later years. We'd hide in my parent's car and literally hit the cloth station wagon seats if we saw someone coming. We were found a couple times and apparently that was still burned in my brain. But no one followed me to the Uptown Whole Foods to drag me back to a voluntary silent retreat. I locked my car, and walked into the welcome embrace of the enticing-smelling healthy foods and air-conditioning, out of the sweltering heat and strong sun rays. I loaded up a medium-sized soup cup with their fabulous penne mac and cheese, a box with kale and dill carrots, grabbed a piece of corn bread and an organic root-beer.

On the way home I called Felicity to tell her of my recent adventure. Of course her response was, "How much did you pay for this retreat of yours?" I told her I'd paid $150 for the Thursday through Saturday night stay, and of course I only made it to Friday late afternoon. I told Felicity about the yard work and my sleeping accommodations. "You paid $150 to pull weeds?!?!?" her voice creaked into the phone with a chuckle. That was all I needed, to hear the authentic laugh and understanding of my Rachelness. I smiled, hung up and pulled into my driveway.

I hadn't called Grayson to let him know I'd be home earlier, as I wanted to surprise him. I grabbed my food and purse and headed to the front door. I pulled on the screen door and it was locked. I looked at my keychain and remembered I did not have the key to the side door; I'd given it to Grayson. I knocked on the door, then after a minute of not hearing a response, banged on it harder with my fist. No answer. I called Grayson, thinking he must be taking a nap. He answered after several rings and told me he was having lunch with a friend across the Cities, and wouldn't be home for at least an hour and a half as they'd just ordered their food.

There was no way into my house. I grumbled into the phone at Grayson and accepted my fate for the moment. I sat down in the shade to eat my food. I reached into the bag for the mac and cheese and fork as I took a sip of my soda. Except there wasn't a utensil in there! I hadn't taken a fork or spoon - I'd assumed I'd use one at home when I got there. I huffed and puffed for about twenty seconds then took those lemons and made lemonade. I ate mac and cheese on my front porch with my fingers and drank root beer, smiling to myself after escaping from a Buddhist silent retreat.

~

In May I'd bought tickets for Grayson and I to see U2 at the new TCF Bank Stadium at the University of Minnesota in August. I'd been listening to U2 since I was little, and was geeked to go. For some reason I felt it in my bones that I wasn't supposed to go to that concert with Grayson, he was supposed to go with his best bud. I gave my ticket to Owen when he came over in July one day. He was certainly surprised at the offer, asking me three times if I was sure. I told him yes, that I knew it would be a special thing for them to do together. It had been nearly two years since they'd been able to go to a concert together. They had a blast, listening to Bono belt out his tunes as the rain soaked them to the bone for the majority of the performance. Grayson told me that despite the eighty-degree temperature he was freezing because his immune system was so low. He said that his hip killed him after standing so long for the show. Owen had gone to get the car as Grayson shivered for the thirty minutes it took his friend to get to him. Nonetheless he was grateful for the experience and the memories they created on that rainy summer night.

~

Holy Quiet Times

The second week of August brought another welcomed respite for this cancer wife. I needed it as badly as a dental patient needs Novocain for a filling. I really wanted to find a nice Lord of the Rings-like little hut, but couldn't afford those, so I booked a quiet weekend at the Franciscan Spirituality Center, thirty miles south of my home. I was willing to go anywhere at that point and was thrilled to find a quiet little haven where I could rest, reflect and pray. I was greeted by a brown-robed Friar upon my arrival, settled into my JFK-era hotel-esque brown and yellow room with fake wood paneled curtains, then walked around to check out the grounds. I felt a sense of peace and safety despite not knowing what the next days would bring. God had placed me in that place, at that particular time, for a reason and I was ready to listen to what He had to say.

That evening we gathered together as the Friars told us the history of the center and reviewed the retreat schedule. After a quick Q&A, they rang a bell and the silent weekend began. We ate dinner in the little retro cafeteria, black beans and salad for me and ham sandwiches and Jell-O for the other attendees.

Aside from one other older lady with thick glasses in a tee shirt with appliquéd flowers on it, I was the only one who wasn't part of a couple among the twelve attendees, and was by far the youngest by at least twenty-five years. As I ate, I looked around and wondered what their stories were and what brought them there. After dinner we prayed in the sanctuary, me with my hands in my lap, as everyone else made the sign of the cross before closing their eyes.

I looked at the colorful stained glass windows, the wooden Jesus statue up in front, and took a deep breath as I prayed for days of solace and refreshment. I later went to the small basement bookstore where I perused metal racks of books, DVDS, Bibles, crosses and bookmarks before I paid for my purchase, putting a check in the lockbox by the door. I bought a book on St. Francis of Assisi and a bookmark that showed the Stations of the Cross, then headed back to my room. That night I stayed up late engrossed in the true story of the young man who went from being an arrogant lush to a minimalist who lived only to serve the Lord and teach others how to live more like Jesus.

The next morning I had a very dry bran muffin for breakfast, prayed and reflected in the sanctuary for an hour, then went for a walk in the adjacent forest for an hour. I came across markers along the trail in the form of crosses, ceramic angels and a beautifully painted Jesus in a wooden box with a glass front to protect Him from the Minnesota elements. I'd spent so much time indoors the past year and felt so alive amongst the greenery and fresh air. That afternoon I attended a service on serenity and peace through scripture reading, while having hands laid on me for a healing blessing by one of the Friars. I thought, "God, give me all you have, I am here, I am listening and I need hope, inspiration and healing in this journey of mine, and in my life with Grayson, and all we're faced with." That evening I made a burrito from the beans, salad and tortilla I was given before spending an hour reading on the grass outside by the pond. Around 8 p.m. I went back to my room, made a quick call to Grayson, breaking my silence to make sure he was okay, then stayed up late reading more about St. Francis.

The next morning, as I ate my blueberry muffin, I reflected on the peace and serenity I'd gained in the last couple days. I attended one last prayer service then thanked the Friars, and headed back home to my Grayson. I drove down the country roads with the wind in my hair as I blasted Peter Gabriel.

Chapter 14:
Here We Go Again and Not Off Into the Wild Blue Yonder of Bliss

It happened again. It really did. Believe it or not, as I was loading items into my car at a Target on the way home from work, my phone buzzed; I'd missed three calls from Grayson. I called him right away as I sat in my car, cranked up the AC and heard him say, "Rachel I went to the doctor and it's bad news!" in a teary voice. I stared at the red and steel blur of the cart corral next to me as I heard my husband say his cancer had returned. I put the phone on my lap and talked to him all the way home, telling him he would be okay and we'd face it all together. Oh. My. Gosh. What now? I breathed deeply and asked God for help.

When I got home I found Grayson sitting on the edge of the couch petting Greta. He looked lost and as I sat down next to him, enveloping him in my arms, he cried and told me he was so scared. My husband looked like a sad puppy and there was nothing I could do to fix it. This reoccurrence of leukemia meant that chemo wouldn't be enough this time; he had to have a bone marrow transplant. Grayson threw his head full of dark brown hair against the couch, sighed, then looked up and said with a crack in his voice, "Pony, I don't want you to have to go through this again. I don't want you to have to do everything for us both again, and work all the time, going back and forth to the hospital."

I replied, "Grayson, we can do this. I love you and I'm not going anywhere. We did this before and we have to do this again. We don't have another choice." He said "I can't do this, I can't. It's too hard and I can't do it again."

I told him he could and we would. I didn't know how at the moment, but we would. I made us both a cup of lemon ginger tea, his favorite, and tried to imagine what was next. That night we lay in bed and prayed for God to protect us and guide us along the journey ahead of us, and peace to sleep that night.

The next morning we delivered the news to our parents. It had mixed reviews. Mine told us that we were an incredible team, had faced this once and could do it again. Victoria, on the other hand, sobbed and wailed as we listened to her say on speakerphone, "Oh no! This is our last chance. This is it or you're going to die! This is our last chance. This is our last hope!" I face palmed, gritted my teeth and redirected the conversation by saying, "Grayson is going to get the best treatment possible at the U, this is our life and reality, and we're going to give it all to God and be as positive as we can!"

Caring Bridge: Aug. 18, 2012: Hi there, Team Graysoners and Rachelers! It's been a long time since my last update, but then no news is good news. First, the good news*: Rachel has been enjoying her new job. My hip and leg pain have been in check so far. We are thankful for these good things. Now the bad news* My cancer has returned. 5-6% Leukemia cell blasts were found in my last bone marrow biopsy. It's a low number but enough to cause alarm. This is a tremendous blow to Rachel and I, and a shock to our systems. I have to have a bone marrow transplant, if I am going to beat this and stay alive! Rachel has been my best friend throughout our 11 years together, and she has been the most amazing wife and caregiver that anyone could ask for, throughout my struggle with this disease. Now my heart is heavy with sorrow at the thought of once again asking her to join me as we take a turn down what might be a very rocky path. Despite uncertainty for what the future holds, we are trying to stay upbeat and positive, and I am going to keep fighting until I beat this! I ask, that on Monday, on our 8th Wedding Anniversary, for your prayers and positive thoughts as I go back into the hospital to begin intensive chemotherapy. With all my gratitude, thank you for your love and support. –Grayson

Sunday evening before his next hospitalization, Grayson began to cry and tell me, "I can't do this! I can't do this again!" My heart broke as I looked at the face of the person I loved most in the world. There was nothing I could do. I prayed for God's peace and protection over Grayson, us and for the medical staff that would treat him. We went to bed, Grayson taking Ambien, me Benadryl, and shut out our reality for a few hours.

That Monday I dressed in a cute red, white and black beaded shirt over jeans and sandals, with Grayson in a short-sleeved green polo, jeans and his standard Vans sneakers as we went to his clinic pre-admission appointment. Word had gotten around quickly to the oncology staff of his relapse, and everyone we saw from the front desk to the infusion floor, gave us hugs and condolences. Grayson used his humor to try to get through it all by saying that this was our anniversary present, albeit one we didn't want. Soon he was back in the oncology ward and headed towards weeks and months of more grueling treatment. I was comforted in knowing my parents would be there by Friday to start caregiving shifts again.

Facebook: Aug. 23, 2012: Grayson is home!!! After 4 days of day long chemo treatments, he is home for now. Next week he will have another bone marrow biopsy, then who knows. We are just trying to take it day by day. We will be setting up a bone marrow registry day, stay tuned. Grayson, I am so proud of you!

~

Bone Marrow Transplants

Bone marrow transplants are a lengthy and difficult process that are a necessary evil when chemo and radiation are not enough. There are two types of BMTs: allogenic: where the patient receives stem cells from a donor via blood, bone marrow or umbilical cords, and autologous: where the cells from the patient are filtered out, treated and put back into the patient. We were very fortunate to be at the U where the first BMT in the world was performed in 1968. Grayson's lead MD was world-renowned and the head of the BMT department. That was not a coincidence, it was God.

We had an entire BMT team to help us navigate the process that included BMT doctors, attending physicians, consultants, fellows, residents, NPs, PAs, a BMT coordinator, a clinical social worker, PT, OT and a dietician. It appeared we would not want for much with this well-oiled machine.

On August 31, Grayson gave consent to the National Marrow Donor Program (Be the Match) and the Center for International Blood and Marrow Transplant Research to take a pre-transplant blood sample to be stored in their research repositories. This would allow researchers to work on improving matching techniques of all of the blood products that are needed to find a match for those needing transplants. Natasha, Grayson's sister, was not a match, so we depended on the Be the Match registry to find us one from the millions of donors. We were shocked to find out that the acquisition of bone marrow or blood cords was anywhere from $28,000-$40,000! Thank God for our great insurance coverage and the fact that we'd already met our out of pocket maximum for the year!

Bone marrow is the spongy tissue inside the bones where blood forming cells are made that turn into red and white blood cells. Imagine holding a wet, soapy dish sponge. Now imagine squeezing it and soap bubbles gush out of it. That is just like bone marrow holding blood cells. Red blood cells carry oxygen from your heart and lungs to the rest of the body and white blood cells help fight infections. Grayson's blood and marrow had been infected and infested with millions of cancer cells that took over his marrow, and he had to have his replaced.

It was decided that Grayson would receive umbilical cord blood, which is donated from parents at the birth of their children, then frozen and saved for patients like him. He would receive the stem cells via an IV transfusion that would only take a few hours, and change our lives forever.

CaringBridge: Aug. 28, 2012: Grayson is doing okay. He had labs and transfusions this week and is very fatigued from his inpatient stay. His medical staff continues to be heartbroken by his relapse, but believes he can beat this. We have a huge stack of info to go through which is tedious and scary. Please continue your prayers!!!   Grayson and Rachel

On Friday, August 31st, I went to the hospital to spend the night at Grayson's bedside to boost his morale, and to try to get him out of his cantankerous mood. I brought pjs and a hoodie in addition to the tank top and jeans I wore. Our incredible neighbors behind us were watching our animals so I was able to focus on just us, relaxing after a crazy work week.

On the elevator ride to his floor I realized that the Women Rock 5K I'd signed up for months ago was the next morning. I was ill prepared and had none of my race gear with me. After I gave Grayson a hug, I told him about the race, ran to the café, picked up dinner, then ran to the U collegiate store two blocks away where I purchased some shorts for the race. They only had men's shorts, but they fit me okay and would have to make do. I remembered I had my running shoes in my car, and my race shirt and bib in the race packet in the backseat, but would have to wear the same undies and socks and run/walk in my regular bra. "Classic Rachel," I thought to myself and sighed.

The next morning I rose at 6:30 a.m., put my hair in a ponytail, cinched the new shorts at the waist and hoped my regular bra would hold me. I kissed a sleepy Grayson, who wished me good luck, and headed to the race. Once I'd parked and reached the race area, my spirits lifted as I saw the plethora of pink banners, thousands of participants in their pink race shirts, and pink tents for the after party.

On this morning, the first day of September, I took in a deep breath and looked around at all the beautiful trees along the St. Paul river line and thanked God for another day. I got in my paced line and prayed for a great race for myself, and a good day ahead for Grayson.

The gun went off, causing hordes of runners to fly by me and within ninety seconds, I'd crossed the start line, shuffling ahead with the masses. My mind tried to psych me out again but I wouldn't listen to it. I'd come to learn that these 5K races were the most fun ones to do as they draw people of all ages, sizes, and athletic ability. I enjoyed seeing all of the little girls that walked and ran along with the teens, adults and senior women. One of the coolest parts of this race was seeing the cheering groups of dads, sons, husbands, brothers and friends all there holding handmade signs to support the ladies in their lives. I finished the race within fifty minutes underneath an arch of pink balloons. I was handed a box holding a silver "W" necklace with a pink crystal from a silver tray held by a shirtless firefighter in his gear. I don't like beefy guys or think it was at all sexy, but found it all quite comical. I walked to the party tents, collected my champagne flute filled with pink champagne, took a few sips, poured it out, then walked to my car. I went home to shower, nap and then went back to the hospital to spend another evening next to my guy.

Facebook: Sept. 2, 2012: Gah! Grayson is in the hospital a few more days. Am getting house ready, and trying to relax. Bathed 2 cats and a dog- that gets your heart pumping! Grayson, you are my hero, and am head over heels in love with you! Hang in there. Eye of the Tiger, dah, dah, dah, dah!!!

~

Becoming a Donor:
- By volunteering to be a bone marrow donor, you are literally willing to save a life. Your number may never get called, but if it does, you could save someone's life and provide years of love and life to them, their family, friends, and loved ones.
- There are excellent organizations out there that provide easy to use bone marrow testing kits for anyone who is willing to do this.
- It is a simple cotton swab test in your cheek that you send back in the mail in a prepaid envelope.

- Please take a second and go to https://bethematch.org & www.dkms.org
- You will not regret it. A majority of patients who need a match cannot find one with an immediate family member; therefore they have to go to a bone marrow registry to find a match. Depending on the timeline of the illness, finding a match sooner than later is key. These organizations that I listed above have large databases that can work toward accurately matching all the needed markers per patient. Give it a whirl; step out in your faith for the good of the world!

CaringBridge: Sept. 6, 2012: Grayson is home after 5 nights in the hospital for low immunity and fevers. Tomorrow Grayson gets platelets, and possibly a blood transfusion as well. He has to have more extensive chemo, which will most likely mean hospitalization. We meet with Dr. Lazar next Thursday to go over the BMT process, but for now we know he will have 2-3 clinic days a week for transfusions. Once a marrow match is found, he will be put into a "preparative regimen" for two weeks to wipe out the bad marrow and immune system via IV transfusions. For the actual BMT he will spend around 90 days inpatient. It's all very cumbersome and overwhelming, but we're taking it day by day. Small blessings are eating dinner together, sleeping in the same bed, and being able to laugh at his hair falling out.

- I send you lots of love. I care for you both, and hope you feel the support of others around you. Let me know if you need anything. Xo
- God's grace is in the blessings and your strength is in your faith in Him. Thank you for sharing this journey with us. We are with you each step of the way.
- Hang in there guys, everyone's thinking of you.
- {{{{HUGS}}}}
- Sending lots of prayers to you guys!
- So sorry to hear all this. Lots of prayers and thoughts to you guys.
- What a blessing you both are! It takes strength that only comes from God to go through this journey. My cousin has been through all of what you are preparing for and he is going through even more as I write. He and his family live a few miles from Grayson.
- Jake and I are sending lots of positive vibes your way. Love you guys!
- You both have amazing spirit and positive attitudes; I believe God's hand is on your shoulders as you continue on your journey through treatment and good health. Feel his strength as you support each other!! We all pray for the best outcome! God bless!!
- Positive thoughts are constantly being lobbed over our fence and into your yard. We were throwing them at your house but I was afraid of breaking a window. So you'll just have to pick up all the positivity in the yard along with Greta's stuff she leaves behind, lol.

On September 13th we met with Dr. Lazar to get the info on Grayson's current state and what was to come. During this process Grayson would get six different drugs, four of which he'd never had, then the actual transplant. He would start the chemo, then have his heart, lungs, liver and kidneys tested for toxicity levels, take Neulasta, a white blood cell-producing drug if needed, then rest for two to three weeks and see if his body was BMT ready. Within one week Grayson's blood had been analyzed and two of the six factors needed to match with a donor had already been met. Hallelujah! Such good news! We were told that GVHD, Graft Versus Host Disease, usually only occurred in 25 percent of cord blood transplants, with only a 10 percent chance of graft rejection. He was going to receive cells from two different umbilical cords which would create more BMT success and less chance of disease reoccurrence for ALL patients, according to a recent study. The meeting was sobering as we were more informed of the upcoming challenges, while also empowering- in that we had info mapped out in a more tangible way.

Grayson went to the world-renowned Mayo Clinic in Rochester with his mother for a second opinion. He and I were comfortable with the expertise, care and plan at the U, but after much prodding from his mother; he acquiesced for this day trip. He spent several hours there, coming home with a detailed report listing his diagnosis, current health status as relapsing with ALL, and that yes, in fact, he did need a BMT. Grayson excitedly told me about the giant blood cancer resources room at Mayo, sharing with me the plethora of materials he picked up including a pen that had floating white blood cell-looking gels that turned red when you clicked on the pen. He was told that his past, current and planned treatment at the U was optimal for survival, which was the reassurance he needed to hear.

CaringBridge: Sept. 23, 2012: My mom and I attended Light the Night last night in honor of Grayson, and he was super bummed to have to stay home. It was very humbling to see so many survivors, many small children, and those honoring loved ones who have not survived. Grayson update: outpatient clinic chemo tomorrow, then blood products later in the week. We're having a tough time individually and together with this cancer battle. Please keep up the prayers and love!

CaringBridge: Oct. 9, 2012: Life's challenges never stop: Hello Team Grayson and Rachelers: He has 4 days of outpatient chemo, then a biopsy. I'm having tooth issues, need a root canal and have extreme ovarian pain. We have had difficult talks about our future, hopes and plans. I tell him he is my future. We feel grateful for all of you. Love and sincere thanks, Rachel and Grayson.

During this time Grayson's hair began to fall out, this time in large clumps. The first time it did, we were both at home. He came up to me where I was sitting in the living room reading, grinned and said, "Look at how my hair is falling out in clumps? What if I went to McDonald's, stood in line and took ahold of my hair like this pulliing at his hair as clumps came out) and said "I can't decide!!!" He could not stop laughing at his own wit, and I was so happy to hear him have humor during this awful time. It was scary and tragic and he was making us both smile. We kept trucking on between my work, his appointments that my mom took him to, and tried to remain as "normal" as possible. We still felt so blessed to have that time together and held onto each other in the storm.

Over the course of the next few weeks Grayson had outpatient visits several days a week and was hospitalized for fevers. We sat in a waiting game to give his body time to recover before further BMT prep could happen. We lost our friend Izzy whom we'd met at the Stupid Cancer conference- to her battle with cancer. It cast a dark shadow of what was to come for Grayson. It made it all more real and ever so frightening. That was not going to be us.

Chapter 15:
Fall into Winter 2012

CaringBridge: Nov. 18, 2012: Grayson has been exhausted for days, but is hanging in there with lots of rest. Friday he had his bone marrow biopsy, so hopefully it will be clear and we will be onward soon! Bless this day and each day Grayson and I can be together at home!

CaringBridge: Nov. 20, 2012: Update: Grayson and I got some craptastic news today: his cancer cells were .08% before the last round of super intensive chemo. His bone marrow biopsy came back with 3-4% leukemic cells, so more chemo we a-go-go. Please pray for our strength, courage, patience and general well-being. Grayson will get hospitalized Saturday for the next round of chemo. Then another two week wait, test for cells and hopefully this darn transplant can start. Same old rinse and repeat. Gah! Everett Grayson, you are amazing, my star, I am so proud of you, and sorry this $(:& is happening again!

Facebook: Nov. 21, 2012: I just talked to my 73 yr old dad who shaved his head for Grayson!!! I haven't seen my dad in 6 months, the last time was only for a day, so I've missed him tons. On Monday he will be here to start his shift. I'm so blessed and feel like it's Christmas!!!

Facebook: Nov. 24, 2012: Grayson starts round 3 of inpatient chemo since his August relapse. We have heavy hearts and minds at this setback. Please pray for our strength, courage and patience. Everett Grayson, you are my superhero!

- Praying for you guys. Keep Strong - Keep Positive - Keep fighting - You both have the will and attitudes to make this happen again. You will get to the point of the transplant and defeat this!! You have many behind you and praying for you daily.
- This will be the magic chemo, I feel it. Prayers and good thoughts coming your way.
- Prayer is in full force. Sending good vibrations your way. Grayson you can do this.
- I continue to pray for Grayson daily. What courage and determination. Hang in there, Rachel and Grayson, and feel the love.
- We all send positive thoughts and keep praying for you every day. Stay strong!
- You and Grayson are a Super Couple....you WILL beat this.

CaringBridge: Dec. 6, 2012: Sorry it has been so long. On 11/22 we found out despite the intensive chemo (the hardest he had ever had) he still had cancerous cells. Sigh. Each time we have a setback, albeit knowing being blessed and supported, we are in this tiny bubble in which we feel so alone and isolated on our little island of doubt. We had a couple nice days at home, and I made a big Thanksgiving meal for the two of us, before he was admitted for that last round of chemo. He's home now, but has clinic daily still. We thank God for the love and support of our parents. He will have yet another painful biopsy in a week, please pray for cancer free results so we can get this show on the road. Our marriage is rock strong, and we are in this for the long haul and rollercoaster of ups and downs of this serious illness, but we need your prayers for strength, courage and patience.

- *Hugs*
- Lots of love to you both.
- Prayers every day, prayers for healing and 100% no cancerous cells next biopsy. If tears help with prayers you have mine.
- More prayers coming your way.
- Your strength in the face of all of this is amazing and inspiring. Know that there are always so many people thinking of you two, you are never alone.
- You two are amazing! Sending my love and prayers!!!
- More love and prayers from me to you and Grayson. Xo
- I know it's easy to feel alone in this but you're not. Hoping for the best outcome on the next biopsy.
- The courage and strength of you both is amazing and a true testament of your relationship.
- I will continue to pray for strength, courage, patience, love, and cancer free results. You both are always in my thoughts and prayers.
- Many prayers!
- My thoughts and prayers are with you both. You are not alone. I love you guys!

CaringBridge: Dec. 16, 2012: Update: Grayson came home from the hospital Friday afternoon. Grayson's sister Natasha visited Monday-Friday (blessing!) and kept Grayson company, along with their mom, during the hospital stay. Grayson is on day 2 of 7 days of outpatient IV antibiotics and blood products. My sister Diana is here this weekend (blessing!), busy, stressful times, but blessed to have him home!

~

It was clear at this time that Grayson wasn't going to be home for Christmas, so I decided to bring Christmas to him. I brought a baby, foot-tall Christmas tree with a strand of lights and ornaments, hoping he would want to decorate it with me, but took over when he was too fatigued. I also brought a gift from my mom- a reindeer in a rocking chair that played "Grandma Got Ran Over By a Reindeer," which he would have me push every time someone came in the room. He would laugh as his shoulders shook, every single time.

The next day as Grayson, my mom, Grayson's Aunt Anna, Victoria and I were talking, the oddest thing happened. Anna, who was visiting from Louisiana, asked my mom how Diana was. A few minutes later Victoria left the room, then returned about five minutes after that with a huge grin on her face. She leaned against the closet fidgeting and wiggling until apparently she couldn't take it anymore and blurted out, "Are we done talking about Diana yet?" to which Grayson, Anna, my mom and I all looked at her, shocked at the very rude interruption. Grayson cleared his throat and looked at me with an arched eyebrow as I sat at the end of the bed with my feet up touching his.

Victoria said, "Oh, my gosh! You'll never believe it. I accidentally walked into the men's room instead of the women's!" then proceeded to fall over laughing while slapping her leg. We all looked at her, then returned to our previous topic.

An hour later my mom and I left to see the Basilica of St. Mary all decorated for Christmas before going to the Christmas Eve service at our church. Once we got into the privacy of the elevator down the hall my little mom blurted out, "I wanted to say "No! We are not done talking about Diana yet, and I will talk about her as long as I want!" as she pulled her red fleece hat down tight over her ears. Oh mama.

That evening I sat down in the back of my church's Christmas Eve service with my beloved mom at my side as we sang carols and hymns by candlelight. Weeks earlier, our pastor, who had been making weekly visits to Grayson in the hospital, called and asked me if he could talk about Grayson in this service. That evening he talked of peace and how despite the struggles that Mary and Joseph faced when finding out that they were going to parent Jesus and the uncertainty they felt, they were able to remain calm and open-minded due to their trust and faith in God.

He then started to talk about a man that he'd spent many hours with in the last year since he'd been diagnosed with leukemia. In a short amount of time he'd lost the life he knew in regard to being able to work, do everyday tasks and chores around the house, and could not go out into public. How this man went through a very difficult and intensive hospitalization that led to remission, followed by months of grueling chemotherapy and clinic appointments. This man was so discouraged to find out he had relapsed and felt at a loss at what to do. He delved even deeper into his faith and prayed every day as he had been, this time asking for peace and grace. He went on to say that this man did this and even though he was unable to receive the needed and lifesaving transplant yet again, due to having fevers and an unstable immune system, he still showed everyone kindness, grace and thankfulness.

Pastor David closed the sermon, stating, "May we all strive to face each day and wait for what comes instead of making rash decisions like we all do when we are impatient. We need to learn to be content in the here and now. May we all be more like Grayson." I was dumbfounded. Absolutely dumbfounded. As he had been speaking about my husband, I rubbed the "Grayson" tattoo on my wrist and looked around at all the other worshipers. They had no idea that was my husband! My Grayson! My husband was in the hospital hoping to live and I was sitting here listening to the pastor talk about him! It was incredible and surreal. I could not wait to tell Grayson when I saw him later.

That night Grayson and I had cafeteria veggie burgers and onion rings amongst the lights of the little tree I brought while we watched "National Lampoon's Christmas Vacation," and "A Christmas Story." Nurses and staff came in every thirty minutes or so, but we were happy to be together, holding hands from our respective beds. We fell asleep happy and knew God would provide, no matter what.

The next morning I woke to an unpleasant rumble in my stomach that resulted in so many trips to the bathroom down the hall, that the kind phlebotomist who had seen Grayson, offered to go to his car to get his Imodium for me. This kind stranger ended up buying me a box as he'd run out of his own supply. Merry Christmas, Rachel, don't get those onion rings again!

Later that morning I went to visit my buddy Wyatt for an hour because he lived so close and we wanted to have a quick celebration. When I returned at noon, Victoria, Bernard and my mom had all arrived. We had lunch and exchanged gifts before receiving the biggest gift of all, the news that Grayson could go home that same day! We held hands from the front to back seats in excitement on the way home. That evening we rested over cups of tea in the comfort of our home, thanking God for our blessings.

Over the next week Grayson continued to have many appointments and tons of fatigue and tiredness. He'd begun to have reoccurring nightmares that he was being chased by a dark cloaked figure with no face and a sickle-like hammer. He said he tried to hide in the dream but couldn't find refuge, causing him to toss and turn all night, and wake up feeling frustrated and drained. I thought it must have been the stress of the continual pushback of the BMT, and the unknown future since his body wasn't strong enough and ready to take it on yet. Oh Lord, what next?

Facebook: Dec. 29, 2012: Grayson has clinic visits every day which is tiresome, yet he is chugging along. He is on a really crappy drug for an infection which causes extreme fatigue, visual hallucinations and scary dreams. Prayers for my lovey please!

Owen came over on the 30th to have pizza and to watch the Vikings play the Packers with us, and on the 31st my mom and I did a puzzle Diana's mother-in-law had sent us while munching on some incredibly good pretzels. We all watched Dick Clark's Rockin' New Year's Eve show, counted down at midnight, hugged and prayed for a healthy new year, then we all fell asleep quickly. The next morning I participated in the New Year's Day "Polar Dash" 5K in three-degree weather. I was super stoked to bundle up in all of my layers and walk the 3.1 mile race to receive my cool medal with a snowflake on it, to add to my growing medal collection.

~

2013 and Onward We Go

CaringBridge: Jan. 7, 2013: The BMT date is finally approaching. Grayson's had to go into the clinic every day since his Christmas Day discharge for IV antibiotics, uses a nebulizer 2x day, and of course takes 15+ pills a day. I don't know how, but he musters up strength from deep down, and goes in every day without whining, or being angry, as most of us would. Last

Thursday we learned that he will be receiving BMT prep that involves chemo and radiation, and he will be added to the list of the only 50-60 people in the world that have had what I call "Space Age Radiation." He will have a regimen run by physicists that are pioneering a protocol specifically for tricky diseases like leukemia. They will use a multi-million dollar machine to deliver the radiation to targeted areas of his body without hitting his vital organs-lungs, liver, heart, kidneys, brain. This has only been done in Los Angeles, California, Genoa, Italy and Heidelberg, Germany. We feel blessed to have these treatment options, but it's daunting to know he has another 5-6 weeks in the hospital coming very soon. He's fatigued and downhearted. Please pray for us as we need you now more than ever, TEAM GRAYSON. Thanks, Rachel

CaringBridge: Jan. 8, 2013: Today was a big day at the U. Grayson and my mom met with his PA Abby and Dr. Lazar who has been called "The Godfather" of BMTs. We could not be any more blessed! Dr. Lazar told Grayson that he would try his best and Grayson needed to try his best as well.

That day I met with Grayson and my mom halfway through his lengthy day of being mapped for the radiation. He'd been scanned for hours, unable to move, and measured for a mesh mask that would be screwed down during the actual radiation sessions so he could not move even a millimeter. It reminded me of something you'd see on Halloween, and the whole thing sounded like a nightmare to me, but I kept that to myself. The radiation oncologists and physicists spent forty hours mapping his body, literally day and night to align everything for the planned treatments. We felt blessed and blown away by this. Grayson was exhausted by all of this, and had to be taught breathing techniques to not freak out when in the mask and leg holders for six, one-hour segments in coming weeks. I prayed for him and the medical staff. This had to work.

A week later I left work early to attend the last major meeting with Dr. Lazar before the BMT. I battled the frigid winds biting my face, yet felt hopeful at the bright healthy future I was projecting for Grayson. Victoria joined us, sitting against the wall by the door. Grayson and I held hands, seated together across from the doctor who was at that time Obi-Wan Kenobi, aka- our last hope. I furiously took notes, writing down as much as I could, wanting to be aware of what was to come.

It was at this meeting that Grayson and I would hear something I wouldn't share with anyone, not even my parents as we ventured into this foreign land. With Grayson's numbers, immunity issues and body condition, there was only a 19 percent chance that it would all work. 19 Percent. We'd just been told that there was only yes, I'll say it again…a 19 percent chance that it would work and Grayson would live. I stomached that information, internalized it and let it fly to the sky. We were in this for better or worse, and the Grayson and Rachel team were going to fight it hand in hand.

After Dr. Lazar was done explaining everything, he gave Grayson and I each a hug, and told us he was pulling for us and knew this was the best possible option and course of treatment. I looked him in the eye and thanked him for his kindness, continual support and expertise. As he left the room to go get the lead scientist to introduce to us, Victoria said, "Did either of you get any of that?" to which we both replied, "Yes." She replied, "Good, because I didn't get any of it." As we drove home we didn't speak of anything medical, cancer or of the future. We talked about our animals, my work and stories of random things we'd seen online. We had to take steps back from the immersion of cancer life that sucks out your soul and being, even if it was good news at times. It is a kind of exhaustion you can only understand if you are the cancer patient or the spouse/significant other. After we got home, we called my parents and gave them the run down, then watched some TV and rested for the next day to come.

CaringBridge: Jan. 16, 2013: Hard times: Grayson has one last big appt. before his Monday hospitalization. Today I decided to schedule a surgery to have the cyst on my ovary removed before it ruptures, as I cannot stand the pain and uncertainty anymore. It will be on the 25th, which means I won't be able to be with Grayson for a few days. It's so disappointing this is happening now, of all times. Prayers for us please. Thanks. R.

Chapter 16:
Last bit of "Normal"

Thursday afternoon I worked a half day, picked up Grayson and jetted to my gyno-surgeon's office to discuss my intolerable pain. I'd been poked and prodded seven times in the last few months at my doctor's office and was told "You've had a gigantic cyst on your ovary that's been cooking for quite a while." Grayson gently rubbed my back as we discussed the upcoming surgery.

After that we spent the next hour perusing the aisles of the Whole Foods across the street from the clinic. He hadn't been shopping in months due to his immunity issues, and reveled in the aisles of tea, coffee and fancy crackers as we looked at each other and giggled. This was a hot date for us.

Friday we met with the bone marrow transplant social worker Nora, who was very kind and knowledgeable as she walked us through the BMT process regarding emotional and mental health. We were given a three-inch binder on BMTs, and graciously gifted gasoline, Target and grocery cards. She informed us how difficult a BMT can be mentally and emotionally and asked about the planned daily support for him; as it was a mandatory requirement for all BMT patients. I felt so relieved and at peace, knowing my mom and dad would be holding down Team Grayson.

Jan. 20, 2013: The night before hospitalization Grayson was cool as a cucumber, while I was a nervous wreck, as if I had a huge exam the next day. We slept in, had breakfast, prayed and just spent time being us, not wanting this cocoon of ours to end. He wore his "Keepin' It Real Since the 70's" Muppet t-shirt, jeans and a white, brown and green flannel shirt from my dad. He backed up his computer, returned emails and spent time with Rufus, Puddin' and Greta, while my parents made themselves scarce, giving us time alone.

Grayson happily sat in a vintage leather chair we'd recently inherited, as he drank tea, relaxed his long legs on the matching ottoman and looked around our home, taking it all in, reflecting on the coming days and weeks in which he'd have to be away. Due to having such heavy feet and neuropathy, Grayson wore socks inside his Birkenstocks, "Jesus Sandals" as I called them, so he wouldn't trip. As he changed his clothes that night, he danced in just his Muppets t-shirt, shorts and socks with sandals while winking at me. I could not believe the joy that this goof would display to me, when he knew the hardships that the near future would bring. When we were together, we were in a world of security and warmth. Our little corner of the world was like a snow globe. Things and times may change but we would remain glued to the foundation of our love, marriage and faith in God, while the snow of life moved all around us and above our heads. We held hands, prayed and went to sleep.

The next morning I felt anxious as Grayson left our home to start the BMT process on January 21, 2013. We'd met on September 21, 2001, eleven years and four months before this. He looked around the house one last time before heading out the door, gave me a hug and a kiss, and off he went with my parents as I went to work.

Each day I called my parents between clients to get the update, and visited each evening after work. My angel of a dad would get to Grayson's room by 7:30 a.m. at the latest, sitting there quietly with his coffee, sometimes in the dark, until the patient woke up, ready to keep him company and take notes when the medical staff started their parade for the day. I had my parents and Victoria write in the "Communication Notebook" I created as a central place to write all of Grayson's stats, updates and info from the doctors.

From January 22nd to the 25th Grayson had extremely high doses of chemo to wipe out his entire immune system, making it like that of a newborn baby. All visitors had to wash their hands and hang their coats outside before they could enter his room, then use hand sanitizer once inside in order to keep him safe, while his body prepared for the new life of the stem cells. By this time he had mouth sores that made eating difficult and had to swish "magic mouthwash" with lidocaine to numb the pain, but his major organs were doing okay, despite the high doses of radiation. I spent the night before my surgery beside him. Although he couldn't sleep, he told me it was comforting to have me there.

CaringBridge: Jan. 25, 2013: My dad picked me up at 5:15 a.m, and we jetted over to Abbott Northwestern Hospital where I had a 7:30 a.m. laparoscopy surgery to remove an ovarian cyst. It turns out I had huge adhesions, cysts and growths all over, thus the diabolical pain I've been in. I'm taking 2 Percocet every 4 hours and being well taken care of by my dad. I miss Grayson. R.

As my dad dropped me off to park, I thought of running away as I walked to the door in the negative ten-degree weather. I signed in. As I waited with my dad I looked at the giant fish tank and thought how odd it was that my husband and I were both in hospitals at the same time. Within the hour I was in a gown, doped up and headed down the hall, telling my dad, who was walking behind the gurney, as we passed the lit-up red and green hall sign that listed patient's names- "Look! My name is on the board like at the airport!" I saw him chuckle and shake his head. Minutes later I was out cold.

Ninety minutes later I woke up groggy and as I attempted to tell the nurse I could not hear her discharge instructions with the curtain open because there were people loudly talking behind her, she clapped her hands loudly together and said "Focus, Rachel! Focus." To this day my dad teases me at times and will randomly say, "Focus, Rachel! Focus!" as he claps before falling over laughing. On the way home I looked at photos from the surgery my dad had been given by my doctor that showed twenty-six adhesions. My dad told me it seemed no matter what I may try holistically to feel better, it looked like there was no stopping these endometriosis issues from happening again

~

Friday the 25th- Monday the 28th: Grayson started the space age radiation, listening to a mix CD he'd made for each of the six sessions. He told me the mesh mask hurt his neck, and he could feel a slight tingling of his skin and hair during the sessions. He was too weak to get up and go to the bathroom so he had to use a catheter, to his chagrin. We talked on the phone for a long time like we did when we first met, which was healing to us both. He was my hero and I let him know it every darn day.

CaringBridge: Jan. 28, 2013: Transplant Week! To prep for the BMT, Grayson was given immunity boosting drugs to help white and red blood cell production and the prevention of GVHD: Graft Versus Host Disease- (When the donor cells attack the recipient.) He finishes up his radiation these last two days then has one last bone marrow biopsy. We are excited to be this close to the big day and feel so blessed for your love and support! Love Rachel and Grayson

Chapter 17:
Mission Control: Countdown to Moon Touchdown

CaringBridge: Jan. 31, 2013: Transplant day! Grayson had a 9:30 a.m. bone marrow biopsy and 1:30 p.m. transplant. We now pray and wait! Thanks for all of your love and support! R & G.

Although this was the day that TEAM GRAYSON had been looking forward to, Grayson felt excited, while also scared and nervous. We'd been told that the bone marrow transplant is known as the "Second Birthday" as it's the day the patient receives new life from the donor. Nurses told us that BMTs came with interesting changes as the patient takes on some of the genetic traits of the donor. A former patient had had jet black curly hair and after her BMT, had blond straight hair; another patient had loved Mexican food pre-BMT, and hated it afterwards. When you take on the stem cells of the donor, you are literally getting an entire new blood type as well. It was all so fascinating!

That day Grayson wore a bright green shirt with white lettering he'd gotten from one of my sisters that said, "I Would Cuddle You So Hard." His mom and my parents all sat around his bed awaiting the transfusion. We took several photographs of him and me, him in his funny shirt and a pair of black sunglasses that had a sparkled hanging mustache from Diana, and me, a hot mess in a bright orange hoodie and purple yoga pants. We each groaned in pain from our separate health conditions, both taking painkillers, then laughed at the boat we were in together. We snuggled and looked each other in the eyes when we had a quick private moment and said, "Ready or not! Here it is: the day we've been waiting for!" Grayson made a blasting up to the sky movement with his arms raised in the air, in one of his cartoon voices that I adored so much. "Here we go, Pony, blastoff!" he said, then yawned and awaited the parade of people that would come in and out in the coming minutes and hours.

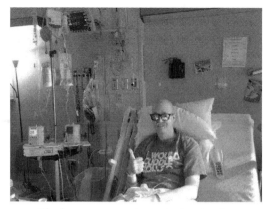
The bone marrow transplant going in.

Our pastor anointed Grayson with oil on his forehead as a rite of passage for this new life, then said a prayer. The two bags of umbilical cord stem cells were hung from his IV pole that would take only two hours to infuse into his body. We learned one baby was born in Eastern Standard Time, the other one in Central. We were told that one of the umbilical cord blood donors would eventually take over his system, as they'd compete to see who won during the process of attachment. I thought to myself, "Go, Gadget, Go!" like from Inspector Gadget, the show I watched when I was little. We had birthday cake that Victoria had brought, as we all said aloud our wishes, prayers and Miss America speeches worth of world peace wishes into the life and health of this man that was my husband.

When the process was done, Grayson was exhausted from his chemo and radiation over that last week and became irritable after our parents left and we were alone. When I thought he'd been in a good mood like he had outwardly portrayed, he said, "I wanted to say, "No I don't want a freaking piece of cake! I want to take a nap and magically wake up in six months feeling better!" He threw his head back in frustration against his stacked pillows. I told him I was proud of him, and to just keep looking toward his healthy future. We took a nap and held hands in our little corner of the world between the frequent nurse visits.

~

Till it All Hits the Wall
The next day I dragged my exhausted behind to work, while my dad went to sit with Grayson. The fanfare had ceased, and this was our new normal.

My dad had told me when I checked in with him mid-day, that Grayson's body had just started to fall apart. He was in a hurricane of hurt and illness that was hitting land at magnitudes we could never imagine, despite us all being informed of what would and could happen with all of the chemo and radiation prep pre-transplant. He had chills, slept terribly, and needed blood transfusions. Somehow, miraculously, he was able to get his biscuit on the stationary bike in his room. He was told he would only feel weaker by the day before things got better as the transplant process went on.

When I got home from work, my dad told me that Victoria stated to him at the hospital that afternoon, "They never told us this would happen!" to which he replied, "Yes, actually they did. This is exactly what they said would happen. All of the hard work his body has gone through and this new immune system is going to make him sick and fatigued." He laughed and told me, "I guess she thought it was cake time, then leave and it's all okay, over and done, smooth sailing from there!"

I felt terrible that there was nothing I could do to help him. I felt so alone and isolated as his cancer wife, while my husband was fighting for his life.

CaringBridge: Feb. 1, 2013: Update: the BMT went well, but now the side effects are really starting to hit Grayson hard. Please pray for strength, faith and courage. I'm so thankful to my Dad for taking care of Grayson and I. Love Rachel, the tired cancer wife.

- God bless you both, Rachel.
- Thinking of you always!
- We know this is hard, harder than anyone can imagine. Just know we are with you.
- When this is over, and it will be, I think your Dad should test for his RN! You will begin to heal and feel better each day-which will help you endure. I am proud of you. You have become a STRONG woman! You will endure. Some day when this is behind you, you and Grayson can look back and marvel at your victory over cancer! Godspeed!
- Blessings to you Rachel and Grayson.
- Thinking of you guys always through this, my family went through it with my uncle (the bone marrow transplant and the toughness after) stay positive, focused, and motivated (I know easy to say). But keep trying. Let me know if there's anything we can do- hang in there Rachel and Grayson. It's a difficult journey but one that can be done. For my BMT, I had to get heavy duty pain medication for a sore throat and be put on nutritional support so I know how it goes. Just remember Grayson will heal in time
- Sending my love and prayers!!
- Thanks for the updates! You're both an inspiration. Sending hugs and warm thoughts for a fast and easy road to recovery now. You deserve it so much.
- What if the blood he got turned him into a tiny purple man? Or Yoda? Who knows what the drugs could do, but I'll tell you what...if he turns in to Yoda, I am totally coming to live with you two. Now that would be science at work.
- Rachel, your love is so healing for Grayson. You two are in my thoughts in prayers at this time.
- Sending healing thoughts to both of you!
- Thinking of you both.
- I'll keep the prayers coming!
- Rachel, I admire your strength and the love and support you are giving your sweet love!! I pray The Lord blesses you with continued undying strength and the blessing of a great outcome!! Thinking of you two always!!

Grayson was on a constant stream of painkillers, had complications like bladder infections, blood in his urine, and throat pain so severe he was offered IV nutrition. To my delight, my friend Esther from freshman year of college was Grayson's BMT nutritionist. She was able to provide him with sound dietary advice, cheer, humor and empathy. She had him eat calorie-packed ice cream-like "magic cups" when he couldn't stomach anything else. He went from being relatively healthy sitting in our home drinking tea on January 20, to having his bowels fall apart on February 2. That required several tubes to help him. It was all frightening and humbling at the same time. I'd tell myself to smile, suck it up and not let him know how worried I was. I prayed to God for peace, comfort and understanding. For such a chatty girl, I was speechless.

CaringBridge: Feb. 4, 2013: Fevers of 101.4. He is on antibiotics. Grayson has lost his appetite and is in so much pain they have brought in a PCA, which is a med machine where he can push a button every 10 minutes to deliver pain meds. My guy is so strong and tough. You can do this honey! You amaze us all!

Grayson often met with the hospital chaplain who helped him learn how to do meditative breathing, as he'd been diagnosed with the "BK virus", no not Burger King like it always made me think of, but a virus that stripped the walls of his bladder, causing painful blood clots that had to be flushed out with continual running bags of fluids. He was too tired to get up and do much, often lying in the bed with his eyes closed, looking so angelic despite the war zone he was living in. I helped bathe him at his bedside several times. He preferred me to help if possible when I visited after work. I'd gently clean his pale, ashen skin as I'd hold him up by his arms as he sat up, reaching his body around all of the tubes and wires. He'd look at me with his puppy dog eyes as I dressed him and say, "Thanks Rachie," in barely a whisper. I wanted to scoop him up and run far away.

Facebook: Feb. 6, 2013: Grayson is very ill. Fevers, barely eating, (is on IV food) and in so much pain. Transplant wise on track. In the meantime, all the comfort in the world cannot keep my heart from breaking at watching my husband, my world, this sick. ~ Rachel Loves Grayson

That same day we found out the BK antibiotics were starting to cause permanent kidney damage. Lovely. What else could happen now? He had lost his eyebrow hair and had begun to have a smatter of freckles appear across his nose and cheeks instead. It killed me to see my 6'2, thirty-seven-year old husband now in adult diapers, but I loved him and helped him no matter what, even changing his diaper when he had peed, unbeknownst to him, as he slept so soundly.

Facebook: Feb. 8, 2013: Grayson pretty much has pneumonia. Had my doctor fax anxiety meds to the hospital as I am having panic attacks. Spending all weekend here. Supersonic prayers please!

I received an urgent voicemail from Victoria that day as I was kicking snow off my boots, getting into my car between clients. I called her back and she told me Grayson had pneumonia, which could be fatal. I somehow managed to get through my next two client appointments, then raced to the hospital. I called my doctor to get a prescription of Xanax sent to the hospital pharmacy; I was panicking. When I checked in with the BMT doctor I had paged, I was told that when immune systems were as weak as Grayson's, lungs have to be continuously checked for infections. For now, he only had a small infection that would be treated with antibiotics, and did not in fact have pneumonia. I face palmed and knew next time to get the update from either my parents or directly from the medical staff.

~

The Dilaudid Days

Grayson had been put on high doses of the painkiller Dilaudid to help manage the pain he was experiencing. It did help, but when it was combined with his other meds and his extreme fatigue, it made him bonkers. He had zero awareness of his actions or words, almost like he was sleepwalking while telling me nonsensical dreams. Victoria told me when I arrived after work one day that he'd told her, "Don't wear anything stupid," when she visited the next time. After she left, he insisted there was a soldier hiding all around the room. He looked with wide eyes around the perimeter of the room as I assured him no one was there. He looked at me, telling me, "Rachel is awesome sauce." I think he did not know at that point who I was. He told me about his friend Lacey from high school, whom he hadn't seen in over a decade, like it was yesterday.

Later he asked me where the water machine was, and was firmly convinced that our cat Rufus was on the "veranda" outside his hospital room window on the fifth floor. I decided to play along if he was going to have such wacky thoughts, asking him "Who is Rachel?" He replied "My best friend, she is on a boat." When I asked where she was, he said, "The island of Mira." One of the nurses told me he said "that he would not be taking the job, as he would be hanging out on the beach instead". When I asked again who Rachel was, he said, "My sleeping buddy! Rachel is there with Grayson. I'm waiting. What is going on with pneumonia and all that fun stuff?"

I decided to ask him about our siblings. "Where is Diana?" "She's with Slim Jim." "Where is Natasha?," "She is with Beef Stick!" Then he sat up and told me what he seemed to think was a genius idea, "There needs to be a jacket for diabetes. You can it, then put fat in the carpet. You can see it, not eat it. If kids eat it you are kinda screwed. Like a Jeep Cavalier?" Tears streamed down my face and I shook in silent laughter as my husband muttered gibberish. I took this moment to laugh instead of cry at our reality.

That night he had a diarrhea blowout from all of his meds and had to be cleaned up. The on-call BMT doctor came in to tell me they'd detected densities in his lung that could be from unseen bleeding or fluid. Something abnormal was present and things were not so funny anymore. I wondered what else could happen, to only shortly later find out from a nephrologist that his kidneys had gotten worse, there was definite constant bleeding in his bladder and they had to continue to measure his creatinine levels to make sure he didn't go into kidney failure.

Alarms went off in my head for hours, much like the bed alarms Grayson continued to set off every hour on the hour as he attempted to get out of bed in his aggravated, confused and delusional state. One time as he took deep breaths and tried to fall asleep he told me, "Rachel is hiding inside a bag of moose," then said in his own amazement, "Remember that time we got stuck in Indiana?" He asked "Where is Ryan-boy?," meaning my dad, right before he conked out. An hour later as he was calming down again he asked me in paranoia, "What is it about being down here? I feel like I am in Korea! Do you feel like that?" I was exhausted from this naughty monkey that was acting like a toddler, through no fault of his own. The night nurse told me the night before he'd set off the alarm saying he had to go, as he'd be late to his photo shoot.

At 4 a.m. I awoke to the sound of shuffling feet, seeing and hearing as I pulled off my eye mask and took out my ear plugs, that in his high-as-a-kite state, he'd accidentally ripped out his IV as he tried to get out of bed. Blood had spattered all over and he had pooped and tried to take off his diaper. It was a literal mess with several nurses and aides running all over. Unfortunately some blood had gotten into one of the poor nurse's mouth and she had to be tested for HIV later. Oh sweet Grayson, one step up, and you run thirteen feet behind. His therapist later told me that the delusions, although concerning, are "Mother Nature's way of helping you not remember and get through," which I was beginning to understand. From that night on he had a nursing aide sit with him to curb incidents like those from happening again.

The next day Grayson slept part of the morning in a recliner. He'd become very ill with fevers and said he felt like crap after what I sarcastically described as his night of partying. My dad and I watched the NCAA basketball championship as we read the paper. I accidentally stepped on Grayson's catheter tube on the floor and he awoke with a roar, stating, "Aw, man! Come on! If my penis hurts forever I'm going to blame you!" I fell backward on his bed collapsing in laughter with tears running down my face. Dad covered his face higher with the paper, attempting to pretend he hadn't heard a thing. Oh, sweet Grayson.

That afternoon while we watched "Police Academy," Grayson asked me to get his phone for him. I retrieved the device he hadn't used in weeks and handed it to him, asking what he wanted it for. He told me he wanted to know how many barnyard animals were in this movie series. He attempted to fiercely push and punch at the screen, not comprehending how to use his phone, which brought me to tears. I took the phone out of his hand and pretended to look it up on my phone, then gave him a random number, which seemed to satisfy him. I applied lotion to his itchy hands that had begun peeling layers of skin as he was shedding the old skin and getting new skin from the new baby cells he'd received. When my dad came back, I hugged Grayson, then went home to crash.

CaringBridge: Feb. 10, 2013: Update: Day 10: Today Grayson had stints put in his kidneys to try to help his bladder drain out fluids. It's becoming scarier by the day with all of the complications. Hopefully this will clear out any obstructions and allow him to heal and get better. His medical team is doing everything they can. Please pray for us. Rachel.

Feb. 13: Ash Wednesday: Grayson's skin hurt badly; he'd gained thirty pounds of water weight, causing his skin to stretch to unattainable boundaries. He had a shadow in his lungs, bruised eyes, and despite all of that, the BMT doc told us there is no reason why the BMT wouldn't work. Until then it was just a crap show of side effects that poor Grayson had to deal with, while we waited for this song and dance of the new cells to breathe new life into his system.

~

Hearts and Everything in Between

On Valentine's Day I visited Grayson after work feeling mentally and physically wiped out, but knew it was nothing compared to what he was facing. He instructed me to get two cards from his bedside end table that had my name written on them. I was immediately brought to tears as I saw my name in a barely legible scribble, compared to the beautiful handwriting I'd come to know over the years. I thanked him for the cards my mom had obviously bought for him, hugged him and told him how much I loved him as I looked into his puffy, large, sunken eyes. I still saw the hazel in there that I'd known what seemed my whole life. He looked so uncertain from the ravaged sea of cancer that kept sweeping his shores. I gave him my card that made him laugh as it had an inside joke of ours in it, then watched TV in a companionable silence as we ate dinner, a salad for me and only graham crackers and applesauce for him, as he was in so much mouth pain.

He told me that night he liked how I always stayed late, that his mom always left in time to get the valet service before they closed at 8pm. I guess he'd asked her if it occurred to her that even after she left, he was still there and would be lonely, to which she replied it hadn't been something she'd thought of before. I had no idea what it would have been like to have had my child go through this, and knew it was hard for her, however it seemed like she wasn't understanding many of Grayson's needs, despite her being physically present at times. Even though it was so tiring, I tried to stay until at least 9 or 9:30 pm. every night and to spend the night on the weekends as many nights as I could. I knew it meant the world to him, even when my candle was flickering.

CaringBridge: Feb. 17, 2013: Day 17: Grayson continues to fight and put up with doctors shoving scopes up his nose, poking and prodding him, and coming in and out every few minutes. A typical day looks like this: 3:30 a.m.: blood drawn, 4:30 a.m.: nursing assistant, 5 a.m.: vitals: temp, oxygen, 5:30 a.m.: nursing assistant, 6 a.m.: blood/platelets, 7 a.m.: nurse switch time and report, Grayson's caregiver arrives, 7:15 a.m.: nurse, 7:30 a.m.: Physician's assistant, 8 a.m.: ENT-ear nose & throat doctors, 8:30 a.m.: nurse, 8:45 a.m.: phone for meal cannot eat, 9 a.m.: nursing assistant, 9:15 a.m.: Grayson uses nasal spray, to open up passages and coughs up lots of blood clots from sore throat and lungs to suction out, 10 a.m.: urinary doctors/ kidney doctors, 10:30 a.m.: nurse- vitals/ platelets, 11 a.m.: BMT head doctor rounds, 11:15 a.m.: nurse, 12 p.m.: phone rings for lunch not having, 12:30-2 p.m.: possible rest, 2 p.m.: physical therapy, 2:30 p.m.: nurse/assistant, 3 p.m.: occupational therapy, 3:30 p.m.: speech therapy (trying to swallow applesauce, solid foods), 4 p.m.: rest if possible, 4:30 p.m. on: dinner, rest, vitals, checks, transfusions if necessary and sleep later if possible. Holy cats! How does he do it and still remain so kind?! And some good news- Praise the Lord- he lost 17 lbs. of fluid in 2 days. Love R & G.

The above schedule would have been my own version of hell. I decided to take a night off every five days or so, resting at home on the couch while I binged on my Netflix DVDs. I snuggled inside my blanket while snow fell outside most nights and tried not to think about the fact that my other half was in the hospital and should have been at my side.

Facebook: Feb. 18, 2013: It's so hard to leave Grayson at the hospital. He is so sick and looks and is…so fragile. Darn stupid, awful cancer! I hate u!

- Totally understand your frustration, anger, sadness, etc. Since I cannot make it go away, just know we are backing you and Grayson 120%. With prayers, strong thoughts and anything else you need.
- I admire you and Grayson's courage and strength.
- I know this is so very hard for you, sweet Rachel, but Grayson IS getting better and will be stronger. Big hugs for you and give him a virtual hug from me. Much, much love, A.
- I send you hugs.

Over the next few days Grayson made huge strides in getting better, like being able to stand to use the commode and wipe his own butt. Can you imagine being so weak you couldn't do that? We take so much for granted, doing so many things on autopilot, always thinking we will be as healthy as we are now. He needed two nurses to help him stand and use the walker to get to the pot, and when he did, he always towered over them with his tall height. It was the first time in weeks he'd been able to do so- and a big deal for us.

In the midst of Grayson's misery, he still treated everyone with grace and kindness, despite how terrible he felt. I'd look at him as he relied so heavily on the medical devices and watch him as if he was an animal on the Discovery Channel, void of any feelings of sadness or pity. It was what it was, and I knew somehow one day this was all just going to be a memory.

130

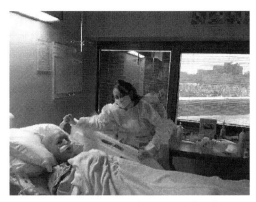
Bone Marrow Transplant Complications

CaringBridge: Feb. 21, 2013: Day 20. Grayson's nursing aide didn't want to wake him so she asked if I would. After 3 attempts I yelled "Hey Grayson there's a hot naked model in your room" ....he opened his eyes! He is still very ill, but getting better in increments and looking more like my husband every day. He is done with ENT and kidney docs for now, but has low white blood cell counts, so it's still a scary time, but I'm hopeful. It'll be weeks before I can take him home, but he amazes me daily!

- Good to hear. I look forward to your updates each day.
- I also look forward to your daily updates. Thank you and I love the fact that the hot naked model thing worked. He is male, after all!!!!
- Love to you both! Great to see your amazing sense of humor always prevails!

CaringBridge: Feb. 23, 2013: GOOD NEWS! Despite being quite sick still, Grayson's most recent BMT results how no results of cancer!!! Hallelujah, Praise the Lord, the winning Super-bowl Team is going to Disneyland! However way you want to put it, I wanted to climb the tallest building and shout for joy. May those demon cells never return! Today an assistant let his ice packs melt on his bed which caused him to wake up in chills. I'm a nice person, but man, don't mess with my guy! I gave them an earful and hope it never happens again! Grrr! Love Rachel

I felt so much like a mom with a baby, constantly checking Grayson over. Instead of bumps and bruises and diapers, I was familiar with every complication he'd had so far as a thirty-seven-year-old BMT patient. I looked out the window at the snow, wanting a helicopter to whisk us away to a foreign land for a vacation adventure of new sights and foods to explore. I hoped one day that would be possible for us. We should have been having babies, going to restaurants and concerts, not cooped up in hospital rooms with Grayson's body falling apart.

131

Chapter 18:
One Step Forward and Two Leaps Back

CaringBridge: Feb. 26, 2013: Huge News! A blood cord unit attached and grafted! Still a long tough road ahead, but hallelujah! Thank you God! I did a victory dance at the end of his bed and let out a breath I'd been holding for the last 26 days, as Grayson clapped and laughed. I hadn't been able to hug or kiss him in weeks, with his immune system so low, and was able to hug him as tears ran down my face at this embrace. He has a long path ahead of him and we miss our "normal" life more than you'll ever understand. At times I feel like we are actors playing a part, but we never get commercial breaks. We pray for strength, faith and courage, R & G.

CaringBridge: Mar. 2, 2013: Day 30 post-transplant, day 40 in the hospital. Tonight as I lay in bed I am crying, saddened by missing my husband, my zany best friend and the sense of security in life, let alone any sense of normalcy. His white blood cells are up, he's lost 27 lbs. via dialysis, but he has a new marrow virus. I wanna beat away those stinkin' viruses, punch cancer in the face and take him away on a vacation. On a more pleasant note-he was able to do a short trip down the hallway with a walker for the first time ever! Thanks to my brother Jack and his wife Maddie, for driving so far to see us. I need my lovies to keep this gal from shattering in a million pieces. Thank you all, please stick with us, Rachel and Grayson.

CaringBridge: Mar. 4, 2013: ICU - Storm heaven with prayers please. Grayson could not breathe on his own- so he was moved to ICU for help. Kidneys and lungs in danger, new level of scary.

I received a 6:50 a.m. phone call from a nurse that took me from my peaceful sleep, to a place of panic. She told me Grayson hadn't been breathing well overnight, and within the hour would be put on a ventilation machine. I hurried to get ready, woke my mom up early, and headed out the door while trying to wrap my mind around the fact that my husband was going to be put on life support. Thank God I didn't yet know how scary that would be. I half listened to the morning jabber on the radio, called Victoria who said she'd be there soon, and drove as calmly and quickly as I could without getting a ticket. As I exited the highway, I called Grayson to find out where he was. Over the noise of the loud oxygen machine, he told me he couldn't breathe well, we exchanged I-love-yous and hung up.

I practically threw my keys at the valet and booked it to his room only to find him not there, as he'd already been moved to the ICU. By the time I reached him, he had been intubated and had a fever of 102.4. I stood over him petting his head, and said quietly over and over, "Please Lord, don't let him die." He was heavily sedated and had his wrists tied down so if he woke up he wouldn't accidentally rip out the vent. His BMT PA Mallory came in and told me she was scared for him. As I looked at her with her cute, curly, short brown hair and bright rainbow sweater I asked her if he could die. She told me it was possible, that he was in a very dangerous state and that the next twenty-four to forty-eight hours were critical, but yes, it could kill him.

I was so upset with Mallory! She had been so helpful and cheery on the BMT journey, and now she was telling me news I didn't want to hear, deflating my hopes and dreams of Grayson getting better and living to old age. She was just the messenger, but told me news no spouse/significant other wants to hear. I prayed like I never had before, begging God to not let my husband die, then said the Lord's Prayer two or three times.

Within an hour my mom arrived, looked at Grayson with tears in her eyes, and said as she death-gripped my hand, "Grayson will be ok. We will not lose him now, he will be okay." Victoria showed up three hours after I called her, stating she had an obligation at church she'd had to attend to first. I bit my tongue to keep quiet while I absorbed her words.

CaringBridge: Mar. 4, 2013: Now totally moved to ICU. His lungs are bad. He is still not getting enough oxygen and either has bleeding in his lungs or a virus/infection. He's about to have a bronchoscopy to find out. I'm thankful my work is letting me use unpaid time off while keeping our health insurance. Please pray like you never have before, as my life lays in this scary bed.

The next week was a blur. I slept every night in the recliner chair next to his bed. When I wasn't attempting to distract myself with the season of "Drop Dead Diva," I'd purchased on Amazon video, or reading Cheryl Strayed's "Wild," I went for walks around the halls, or held Grayson's hand. The endless stream of medical professionals kept me alert and on my toes during the day, and I was so grateful for all of their knowledge and expertise.

One day my friend Cassie, who I'd met while cheering for a TNT race months before, came to drop off a card from Tony, a new widower who had lost his wife the December before to BMT complications. Inside the card were the nicest and sweetest words of encouragement and prayers, a phone number and an offer to talk if I had questions or just wanted to talk to someone who had been there before, and five one hundred dollar bills. My jaw dropped at this kindness when I needed it most. That night I caved, springing for a hotel room two blocks up from the hospital. I walked in the falling snow past the markets and buildings I'd frequented in undergrad so long ago. I passed all of the young babies walking around campus without a care in the world. I paid for a room, passing the couples drinking and laughing around the fireplace bar and went to find my room. I filled up an ice bucket, bought Cheetos and root-beer, watched Conan O'Brien, took a Benadryl, cranked up the AC and fell fast asleep.

The next day was a whirlwind of medical staff again, who told me there was little improvement. I didn't know whether Grayson would get better or this would be the new temporary normal.

I had dinner that night with Vera and Owen at Sally's where we munched on sandwiches and waffle fries as I told them he might improve, but there was a chance he may die. It was so surreal how calm I was, accepting the possible fate. We attempted to talk about funny things for the rest of the meal before we gave hugs and headed home. Outside on the street Vera went one direction while Owen and I stood in the falling snow in silence. I looked up at him in the glow of the streetlight and asked him if there was anything he wanted to know. He gravely shook his head with tears in his eyes, so sad at the prospect of losing his best friend of twenty-three years. We hugged and walked our separate ways. That night I felt a little less worried as I fell asleep feeling God's embrace, knowing tomorrow was a new day and God had a plan, even if I didn't know it. I just had to trust Him and wait.

Over the next few days I would see and hear illness, death and grieving all around me in the ICU. I saw other patients hooked up to machines, and families crying in and outside the glass partitioned rooms as Blue Oyster Cult's "Don't Fear the Reaper," played continuously in my head.

CaringBridge: Mar. 9, 2013: Day 6 ICU, Day 37 post-BMT, 47 in the hospital. He seems to have stabilized a bit. He has so many cords all over him; he's lit up like a Christmas tree. I want to spring him out of here so badly. This is a longer process than any of us thought, please PRAY! Love Rachel

On this day I started to play music for Grayson from the iPod dock I'd brought from home, hoping he'd hear it. Felicity flew in to keep me company. I'd been having a lot of one-way conversations with Grayson after my mom left for the day. On the second day my sister was there, I went to give Grayson a hug before we left to go to lunch. He must have been upset I was leaving, because he tried to sit up and stop me with his arms, accidentally ripping out his feeding tube in the process. It splattered all over my black coat sleeve and the bed. Once he'd been cleaned up and sedated, I pet his face and told him I'd be back soon before I ran down the hall and collapsed crying in Felicity's arms. It was a nightmare. It really was.

CaringBridge/Facebook: Mar. 10, 2013: Day 7 ICU: HUGE update! Grayson is still critically ill and certainly not out of the woods yet, however his white blood cell count is 1,600 today and there are zero traces of the virus in his marrow anymore, which means the transplant is working! He's now able to shake his head to confirm if he wants something, and was able to tell me he heard the music I'd been playing him. Thank you to my angel parents who have given up so much to be with us all the time. My dad just drove 1100 miles from Georgia to be here. Please keep storming heaven with prayers! Love, Rachel

- Thanks be to God!
- Yes! Ask the nurses for a communication board for him. He can point and spell if he can have a hand free.
- Awesome! Keep fighting you guys!
- Great news. Stay strong Lots of love sent your way from us.
- That's awesome
- Oh praise The Lord. That white count is so important. I am overjoyed.
- Happy Day!
- This IS the news we have been praying for. With the hundreds of people petitioning God the Father- a miracle from one week ago is before us. Please tell Grayson from us that we have been praying every day and more. I am just so happy.
- Thank God.
- So exciting to hear Rachel- best news I have heard in a while.
- Trinity Lutheran church Vermilion, OH- will be so excited to get this news. We're keeping on keeping on with prayers.
- Almost in tears reading this - you both needed some good news. I know things are only going to get better from here! Hugs to you both!
- Yeah!

~

Miracles are Real

CaringBridge: Mar. 11, 2013: Miracles do happen! White count is 2700 and he's coming off of the ventilator day! Dr. Lazar and his ICU doc said he is headed in the right direction and his BMT PA Mallory said she is "Pleased as punch," that his transplant is working despite the organ issues.

I held Grayson's hand as he was taken off the ventilator, which was traumatic to watch. He had to continually cough as they pulled the long tubing out of his throat. Of course, at that same time the bandage on his leg where he received dialysis decided to spring a leak, spurting blood up in the air as well. He kept coughing with tears dripping down his face until the tube was out. It was really hard to watch, but I was so relieved when he was able to speak in low raspy voice for the first time in seven days, after some sips of water. Twenty minutes later Victoria walked in and upon hearing the news, said, "We've done it! Look how far we got!"

I decided to walk away at that moment towards the window so I wouldn't say something I'd regret. She'd just missed the trauma her son went through. I glanced over my shoulder for a second to see Grayson raise his eyebrow, roll his eyes and shake his head in shared annoyance.

Over the next few days Grayson became more aware of his current health status and how his organs had been failing him. He wanted to be up to date on everything, but often did not want to know things that happened he wasn't aware of, such as the Dilaudid wacky times or

136

while he was sedated on the vent. I think it was all just so the opposite of optimal health and where he wanted to be headed, that he'd rather be in the dark about it unless it was pertinent to know.

He was unaware of how long he'd been hospitalized, asking my dad during the days if he could go home. Now he said to me, "Rachie, I want to go home," with his sad puppy dog eyes. All I could do was remind him how far he'd come, and how he had to still stay there and do his job. I showed him on the room's whiteboard what his different organ levels had been, what they should be, and how far he had to go to get there number-wise. I went over how long he'd been there to try to help him understand the situation more. That same week we were told that he'd had an alveolar hemorrhage in his lung that one in a million people recover from. Now that my friends, is God.

CaringBridge: Mar. 13, 2013: Post written by friend Olive:

When I taught summer camps at the zoo in 2003, I befriended one of the interns. Rachel and I became fast friends and were a good match in our young single days. We did all kinds of girly things together: movies, shopping, dinners out. I'd say our most successful outing was a Bruce Springsteen concert. He was performing a one man show at the Northrup Auditorium. To this day, it's still the best show I've ever seen . . . by leaps and bounds.

Rachel dated Grayson for the whole time we have been friends. They married in 2004 and danced their first dance to "The Luckiest" by Ben Folds. It was a beautiful celebration. As they started their new life together, they met the challenges of making ends meet. Rachel was in graduate school and worked as much as she could. Grayson worked second shift and got home in the wee hours of the morning. The time they had to spend together was extremely limited. Even so, they made it work and they were very happy in their relationship. The little time they could spend together was treasured.

In January 2011, at the age of 35, Grayson was diagnosed with acute lymphoblastic leukemia. It was right at the time that this happy couple was planning to start a family. As cancer does, it ebbed and flowed. It got bad and then it got a lot better. Cancer is such a trickster. It gives the false hope of overcoming the disease and then it strikes back even worse. It's a horror story that you can never escape once you're afflicted. Even in remission, it changes the way you live and it always makes you wonder if, how, and when it's going to attack next.

Grayson was in remission for a while. He suffered bone loss from his treatments that would be a permanent hardship in his life, but the disease itself was gone. Or so we thought. Last fall, things got bad again and the recommended course of action was a bone marrow transplant. Thankfully a match was found and Grayson received the transplant in January. As of today, he's been in the hospital for over two months in preparation for the transplant and then recovering from it. During that time, Rachel had medical issues of her own that required surgical attention. The stress in their life was compounding. You can imagine getting by on one income and accumulating infinite medical bills. To add to that, Rachel recently started a new job and has not yet worked there long enough to be eligible for FMLA time off. Not only was her husband critically ill, but she had to keep working to maintain the medical benefits.

Then last week happened. Last week, Grayson was admitted to the ICU because his kidneys were failing and he wasn't breathing well. He was put on a ventilator and started dialysis, all while trying to replenish his white blood cell count. It got really bad and Rachel thought she might lose Grayson. We all thought she might.

As of today, Grayson is improving. He had several days of uncertainty followed by a boom in his white blood cell growth. His tube was removed and Grayson continues to recover and even communicate with his wife and family.

My way of supporting them is sharing their story with you.

I can say now that I'm confident in Grayson's survival. He has a long, long journey of recovery ahead of him, but Rachel and Grayson are fighters. They will do everything possible to get back to a normal life.

~

Chapter 19:
The Balancing Act of it All

Once Grayson was off the vent, I reluctantly went to work, getting updates from my parents and calling the night nurse before falling asleep. I was able to keep it together and visit my clients while my husband was in the ICU, only by the grace of God. On one hand it was hell, and on the other it was nice to have a sense of normalcy and a distraction. Grayson continued to ask my mom if he could go home, which broke her heart as well. She'd tell him he needed to get stronger and that he had to get all of the fluid out of his lungs first.

CaringBridge: Mar. 15, 2013: Sorry to not update sooner-crazy busy with work and hospital running. Grayson is still in the ICU. His kidneys are not great but he is doing ok. He has daily dialysis for 3.5 hrs, as he's back up to 200lbs. I wish I could take him home like he continues to ask us to do so. Oh how I wish that was a possibility. The family next door here, is crying because their family member is probably dying. Lord please let this not be us, Love Rachel

CaringBridge: Mar. 15, 2013: Please pray for my guy as he is having a rough time emotionally. It's all wearing and catching up on him in fear, frustration and anxiety.

I skipped my planned St. Patrick's Day "Get Lucky" 7K walk with Owen; Grayson was frustrated, crabby and sad. The three of us spent the weekend doing MadLibs, watching movies, Seinfeld, and eating sub sandwiches while Grayson got used to his high-flow oxygen mask that had bright blue toy-looking tubes coming out of the sides. He was not happy, stating it was so loud, like he was riding on the engine of a Boeing 747 -24/7.

That Sunday, St. Patrick's Day, as he watched the aide empty his urine output into a plastic pitcher, he said, "I know this sounds really weird, but when my pee foams in that container, it looks like a cold frosty one! Man, I really wish it was real and I could drink a beer right about now!" I thought he was cute, nuts and delusional, but his nurse looked at him and said, "I will see what I can do!" Soon after that Dr. Lazar ok'd having a beer. Unfortunately it was Sunday, and the liquor stores in Minnesota were closed so we had to go with Angry Orchard Hard Cider from home. I offered to drive to Hudson, Wisconsin, to get him his beloved Sam Adams or Summit Ale, but he said the hard cider was fine. An hour later my mom had smuggled in the drink, which Grayson happily drank while wearing the felt hat with a shamrock on it Felicity had brought him days earlier.

CaringBridge: Mar. 20, 2013: Grayson is out of the ICU, his transplant baby cells have taken over and are working!!!!! His blood is now new baby blood and he is down to 193 lbs. He has teeny bits of red hair coming in on the top of his head and face as well as light brown freckles. Craziness!

CaringBridge: Mar. 22, 2013: Day 50 post-transplant! Day 60 in the hospital. Grayson is now all moved in and cozy in his small BMT unit room. He is working hard with physical therapy to get strength back. Baby steps each day. The feeding tube came out yesterday, so he can have pureed baby like food. He does have GVHD: Graft Versus Host Disease, but is on meds to help with that. It can be par for the course, so we aren't too worried.

~

Spring Brings New Life and Healing with a Side Order of Pain

CaringBridge: Mar. 25, 2013: Thanks Be to God: I know not all of you are believers, which I respect, but my God has given us a miracle indeed. Grayson will need to be on oxygen for weeks, but his lungs are healing! He is down to 165 lbs., having lost 75 lbs. of fluid via dialysis since March 13th. He has lost a ton of muscle mass, but will be able to regain it when he goes to rehab! Yes, his medical team is thinking about discharging him to move to a transitional rehab care center! Can you hear my jaw hit the floor from here?! Three weeks ago we nearly lost him and now this news! We still have a long, hard and trying road ahead of us, but God has graced us again!

Grayson was such a card in general, but as he got stronger and better, his humor came back in spades. One day when a doctor came in, as he was sitting up in bed using nasal spray over a bin, he began to make a retching sound. The doctor stopped short of the bed, held up her hand and said they'd come back later, to which he lifted his head, laughed and showed he'd pulled one over on them. He also had such quiet grace, patience and kindness. One evening when we were alone he looked at me and frowned. I could tell how tired he was and told him how proud I was of him. He was wearing his "Team Grayson" hat and Stand Up to Cancer bright red t-shirt with the oxygen tubes hanging from his face. He looked at me with his nearly hairless eyebrows, giant eyes and new freckles splattered on his pale face and said, "I am doing this for us! Rachie, this isn't just for me. I am doing all of this for us!" That was the grace and love and the faithfulness of God.

Over the next week I cut his really gross toenails. His feet had layers upon layers of shedding skin. We watched "Curb Your Enthusiasm" on DVD, while I tried not to gag and/or laugh at the oddness of the situation. On Easter I came to the quiet and deserted hospital armed with amazing apple and cherry cheese Danishes for us as well as the nurses. We happily ate as I read the paper, sharing local articles of interest, enjoying time in our little bubble.

On April 1st Grayson was transferred to rehab, an older brick building near the West Bank of the U, where he had less constant care as he had in the BMT ward. He was pushed to the limits by walking one hundred steps at a time, and worked on PT and OT twice a day, to regain strength to stand up and to be able to be upright at the mirror to brush his teeth, comb his hair, as well as toilet and dress.

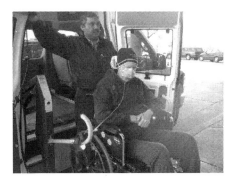
Grayson on his way to rehab

It would have been much easier if the BK virus hadn't come back. He had to have a catheter flush of two bags of fluid pumping through him that had to be refreshed every thirty minutes. The rehab was not staffed enough to meet the needs of the flush system, causing the catheter to back up, resulting in horrific pain. He called me, crying, one day, saying he had to have his catheter changed six times in one day. My dad told me Grayson was so upset by this lack of proper care by the young staff, that the first thing Grayson said to him when he arrived that day was "Get your pencil, I have a lot for you to write down!" It was not the rehab any of us envisioned in many ways. He worked out in a gym working on getting in and out of a car, walking up and down steps, using an arm bike, a stationary bike and walking. He was a fighter and I was proud!

One night Owen, Grayson and I had a pizza party. We watched a Ben Stiller and Vince Vaughn movie, happily chowing down on Davanni's, laughing and spending time together. I left early so they could have some guy time, knowing how much they'd missed each other over these months.

CaringBridge/Facebook: Apr. 8, 2013: Hospital Again: Two steps back. Grayson is back in the hospital BMT unit. Bladder issues are too complex and the medical expertise isn't enough at rehab. Grayson is actually glad to be back in the level of care he is accustomed to. I was just beginning to walk around Lake Calhoun when I heard the news from my dad. Please pray he gets back to rehab soon!!

- Nothing you guys can't handle! Lots of love.
- Thinking of you guys.

I had bittersweet feelings about him being back in the hospital. He was ecstatic to be back with his peeps, so much so- I laughed and told him it was kinda sick how happy he was to be back inpatient, when it was a step backward. My friends knew it was a big blow and step back for us so they began to take me to dinner, out for tea, or bring me treats. My friend Cassie met me in the lobby, handed me a big shopping bag, hugged me and ran back to her running car.

When I was looking at the super-soft quilted blue blanket, Sudoku book and M&Ms in Grayson's hospital room minutes later, Victoria happened to walk in. She immediately told me I was so selfish to go shopping when she was helping us with the mortgage and my husband was fighting for his life. I took a deep breath, told her it was none of her business, that it had been a gift from a friend and that the money she helped us with was from Grayson's late father, to which she huffed and left the room.

The next week I got into a small car accident near a stoplight when I was unable to stop sliding on the ice. Diana came for a visit that weekend, thank God, as it provided some comfort, relief and distraction.

One night as we sat around his bed and ate falafel and gyros, Grayson said something snarky and I replied back just as snarky. Diana told me to be nice to him, that he was sick, just as my friend Poppy had said to me, the fall before when she'd witnessed the same thing. I told her no, that he still needed to be respectful, as I was of him, and just like my therapist said, we needed to be as normal as possible. At the end of the weekend we were told that it would take three to five years for his immune system to fully recover from everything he'd been through, so to be patient. Oh Lord, how the dominos just kept falling.

Chapter 20:

Please God, It's Rachel. Can You Hear Me? Please Don't Let Grayson Go…

CaringBridge: Apr. 17, 2013: Grayson is back in the ICU. Bad lungs and breathing needs help.

Wednesday Apr. 17, 2013 was the worst day of my life. It still is, to this day. I received a 5:45 a.m. call from the BMT unit telling me Grayson could not breathe again and had to go back on life support. My dad drove to the hospital as I sat there in a daze, cool as a cucumber. I called Grayson and talked to him as he tried to yell over the noise of the extremely loud oxygen mask he'd been given. He said, "I have the highest powered oxygen mask on, it looks like one of those WWII masks. I wanted to tell you I loved you before I couldn't talk again." "I love you!" I said back to him, to which Grayson said, "I love you, too!" "I love you!" I said again.

When I got to him, Grayson was intubated in the ICU. I was told he had "cloudy lungs," breathing thirty breaths per minute, to a healthy person's twelve. He looked at me with anxious, giant eyes seeking help or reassurance. For two seconds of uncertainty I froze, then held his hand and started to rub it with the other. I asked my dad to do the same on his other side, and requested Grayson be sedated.

An hour later Mallory came in and gave me a hug. It was 7:30 a.m. By 10 a.m. a BMT doc told me they had never seen a BMT patient survive two blood clots in their lungs. The combination of chemo, radiation, lung issues and the flu all contributed to his now- failing body. Several doctors including Dr. Lazar, who had been with us the whole time, came in to tell me they were sorry. Dr. Hughes, the ICU MD, told me all we could do was wait until that Friday to make a medical decision.

I was numb. My husband was going to die. I took a Xanax and sat there watching medical staff come in and out for what seemed like hours but could have been minutes. It was all a blur. I began to watch Grayson slip away. I thought of Sarah McLachlan's song "Hold On," that I'd heard first as a teen. It was now my reality.

Facebook: Apr. 17, 2013: Broken Heart: I feel super crass posting this on here, but u all have been so supportive. He has another blood clot in his lung on top of the flu and pneumonia and pre and post BMT issues. My husband, my world has 48 hrs then a decision has to be made, on my birthday no less. Please pray for my love and broken heart.

- We are praying and so are many others. We are with you.

- Sending prayers.
- Praying Rachel.
- Hugs your way!
- Sending Strength
- Praying for you all!
- I am, dear.
- Anything at all, we are both here for you.
- I'm praying for you both.
- Sending my love and prayers. Love you guys so much.   Please call me if you need anything.
- Prayers to you and Grayson.
- Omigosh Rachel, I am praying for you both. What else do you need?
- Please call if you need to! Whatever you need!
- Sending super healing thoughts to Grayson.
- Prayers to you and Grayson.
- Prayers coming your way.
- You're both in my thoughts and prayers.
- Praying Rach!!
- I'm praying for you guys!!
- Love you!
- Storming heaven with prayers and sending you both strength and love.
- Sending you all my positive energies. hugs and support.
- Holding you both close, Rachel.
- Thinking of and praying for you both!
- 48 hours filled with fervent prayer!
- Big prayers coming your way!!!
- You're both in my prayers...my love and thoughts are with you right now.
- Rachel, you and Grayson are in my thoughts
- Praying for the both of you Rachel!! Stay strong!!
- Much love sending your way.
- Love and more love and prayers. Thinking so much about you both/
- Praying.
- Praying for you both.
- Please let me know if there's anything I can do/bring/etc. I'm sure I speak for everyone else when I say I'm NOT just saying this. Totally willing to do anything I can, just say the word.
- Holding you both close.
- Prayers for both of you!
- You are in my prayers.
- You both are in my thoughts and prayers.

This was it, what I'd been dreading from the day he was diagnosed. The walls were closing in. There was nothing I could do but love him. I looked at the white metal blinds above the window seat that separated me from the land of the living outside and those dying in the ICU, which now included my husband.

I knew there was always a chance this could happen, but didn't think it would happen to us. That happened to other people, not me. I felt like I was watching myself from above in a weird black and white or sepia tone movie. This couldn't be my real life. I was turning thirty-one in two days and was too young to have my husband die. I didn't plan on this. This was so surreal, that I had to be dreaming. A nightmare in which I fall down an elevator shaft and can't get to Grayson as he's standing looking down at me from the doors that are open above as I fall down the Alice in Wonderland rabbit hole. That has to be it, right? This can't be real. I felt weightless and didn't require much to eat or drink this first day. I was floating on adrenaline and felt so calm I thought I might just float away.

My mom was flying in the next day, getting there as soon as she could. That night after my dad went home, I sat at Grayson's bedside hour after hour just staring at him. His skin was very pale, having lost its usual rosy tone. I rubbed lotion on his hands, finger by finger as I watched TV that I didn't really see or hear. I heard the laugh track but not the lines. I was like a turtle with no shell. I had an existential moment of "I am Rachel. I am Grayson's wife. This is Grayson. The doctors say he is going to die. I have no idea what is going to happen in my life. I know I will be okay somehow. God loves me. I love God."

Fatigue set in and I slept in the narrow gray vinyl chair with my black camping pad underneath me. I put in my ear plugs and covered my eyes with the pink eye mask with black eyelashes painted on it, attempting to block out light and reality for a few hours of rest. When I got up in the middle of the night and returned from the bathroom, I went to Grayson and felt his hand grasp mine in the barely lit room. I told him I loved him, to relax and go back to sleep.

The next morning the nurses told me I looked so cute in my mask that they'd all come in to see me as I slept. I didn't know what to say, so I said nothing. I played Grayson music on our iPod dock again, and had brought a photo of us from our wedding inside a frame I'd recently purchased that had the lyrics to "The Luckiest" on it. I sat there for hours with him, listening to Enya, Coldplay, Jose Gonzalez, Nick Drake and other chill playlists I'd made. There were no real changes that day. Mallory came in and told Grayson, "I am so very sorry this is happening. You've been quite the fighter through all of this." She asked him if he wanted to keep fighting. He nodded, then she said, "Then that is what we will keep doing."

Facebook: Apr. 18, 2013: Grayson is hanging in there. Lungs a little better. Still super critical. I love u all and will need u later. I ask to not be called or texted, it's too much right now. Thanks

- Thank you for the update Rachel

- Gosh darn I have been thinking of y'all for the past day and night... I believe in miracles and he is definitely a miracle. Anything can happen. Stay strong.
- Thank God, been thinking of you guys nonstop.
- Been thinking about you both all day. We're here for you.
- Stay strong!!
- Thank you for the update. Keeping you both in my thoughts and my heart. Stay strong! Stay   positive!
- Stay Strong. Been praying and thinking about you constantly the past couple days.
- Please know I'm praying.
- Thank you for the update. I've been thinking and praying about you and Grayson fervently. You both are loved so much.
- Haven't stopped thinking about you both all week. Love and prayers.
- Lots of prayers!!
- Praying and praying.

Owen came to visit later that morning. He grabbed one of the wooden chairs that was scattered in the room, pulled it to Grayson's bedside, then took one of his lifelong best friend's hands and quietly held it, not knowing what to say. None of us knew what to say. This wasn't something any of us had predicted. We were so young, and not supposed to deal with death at our age. Death was for ninety-year-olds, not those of us in our thirties! Owen told Grayson that he was there and he loved him, as Grayson peacefully slumbered. As Owen went to leave, Grayson briefly opened his eyes and nodded. I'm not sure if Grayson had the capacity to understand what that nod would forever mean.

In the afternoon Dr. Hughes came in, shook my hand and told me they were going to do all they could to support Grayson through medications, platelets and immunity-boosting drugs. He said all we could do is wait to see if his body could repair itself in the coming days. He, Dr. Lazar and Mallory were so calm. They made me feel like I was talking to friends. They showed authentic care and empathy, which was so appreciated.

I sat by the window and watched the blizzard fall, and held my breath on and off as Grayson continued to slip away. That night after a half-eaten veggie burger, some fries and an orange soda, I hugged Grayson across the tubes and wires and went to the hotel across the street that I was able to afford, thanks to Tony's amazing money gift the month before. I called Felicity for a quick chat, shut out the lights and fell into the darkness of sleep.

The next morning I woke up, took a quick shower and thought about how surreal it was- that it was my 31st birthday, and my husband was in the ICU dying. The first thing I saw when I opened the door to his room was "Happy Birthday Rachel!!!," written on the whiteboard across from his bed.

I smiled at that gesture from the nurses, as I slid the gray recliner near Grayson's bed in the darkly lit room, kicked off my shoes, covered up with a blanket and attempted to cop some zzz's before any medical staff came in. The first nurse that I saw told me Grayson had left me the message which made me smile and laugh. This life couldn't be real. Was I being Punk'd?

146

Where was Ashton Kutcher? My husband was going to jump out of that bed and we'd leave the hospital hand in hand, right? That was my birthday wish.

My mom arrived an hour later and looked at Grayson as tears fell down her cheeks. She looked at her son, her convertible-riding, American Pickers-binging, pie and dessert-eating buddy, knowing he most likely would not make it. She took her winter hat off in one hand and grabbed a chair in the other, took his hand and told him she was there.

I left to go get a soda and sugary donuts as a birthday treat. I didn't care about being healthy. He was dying and I needed energy. My mom handed me a small flat paper bag with a birthday card inside. "This isn't the way I wanted you to get this," she said with a frown through tears. "I know," I said with a sad smile and hugged her.

That morning the medical team told me there were no longer any more signs of the flu, but his lungs and bladder were quite bad. He was pretty anxious that morning despite sedation. When he tried to sit up, by lifting his head and shoulders, I popped out of my nested spot and gently pushed him back onto his pillows. He was given more Fentanyl for pain and Ativan for anxiety.

This was it. Today was "The Day," that I was supposed to make a decision. Hey, you're 31 today! Is it the day your husband is gonna die? What a crappy game show. Around 9:15 a.m. Grayson tried to get up again. This time I told him to breathe deeply and to lie back down as I pet his forehead and held his hand.

I said, "You're in the intensive care unit still and can't breathe on your own. You have to be calm to be okay. Do you understand?" Grayson nodded. "Honey, they don't know if you're going to be able to make it. You're really sick and have another blood clot in your lung. This is really scary, I know. I can't imagine what you're feeling or thinking. I'm right here, okay?" Grayson nodded. "Do you understand what this means?" He nodded. "I hate this and I am so sorry. I wish I could take this away, but I can't." Grayson opened up his eyes for two seconds and looked at me, then they flew shut.

"Do you want to keep on fighting?" He shook his head no. I said, "Are you ready to see Jesus, then?" as I wiped tears out of my blurry eyes and snot from my face with my shirt sleeve. He shook his head no. "Do you want to keep fighting?" He nodded yes this time. "Do you trust me?" I said. He nodded, then fell into a sleep. My mom was on the other side of the bed watching this whole interchange. She nodded, then said, "He wants to keep fighting, so we will!"

Victoria got there around 9:45 a.m. and told me that her sister Anna and Grayson's sister Natasha would be there that evening as well.

Dr. Hughes came in to tell us that nothing had really changed and we'd wait until Sunday to make a decision. I felt doom and gloom and also at peace with this news. Nothing was decided, yet I knew that this day, my 31st birthday, was the last birthday I'd ever have Grayson in my life. I knew it in my bones, just like I knew he'd have cancer when he had to do that biopsy after the blood infusions two years and three months earlier. Just like I knew I wanted to be with him when I was a bright, shiny-eyed, naïve nineteen-year-old. I just knew I

147

was going to lose the love of my life. Nonetheless, I was still me and needed to support Grayson as if he was going home tomorrow, so I played his favorite tunes on the iPod and sat there holding his hand hour after hour, wishing for a miracle.

The next day Comcast was scheduled to come and install cable service; I'd scheduled this so Grayson would have more to watch when he came home. I called Comcast and said, "I need to cancel my install, a family emergency has come up and I do not need the service anymore." The representative replied, "Oh! That's just fine. We can reschedule for another day that works for you!" I told her, "No, I do not need the service anymore, please cancel it." She replied, "Oh we can find a plan that works for you!" I covered my face with my hand and told her in severe frustration, "My husband is dying and I do not need or want the service." She actually said, "Oh I am sorry to hear that, we can work with you on a budget plan!" I bit my tongue to not yell back and said, "Please just cancel the install and take me off your customer list, please!" and hung up. Geez Louise, they really will do anything for a buck!

Victoria and my mom left the room later that morning as the nurses lifted Grayson up in the ceiling lift to clean up his body after he'd had a bowel movement. I sat in my chair and looked up at my thirty-seven-year-old husband, so pale and frail, lying on a transfer blanket, among blue and green loops connected to the metal lifting mechanism and wondered "How did we get here?"

Grayson was so weak and just a fragment of who he used to be. I remembered how when I met him and we'd meet up, he'd be across the street or coming towards me from several feet away and as he walked, I always thought he walked funny. It turned out he just had such great posture on his 6'2 frame, and it was the rest of society that slouched. He would laugh so hard sometimes that his shoulders would shake and move up and down as he'd look downward and close his eyes for a second and grin. This man feet above the bed, hanging from the ceiling was not Grayson. I felt like he'd already left me at this point, even though he was there. He was no longer able to get out of bed and walk as I thought he was going to after rehab. I'd already begun pricing walkers and had almost bought one the week before, so I'd have one ready when he left the hospital and came home.

Come back to me, Grayson, come back. I felt like Rose talking to Jack in the Titanic movie when they are hanging on a piece of driftwood in the water, waiting for a ship or rescue boat to save them. I wanted him to survive and yet already felt like he was gone…

That afternoon two more ICU docs came in, adjusted Grayson's meds and the vent, checked his levels, gave me somber smiles and left. The chaplain came in to pray over Grayson and with my mom, Victoria and I. Around 3 p.m. my dad came and switched shifts with my mom and me. I didn't want to leave Grayson. After much encouragement from my parents, I agreed to go home and sleep in my own bed. I pet Grayson on the face with the side of my hand and ran my fingers over his wisps of eyebrows that were growing in darker red. "I love you forever," I told him as a tear slipped down my cheek. I checked out his pillows, blankets, tubes and vents and made sure he looked comfortable and then grabbed my coat, hat and purse, took a last look at my husband and left.

The ride home was a blur. I was so tired, I could barely see straight. I was aware of the snow falling around us and knew the way we were traveling by heart, but I was again floating and barely there. When we got in the front door Greta came bounding toward me and Puddin' and Rufus jumped off their respective couches and came to greet me as well. "Hi guys!" I told them as I collapsed in a puddle of sheer fatigue on the nearest couch. Greta, Grayson's dog was so excited to see me, I thought her tail was going to fall off.

Mom had me come into the kitchen and took the lid off of a Hello Kitty cake she'd gotten me for my birthday. I took a few forkfuls of the sweet sugary delicacy then retired to my bed and fell asleep for the next several hours, out cold to the world. I woke up later and called my dad to see how Grayson was. He told me that he was much the same. At 11:20 p.m. Grayson had a bed bath and rested for the next several hours. My dad spent the night at Grayson's bedside, bless his heart. He knew that Grayson would want to have someone there, and was committed to staying beside his beloved son as he struggled to stay alive.

Throughout the night he had his mouth suctioned and cleaned around the vent, a respiratory treatment, platelets and every two hours had to have those darn bladder fluid bags changed as the BK virus still ran rampant in his bladder. Grayson had a chest x-ray done with results TBD. He was turned every two hours and was given a very early morning insulin drip to control his blood sugar.

Saturday April 20th: Mallory came in at 7 a.m. and said things were the same with no change. My mom and I arrived at 7:15 a.m., switching shifts with Dad so he could go home to sleep. I noticed that Grayson was breathing over the vent which was hurting, not helping his lungs. His mom came in two hours later. By then the staff had to increase his Fentanyl as his breathing got worse. He was up to 209.6 lbs. with fluid in his belly. Everything was heading in the wrong direction. By noon he was finally breathing with the machine.

I went to lunch with his sister Natasha, having the spicy mock duck and vegetable Vietnamese sandwich and spicy fries I adored from the restaurant two blocks over. I told her I knew he wasn't going to make it and how devastated I was. She once again told me, as she had two months earlier at that time from across the room of Grayson's hospital room, as she set down her book on how to get rich, that we hadn't been there for her when she was in her time of need and she, too, had been through hard things. She'd had a messy divorce years earlier. I sent her a care package of a really good chick-lit book I'd read called "P.S. I Love You," nail polish and some candy, and another time when she said she wanted a boyfriend, I sent her a Ken doll.

She sat across the table from me, looked me in the eyes, and stated that Grayson would pull through and that Grayson had asked their mother that if anything ever happened to him, to pay off the mortgage on our house with the money left for him from his dad's trust. I felt relief in that, but also wasn't sure of the accuracy of her words. I let it fly above my head as she continued to rattle on about getting no help from us or her mother, when we'd been "up here" and she was "fighting, kicking and screaming," in Louisiana, comparing that to Grayson fighting cancer and literally dying. I almost wanted to check her for a green monster head coming out of her neck, as if I was punked yet again, but sat there eating, calmly accepting my fate, the impending death of Grayson and our marriage. My life was never short of bizarreness and this was topping the list for recent events.

At 3:30 p.m. I succumbed to exhaustion and headed home, first hugging family members then kissing my prince on the head and petting him on the arm, silently praying for God to protect him. I leaned over him and said the Lord's Prayer. It was so surreal and so odd. I looked at him and knew there was nothing I could do. I left, defeated, to rest at home.

I was called around 4:30 p.m. by Dr. Hughes, asking my permission to drain fluid from Grayson's belly via an abdominal cut on the side. I consented. Two liters of fluid were drained off of him, as my dad again sat vigil by his bedside. I thought of how odd it was that a 2 liter of soda sized amount of fluid was drained from my husband's body. Dad told me that Aunt Anna and Victoria told him as they left at 9 p.m. that it wasn't necessary to stay overnight. But Dad knew Grayson would want someone there, and he wanted to be there for Grayson.

I knew I would sleep soundly after checking in with my dad, hearing that nothing had changed, and knowing he was with my beloved husband. They had to put in some other tubes to prevent fluid from getting on Grayson's skin as he laid unmoving in bed that night. It made me squirm to think of it. Dad said he slept soundly all night and rested well.

Around 10 p.m. I got out of bed, taking myself away from my post staring at the ceiling, sat on the couch in the living room surrounded by my loving pets, and made a "Heaven Playlist" to bring to the hospital the next day, just in case. I carefully put the songs Grayson loved and that we loved together throughout our relationship in order of what I wanted him to hear as he took his last breaths. I was 98.9% positive he would be gone by Monday, and on this night, I wanted to be prepared to give him the sendoff he deserved. I put the playlist together as I drank Grayson's beloved lemon ginger tea. I took a few deep breaths, looked at the chair in the corner of the living room that was the last place he ever sat, then stood up, hugged my crying mom, brushed my teeth, took a Benadryl and went to bed.

~

The Last Day of Being a "We"

Sunday, Apr. 21: At 6:25 a.m. another x-ray of his lungs showed no change, and at 7:25 a.m. my mom and I got to the hospital and switched with my dad. He got into the running car in the frigid morning air; we told him we'd see him later. He said, "He is hanging on and looks great. I love you two," then closed the car door and drove off.

My mom and I took off our coats, hats and purses, washed our hands, then foamed in and went to Grayson's bedside. At 7:05 a.m. Dr. Hughes came in and sat down next to me in one of the wooden chairs. My mom was down the hall getting tea. Dr. Hughes said, "Rachel, buddy, today is the day," as he put his hand on my shoulder and let out a giant sigh, holding his chin in his hand. This kind, sixties-something man in his white lab coat with his stethoscope around his neck, had just told me that today was the day my husband was going to die. My life was going to forever change, and I was responsible to make this decision on behalf of my husband. He said he was sorry and he wished there was more they could have done, but Grayson's body had just reached its limit and could not fight anymore. His body didn't have the capacity or strength to do more, and that it was time to be humane and let Grayson go.

I called my dad, telling him to come back to the hospital that Grayson was going to die. This was one of the hardest things I have ever had to do. Dad was the one person who held out the most hope and projected the most positivity to us all. He'd reminded us that Grayson had made it this far and that God could do miracles. I had to tell him no, that Grayson would not make it and asked him to get there as soon as possible.

At 8 a.m. a hospital staff member from legal went over Grayson's health care directive with me, double checking what I already knew, that Grayson didn't want to keep living if he had to be kept on life support with no chance of recovery. He trusted me as his wife and life, and knew I'd make the call when I had to.

When Victoria arrived at 8:30 a.m., I had Mallory come in to talk to her about the decision we'd made. She said, "I'm not ready!" over and over again. Mallory started to tell her we could wait until tomorrow to see if he improved, but I jumped in and said, "No, today is the day. I am sorry, but it's today." I couldn't imagine losing a child, let alone after losing a husband as she had twenty-one years earlier, but this was my husband and my call to make. Grayson's body was done. He was suffering and doped out on the highest levels of pain killers they could give him. The Fentanyl was keeping him as comfortable as could be in his war-torn state, but he had no fight left in him.

I saw Dr. Hughes standing outside Grayson's room with his back to me, and jumped out of my chair, opened the door and asked him, "I just want to double check, there literally is nothing that can be done to save his life, correct?" to which he replied, "Yes. You are correct. His body cannot fight anymore and if he were to live, he could only do so on life support and the BK virus would never leave his body. He'd have it permanently." I nodded my head ok, reached up and gave him a hug, and returned to the room.

I began to play some chill playlists of songs Grayson put together himself in past years, of his favorite techno artists. He was a former raver, dancing in fields with Owen and his friends Bryan, John and Stan in the middle of nowhere in his late teens and early twenties. I called our church and was surprised that someone answered on a Sunday. I told them that we needed our pastor to come to the hospital as soon as possible. I was told that he was preaching in a service right then but would come as soon as he could.

Several of Grayson's doctors who had worked with him along the way in the oncology and bone marrow transplant departments came in, each telling me "I'm sorry," while looking at me with a frown or sad smile. The last doctor to come in was Dr. Lazar. He had been the expert and doctor with one hundred percent of the information about Grayson at all times, calling even when he was out of the country. He told me he was very sorry that Grayson would not make it and that, "He fought incredibly hard, harder than any of us can imagine. I will be

151

thinking of you and your family." I got up and gave him a big hug and thanked him for all he'd done to help Grayson for the last two and a half years.

I calmly called my siblings and told them each that today was the day Grayson was going to pass away. I called Owen to deliver the bad news, and asked him if he wanted to come to the hospital. He replied, "I think I will just stay at home with my girls and be surrounded by their love." I thought that was awesome self-care.

Around 10 a.m. I signed papers and gave verbal consent to stop all medical treatments, quickly scribbling my name. I only glanced at the paper, as I knew there was nothing more to be done to bring my husband back to life. I glanced at Grayson and saw a man I barely knew. His skin was bloated and had a pale white and purplish tint to it. His eyes were gooey and yellow around the edges. He was gone. My Grayson was there in body, but my baby had already left.

Soon after, someone from the University of Minnesota Mortuary Science Program came in and had me sign the forms to allow Grayson's body to be donated to the school. Being the amazing human being that he was, Grayson not only did extra spinal taps and bone marrow biopsies and other tests in his clinical trial while upwards of ten students stood around and watched, but also wanted to donate his body to scientific research so others could learn from his illness. I was very proud to be his wife for a thousand reasons. Right then and there, sunlight lit me up inside despite my world collapsing. I knew he would live on in that way.

Grayson's poor sister refused to come into the room. She didn't want to see her brother die, as she'd seen their dad do when she was a young teen. She waited out in the hall with their aunt as we huddled around his bed waiting for the pastor.

The nurse had everyone go outside so she could clean him up. She turned off the main ceiling lights, only having the bar light above his bed on, casting a gentler glow in the room. After she brought a bucket of soapy water and a wash cloth to the tray table as well as lotion, I told her I had it covered and asked her to leave.

I pulled the curtains shut, giving my husband and I privacy, and played a second playlist I'd created as the "Pre-Heaven Playlist'" with Joe Cocker's "Beautiful" filling the room. I'd always loved Joe Cocker's voice, but I thought this song was so cheesy, and when Grayson would sing a line or two to me, I'd roll my eyes at him. However this was his literal last day on earth and I wanted to honor him.

I took my time on his face, going over his forehead, eyebrows, cleaning around his eyes, what I could around his tube-filled mouth, then his ears and neck before applying Johnson & Johnson's pink bottled baby lotion to his skin, apologizing to him because he'd always hated the smell. It was interesting as he had half an inch long red hair coming out of his head, red and white coming out of his beard and teeny black mustache whiskers as well. I thought it would have been really cool to see what he would have looked like with the new traits of the donated stem cells.

I left Grayson there and went to the family lounge down the hall. It had light brown lockers on either side of the room, a couch and several chairs. I chose a chair sandwiched between the lockers and the window, plopping myself down into it as I emitted a deep exhale.

Victoria took that as a moment to come up to me, pull me forward, wrap me in a hug and wail, "I wanted to be a grandmother!!!" I thought my eyes would fall clean out of my head. I quickly switched from the floating above us sensation, to feeling like I'd plummeted out of an airplane in the clouds, down to my seat, buckled in and all. I didn't say anything. I was flabbergasted. What I really wanted to say was not something that as my mother would say "Is becoming of a lady," or "The Lord would look kindly to." You get my drift.

Victoria went back to the couch where she'd been sitting and pulled out her planner, asking me when the memorial service would be. I told her I wanted to have it the following weekend, to which she responded, "I can't do it next weekend, some of my former students are singing in a competition and I promised I would be there." I cannot make this stuff up. That is what the mother of the man lying in a bed dying and ready to be taken off life support focused on first. So we went with the next weekend after that.

Shortly after our pastor arrived, my parents, Victoria, Bernard and I went and stood around the bed. My mom and I were on either side of Grayson's head, with the pastor at the end of the bed. He read the Last Rites and said a prayer wishing Grayson grace and peace on his way to heaven. My dad fell apart, gripping the bed railing to keep from collapsing. This just ripped me to the core to see; I knew my mom and dad had become Grayson's surrogate parents in the last two years and three months. I asked each family member to come in one by one, to say their good-byes and to listen to his heart beating one last time. Natasha did not want to come in, but did so as her mom and aunt told her that if she didn't say good-bye she would regret it someday. I was so glad she did.

Earlier I had packed up the closet that held all of Grayson's clothes, cards, and my things from staying over, and gave them to my parents to take home when we left later. The wire mask that he wore for the radiation was at the top of the closet; he'd wanted to take it home. I threw it on the floor and stomped on it before putting it in the trash.

The time had come. I gave the okay and only Mallory, a single nurse and I remained. The nurse turned off the ventilator, took the tubing out of his mouth and cleaned up his face a little bit, as I sat in a chair three feet from his bed awaiting the end. It was time to say good-bye to my love, my life, my world, my best friend and my husband. I wheeled the tray table closer to the bed and climbed in with Grayson. The nurse left and Mallory helped cover me up with my blue quilted blanket and Grayson with the rainbow prayer shawl my friend Julie had given him. Grayson began to breathe loud, snoring-sounding breaths, which Mallory said was normal. His eyes were fully open for the first time in five days, looking upward and not focused. I asked her if he could hear me and she nodded and said "Yes, he can." She told me to give her my phone that I would want a picture of Grayson and me. I said no, and she stated, "Trust me, you will want this, it will help you later." She put the call button next to Grayson's side and told me to call if I needed anything.

I pushed play on the iPod and cradled Grayson in my arms, listening to the music while I waited for his heart to stop. I calmly and evenly told Grayson that I loved him, prayed out loud that God receive him quickly, that he have no more pain and suffering, and that I'd see him again in heaven someday. I was cool as a cucumber, barely crying at this moment, as God had given me the strength of a gladiator. I knew what I was doing, and had to do for Grayson. I pet his eyebrows and forehead, stroked his cheek and laid my head on his head, the whole time holding him in my arms, him in his gray t-shirt and me in my pink and gray striped sweater and jeans while I kept telling him over and over I loved him. "Can you hear me? Give me a sign you can hear me?" I willed him two or three times to give me a sign. I just kept hearing the animalistic sounds of his lungs attempting to breathe, then his breath faded and became quieter over time. I looked at his mouth then looked at his chest as Ryan Adams sang of the stars going blue, and then it became quiet. I lay there with him for a minute, then pressed the call button.

It was 1:52 p.m. on 4/21/13, three months/ninety days to the day that Grayson left our house last on 1/21/13. I met him on 9/21/01, eleven years and seven months to the day that he died. Mallory came in and I asked her if she could confirm he was gone. She took her stethoscope off her neck and placed it on his flat chest, then nodded. "Take all the time that you want" she told me. I closed his eyes, sighing, so sad my life with my love was over. He was one in a kazillion. Mallory left and closed the curtains again behind her.

I picked up his head and it flopped back into place on the pillow with its -no pun intended –dead weight.

I thought, "Grayson is gone! I am out of here!" I climbed out of the bed, slowly put the iPod dock in the bag I'd brought it in, grabbed our wedding photo and got ready to leave, playing his favorite song by his favorite band, "Love Will Tear Us Apart," by Joy Division on the iPod in my hand.

It was incredible, his body in death created a trickling of spider webs running up and down his body right before my very eyes as it became the shell that once was Grayson. It was like watching Spiderman take over and fling out webs. His veins of blue and purple on his now super-white skin popped up in seconds, his body eliminated into the bag on the side of his bed and then became rigid. This was of course the worst day ever, but biologically speaking it was fascinating to see what the body could and couldn't do in life and death. God sure created the human body with such mysteries and complexities.

I saw his beloved Birkenstock sandals peeking out from under the bed and set down the bag I was holding. I put his Jesus sandals on to go meet Jesus in. Part of me wanted to keep the shoes, but knew the sentiment was great and that Grayson was already floating above me on his way up to heaven and would get a kick out of it. I covered up Grayson to the top of the bed covering his head, and started toward the door.

I stopped, went back to him, set down my bag, pulled the sheet off of his head, looked at him, cranked up the Joy Division song again, did a little dance for about fifteen seconds, and said, "You wanted to beat cancer and you did! Then I said one last "I Love You!" covered him back up and left. I grabbed the cold steel handle on the light colored wooden door and did not look back. Grayson was not there.

I stepped into the hall. I was thirty-one and a widow and my life was…..?????

Part 2: ~*Rachel 2.0*~

Chapter 21:
The First Step of Being 1 from What Was 2

I walked out of Grayson's hospital room into the darkly-lit hallway, literally closing the door on my life with Grayson, and what I knew to be my life up to that point, as I put one foot in front of the other. The white with gray specks hallway tiles and the whitish-blue painted walls oddly surrounded me with comfort. I'd spent days, weeks and months within the walls of this hospital, listening to information and knowledge about the human body, cancer and every iota of what Grayson was going through. I knew the decision I made was right, needed, dignified and I felt confident in that knowledge.

As I carried the blanket and prayer shawl that I'd had on the bed, along with the iPod dock and Grayson's other items to the family waiting room to my parents, I felt a sense of relief. Why did I feel so calm? I wasn't crying or weeping or falling apart. I was calm. Just. Simply. Calm. As I opened the door both of my parents looked up from where they were sitting and came to take the items from my hands. My mom was sobbing and enveloped me in a big hug. My dad came around to my other side and hugged me as well with tears falling down his face. I sat down in the room lit only by the winter sunlight for about five minutes, then gathered everything up and was ready to go home.

It felt so odd to leave Grayson there, to leave the human casing of my husband in that bed and just walk away forever. But I knew in my soul that he was already waiting in line at the pearly gates, and had been for the last twenty minutes or so. I wondered how long the line was. Are we talking TSA at the airport long where there are several choices of which checkpoint to try to get into, or options to get into the paid   toll line from different bordering states or cities, or are we talking walking six miles to get water in the desert kind of line? Hmmm…either way Grayson was on his way to be with Jesus, God, his dad, and dozens we'd lost before. It was time for me to go home, lie down and take a nap, then face my new life without him.

As I walked down the hospital corridor, nurses and medical assistants and even a couple doctors, came to give me hugs, tell me they were sorry for my loss or waved and half smiled at me. This gave me so much comfort and peace. I knew they'd done this many times before with other patients and family members. I knew they authentically cared about Grayson, and gave him the best care available from the bottom of their hearts.

My mom and I waited for my dad to get the car from the parking garage, standing inside the front entrance of the hospital, holding Grayson's belongings that he'd never need or wear again. I felt like I was in someone else's body and in my own at the same time. You know that super floaty feeling you get when you're waiting in line to board a plane and it's almost your turn for the flight attendant to scan your boarding pass? I felt like that, with an odd peace that had no name. I felt weightless and grounded at the same time, uber aware of a shift in my life that was already starting. The dominos had been hit and were falling into place and there was no way to stop them. I was on a mission and had no road map or navigational system to guide me. I'd spent so many hours, days and months in this hospital.

After this moment in time, right now today, I would not ever be coming back to see my husband. I had to fight the natural human instincts running through my mind and body to run back inside, up the elevator, down the hall to his room, and ask him to wake up and walk out of there with me. In one breath, I wanted to shout that this couldn't be real, but in the next exhale I was so thrilled that Grayson would no longer be in any pain, discomfort and would be living in heaven now. He would be healed and healthy in a way that none of us on earth could ever imagine.

I called Victoria as she'd requested and told her that Grayson had passed away. She had headed home earlier with her husband, daughter and sister, wanting to grieve in their own space after saying their good-byes. I was glad she took the time to practice self-care. I had no idea how much pain she must have been in after losing Grayson's dad so long ago, and now her son.

I went through the revolving doors one last time and out into the snow, as my dad pulled the car up. I heard the swish by my feet as the doors flipped open in front and behind me. I couldn't believe I was leaving my husband's body there to be studied by students at the U. I got in the back seat, buckled up and turned my head to watch the hospital fade in the distance, as the car traveled farther and farther away. I absolutely adored the grounds of the University of Minnesota in Minneapolis, where I'd spent four years of my life and began my love story with Grayson. We'd come full circle. He picked me up for our first date at Pioneer Hall and died across the street at the Fairview hospital. God had a plan for nineteen-year-old Rachel to be with soon to be twenty-six-year-old Grayson, and today was the last day of our story with both of us alive.

Within a couple minutes of getting in the car, I called my siblings, then Owen, then a handful of other close friends, calmly informing them that Grayson had peacefully passed away and that I loved them. They each told me they were so sorry and to tell them if there was anything that I needed. I felt enveloped in solace and peace, all bundled up in my warm winter coat, mittens, and Team Grayson hat, looking out the car window at the snow-filled highway lanes and buildings that I'd passed by hundreds of times before. I somehow made it in from the car to the house, went to the bathroom, threw on some pajama pants and fell fast asleep for several hours.

CaringBridge/Facebook: Apr 21st, 2013: Angels

Grayson peacefully passed away in my arms listening to our favorite songs at 1:52 p.m. today. Memorial Service will be May 4th at 11 a.m.: Celebration of his life, more details to come. Everett Grayson, I love you forever.

- Sending you and Grayson peace on this day.

- I am so sorry. Words cannot express the sorrow I feel for you and your family.

- I'll never forget you Grayson- you were a great man who always put others before yourself.

- Rest In Peace.

- He was always such a great guy. My heart goes out to you. I'm so very sorry.

- I am so so sorry to hear this. Grayson had been so strong. I pray now for strength for you as you begin to piece your life back together again.

- One of the sweetest people I've ever met, just heartbroken. . . Rachel,   ANYTHING you need let us know.

- Continued best wishes & thoughts onto you and your family. You're surrounded with love and support so please reach out if anything is needed.

- I am so very, very sorry. I will keep you in my thoughts as you navigate these dark waters. I wish you strength. I wish you peace.

- Rachel, I am so sorry. I'll continue to pray for you. Love you!

- He fought so hard. So sorry.

- Rachel I am so so sorry to hear that. Love and prayers to you.

- Sorry for your loss Rachel, Grayson was a great man he will be missed by many. Rest in peace Grayson.

- Oh Rachel, I am so heartbroken for you. Praying for you now and will continue to. He was so lucky to have you and your positive support. You are amazing. Your love and dedication to Grayson has really touched my heart. God knows your pain and in time he will heal you. Sending my love to you!

- Grayson was a wonderful childhood friend; I have such fond memories of him. Our thoughts and prayers are with you and your family.

- I'm terribly sorry to hear of Grayson passing. Hopefully someday the world will be rid of this horrible disease.

- I am so sorry Rachel. You and your family are in our thoughts and prayers. He could not have had a more loving and supportive woman by his side through this battle.

- Oh God, Rachel, I don't even know what to say. As always, the phone is on. I'm not sure what you will need, or if there's anything worth needing right now, but that's all I can offer.

- Rachel I am so sorry to hear this. My thoughts are with you and your family.

- Oh my Gosh, we are both sorry to hear this. You are both in our thoughts and prayers.

- Anyone that knew Grayson was blessed and made better by knowing him. I'm so sorry for what you're going through right now Rachel, and the rest of the family too. He was a genuinely sweet and kind guy when I knew him as a child and in high school. I have no doubt that he was that same guy to all that knew him.

- My heart goes out to you. Like so many others, I'm here for you. Rest in Peace Grayson.

- Am so sorry to hear the news. My heart is breaking with sadness. May the memories of the good times you shared with Grayson bring you some comfort during this time. I am praying for you and your family.
- My heart is broken. What a wonderful young man he was and what faith, strength and courage you both had through this time. Rachel, there are no words to say to let you know how blessed I was to have been able to share a little of life with Grayson.
- I am so sad to hear this news. It's really not fair but I'm glad he had someone as special as you to stick by his side throughout the journey. You both are in my thoughts. Grayson will not be forgotten by any of us.
- We are lucky to have had Grayson in our lives. No words can describe how much the world will miss him. I am so very glad that you were there with him. May peace now come to him and to you.
- Your love story has been such a beautiful and inspiring one, in spite of all the heaviness and hurt you've endured together. I wish you peace during this hard time, and I know Grayson's love will continue to be with you always.
- Oh Rachel, I am so sorry... thoughts and prayers to you.
- I am so sorry for your loss, Rachel. Hugs and prayers to you.
- So sorry to hear. Sending you strength & peace.
- Rachel, I am so so sorry. He was very blessed to have such a caring, wonderful and loving wife throughout your life together.
- Oh how I love you. My heart aches for you. Grayson fought the good fight and ran the good race and you fought and ran beside him every step of the way. I admire you courage and devotion. You loved him well and I am proud of the woman you are. RIP Grayson.
- I hold you strongly in love and prayer sweet friend.
- Rachel, my heart aches for you. Both of you have been in my thoughts and prayers. I pray for peace and strength for you!

CaringBridge: Apr. 21, 2013: Angels Pt. 2: Please keep in mind, GRAYSON BEAT CANCER! As he aspired to, it was the complications that flew him to heaven. Let's be proud his donor cells took and he kicked cancer in the teeth!

That night I woke up around 9 p.m. to find my mom and dad quietly watching television in the living room. I made a cup of lemon ginger tea and plated birthday cake; it was the only thing that I wanted. I took a bite of sweet sugar and sighed as it hit my tongue, then sat on the couch by my dad.

He told me with a frown, "Tomorrow I am going to head back home to take some time away, but I of course will be back in time for the memorial service." I immediately felt a little bit down that he was going home, but could tell that he needed some space and time for himself. I was so used to being encapsulated by both of my parents lately, but knew we all had to do what was best for ourselves in this time.

After a half an hour or so I picked up my phone and saw several missed calls and thirty or so texts from friends and family. My sister Felicity texted to call her right away. When I called her back, she said she'd be there to help me with whatever I needed and would arrive on

Tuesday. I felt a sense of relief in knowing she would be there to help me navigate whatever would come in the following days. She told me she was going to be there for two weeks. It was amazing and so generous, as it meant she'd leave her four year old Ione and husband at home.

I could not believe how tired I felt. I knew how hard the last few days had been, but felt like a zombie in a foggy haze as I sat quietly in the home that was now solely mine. The light brown of the couches and light tan walls enveloped me in the arms of known comfort, as I could only think of the then and there. I knew Grayson was gone forever, but at the same time it seemed like he was so far away and on a trip across the ocean. I hugged my mom and dad, let Greta outside one last time and went to sleep.

Monday: The next morning I awoke around 8:30 a.m. in my dark bedroom, lit only by the light coming in from the top of the curtains. I looked at the clock and then stared at the wall for what seemed like an hour, but in reality was about fifteen minutes.

"It is just me. Grayson is gone. Gone forever," I said aloud. The words shuffled around in my brain in a slow repeat, as if projected up on a screen in the front of my mind. It was odd, bizarre and didn't make sense. I had a strong feeling I needed to go visit him at the hospital like I did every other day, and had to let it sink in that I wouldn't be going back. It was my first full day without Grayson since I was nineteen, and I had to figure out what to do now. I not only had to move forward with my life, but needed to make phone calls and do logistical things like update my employer and plan a funeral.

"Here we go," I said out loud in a huffed exhale as I threw on my bathrobe and opened my bedroom door. As soon as I entered the hallway I was greeted by my pets, then said hello to my parents. My mom immediately said, "Look outside!" I went to the front window and saw it had snowed three inches overnight. Everywhere I looked was blanketed with sparkling and glistening snow. I let Greta outside and looked out in wonder at the lilac bushes to the left of my yard, reveling in the beauty that I felt had been created just for me, on April 22nd, when spring had usually started. It was a sign from God that Grayson had made it into heaven and everything would be okay. Another layer of peace filled my veins and a rush of warmth filled my body, even as I stood outside on the cement porch step in my slippers, in the thirty-degree weather. "Grayson, I hear you. I love you, thank you!" I said quietly to the wind before I unhooked Greta from the tie-out line and went back inside.

Later that morning I gave my dad a teary and temporary goodbye, thanking him for everything he'd done for us. After two years and three months we all had to find a new normal without Grayson. I watched my parents hug, knowing I would never do that again with my husband, and watched as my dad backed out of the driveway. The three of us all had tears streaming down our faces. "He has to get away and take time just being around our house, doing yard work or whatever. He really didn't think that we'd lose Grayson and he needs time to decompress and grieve on his own," said my mom.

Next, I called my boss and told her Grayson had died and that I needed more time off of work. She told me I had used all of my time off, including what other employees had donated, but asked for the funeral info, that she'd like to attend. Apparently this was the first time the spouse of an employee had died at my small company, and they were trying to figure out how to best support me. I took the next two weeks off unpaid. I then called my church to set the date and time of the memorial service, as well as the time to meet to go over my wishes and plans for the service with our pastor. I'd seen people have to do these things in movies and TV. It was so odd, as now I had to do that, too.

The rest of the day I napped, watched TV, and pet my animals while trying to battle out the endometriosis pain, before throwing in the towel and taking a Vicodin. I looked around my house letting the gravity of the situation sink in that now I was alone and financially responsible for everything myself. I'd done the bills for both of us for years, and had taken care of things the entire time Grayson had been sick, with the help from the money left from his dad's trust fund, but now the house and the animals and everything else imaginable was solely up to me to pay for.

I had been living on the assumption that Grayson would come home. I'd help bathe him, make his food, help him with PT and OT, and learn to walk on his own again, to breathe on his own and then once he got stronger, we'd go back to the "us" that we were before cancer hit. In my mind I'd always seen him getting stronger, and us having little feet running around the house, school events, wedding anniversaries and traveling. But now it was just me, me, me, and no Grayson ever to be part of my story on earth anymore. Hmph. What now? I imagined someone sitting at a table drumming their nails up and down, while their other hand held their chin, with one eyebrow arched up in question. What now, indeed?

The rest of the day was a blur. I talked to my friends Bella and Vera, and sister Diana, who would be coming in a week, and went to bed early. I laid awake staring at the ceiling until my cheeks burned from the hot tears that fell, and my snot-filled face was empty. I said the Lord's Prayer and told Grayson I missed him and I'd always love him. Dear Lord, what in the world was my life going to be like? It was all so surreal. My senses were dulled and heightened all at the same time. I fell asleep once my eyes became sore, as I stared at the calendar hanging on the wall where I marked down all the days I'd visited the hospital, spent the night and numbered the days on Grayson's bone marrow transplant journey. Day 90 was the last day checked off on the calendar and it would always remain that way. I played Ryan Adams's "Oh My God, Whatever, Etc.," a favorite bedtime song of mine, on my phone, then fell fast asleep.

Felicity arrived on Tuesday and helped me get down to business, sorting out Grayson's stocks, our finances, and creating a new monthly budget. I planned out how to pay for things the next few weeks and weighed the idea of not going back to work right away as I'd have the life insurance plan, savings and stocks to live on for a little while. I needed time to rest and grieve and decided that was what I planned to do. I had enough money to live on for a year if I budgeted carefully. During all of this I was as cool as a cucumber and calm despite my life completely falling apart and crumbling to the ground. I knew I had to take care of so many things, just as I'd done when Grayson was in the hospital, especially during the last days of his life. I had to figure out all the legalities, finances and logistics now that Grayson was gone.

Later that day Felicity, my mom and I watched TV and discussed what I wanted for the memorial service. My friend Cassie called and said that she was going to have a fundraiser for me at the Mall of America, with the help of TNT friends, which was so encouraging and awe-inspiring. It was amazing to feel so supported. God had blessed me when Grayson was alive and was still blessing me tenfold after his death.

Felicity and I shared my bed during her stay with me, and that night she rubbed my back as I cried and cried. We talked about how Grayson was in such a better place now, not hooked up to wires and tubes, and shared some funny stories of him from the last few years. As I lay there looking at the tall dark wooden armoire in the corner, it hit me that it was full of Grayson's clothes that he would never again wear -- all his shirts, sweaters, pants, jeans, socks, underwear, and belts. He literally left Earth and everything was left behind. He'd never again put on the sweaters I'd bought him for holidays or his favorite jeans or his Vans shoes. He was never coming back, and I had an entire house full of his every earthly possession. It was one-hundred percent up to me what to do with it all. I looked at the ceiling with wide eyes and let out several huge exhales, telling Felicity what I was thinking about. She told me she had some ideas of what I could do with his clothes and that she'd look it up online tomorrow, then let me know what she'd figured out. I thanked her for being there, cried another minute or so, and fell into a deep sleep.

Facebook: Apr. 24, 2013: Grayson's full obituary will be in the Star Tribune on this Sunday and his Memorial Service will be Saturday May 4th at our church.

- We'll definitely be there!
- We ran in the rain tonight Rach for our TNT practice. We all had green ribbons and team Grayson bracelets. Angela spoke and it was beautiful. Love u
  - Cassie, this made me cry. Thanks!

On Friday night Owen came over to have pizza with my mom, Felicity and I. We hugged and talked about his little girls and how he was doing. I hadn't seen him since the ICU. He was now a single dad due to his marriage getting ripped apart, not from his own doing. We'd both lost our best friend, and were solidified in our joint losses, having to start our lives over. We shared memories of Grayson, while watching the documentary about couples that my friend Sage had made when she was in film school. Grayson and I were the young married couple she interviewed, looking so fresh-faced and innocent, staring back at us from the screen. It was fun to see and a kick in the teeth at the same time.

On Saturday the 27th, Victoria called me on her way to her former students' event, the reason we couldn't have Grayson's service that day. Before I could say anything, she said, "Oh I am getting all of these gift baskets and presents and flowers and food from so many people! It is so wonderful!" I thought my eyes were going to fall clean out of my head.

She said she'd decided to have her own memorial service in St. Cloud, on Sunday, May 5th, the day after mine. She wanted to have "my friends, my people that have supported me, and I'd like you to come." I was so shocked and surprised for about ten minutes, then reflected on how I felt a little sickened by the delight in her voice at the attention she was getting, and her excitement about it, after her son had died. It sounded mean even in my head, but I was sick of the "Victoria Show" that I'd witnessed for years, especially the past few months. She treated Grayson and me badly, even in the hospital. He told me that he'd even had to kick her out of his room one day when she'd been so careless and cruel with her words. He asked for the on-call therapist to talk to, when his regular counselor was off duty that day.

Facebook: Apr. 27, 2013: I feel like Grayson is with me all the time. Especially when I hear the Beastie Boys song "Fight for Your Right" and have the urge to have one of our dance parties

I lived in a fog, going through the motions of feeding the cats and dog, showering, eating, making mandatory decisions for the timeline of the upcoming memorial service, and spending time with my mom and sister. I had fits and starts of energy and napped a lot.

Facebook: Apr. 28, 2013: My beloved has been gone for a week. Please pray for a friend I met on this recent BMT journey whose husband just passed too.

Facebook: Entry by my sister Diana: Apr. 28, 2013 · New York, NY: Grayson was one of THE most thoughtful and kind people I've ever known. His grace, humor and determination throughout his journey has taught me lessons I will remember my entire life. One of my favorite days ever was a short road-trip from Minneapolis to Duluth with Grayson and Rachel in mid-October 2011: stunning autumn leaves, Lake Superior, blasting Phil Collins in the car, followed by an amazing dinner at one of Grayson's favorite breweries. WE LOVE YOU Grayson!!

On Monday the 29th Felicity showed me the name tag stickers she'd purchased to go on the clothes and CDs I had decided to gift Grayson's closest friends and family. They were the kind of tags that would go in the back of a little kid's shirt, very cute little purple stickers with a cat on them that said "Grayson." As we started to go through his clothing to decide what to keep, gift or donate, I reflected on how odd it was, as I'd only seen it done in movies and TV before. In the fictionalized versions you'd see the widow or widower often holding on to items for years, then going back into the closet to smell the clothes and collapse crying on them. I wasn't ready to give away many of his things, but I knew I wanted to share some of these treasures with his lovies who would appreciate the gesture. He was gone forever and would never wear the clothes hanging in the closet, sweaters on the shelf or items in the armoire.

As Felicity went through his clothing, I sat on the bed taking my time to hold, unfold and inspect each item before making a decision. I decided to keep several of his sweaters, and a few pairs of pants. For some reason, I kept one pair of his underwear and a couple pairs of socks. I wasn't ready to give away or even touch his shoes, boots or coats, knowing I'd get there one day. That night as we were lying in bed in the quiet, waiting to fall asleep, the covers moved even though we remained still. Felicity said, "Did you feel that?" I replied, "Yes!" We both said aloud how we hadn't moved. "That was Grayson!" she said. I agreed, smiled and fell asleep knowing he was still with me.

CaringBridge/Facebook: Tuesday, Apr. 30, 2013: Fun Grayson and Rachel things.

- We were together 11 yrs and 7 months to the day-September 21, 2001-April 21, 2013.
- When we began dating I was 19 and he was a month from turning 26, so my parents couldn't say anything, because they were the same age when they got married.
- Puddin', Grayson's cat is purring at my side. I knew Grayson was an okay guy when I met him, if he could keep another living thing alive! Puddin' will be 13 soon.
- We also have Rufus a nearly 13 year old cat as well, that I adopted from my sister 11.5 yrs ago. Grayson and I called Rufus and Puddin' "the Boys".
- Greta our puppy is 2. She was a blessing in the cancer storm from Grayson's sister Natasha, who saved Greta's life, healed her and brought her to us. Grayson was "Papa" and taught Greta to high five and shake. Greta and Grayson both had to have blood transfusions.
- Grayson had a weird little cartoon voice he would do for me that would make me laugh so hard my ribs hurt. He loved to make me laugh.
- Grayson took 2x longer to get ready to go out than me, he was very pretty and handsome!
- I asked Grayson on our first date, asked him to kiss me (he was so shy) and asked him to marry me! He also had more expensive lotions and shampoos than me.
- So far I am coping so much better than I thought, (day, by day) I feel like Grayson is with me. The blessings of my faith, my love for Grayson, wearing his wedding ring with mine since before he died, and our many hard talks about what if he were to die, all have provided grace in this earth quaking, life changing, heartbreak.
- Grayson, I miss you! But am so glad you're pain free my love. Tears and love, Rachel

Owen came over that evening to help me go through some of Grayson's music to decide what I wanted to keep and what to gift. We sat cross-legged with stacks of CDs between us on the basement carpet, the same cream-colored tufted carpet where Grayson had made snow angels in excitement the day we bought the house. As we sorted through Anthrax, the Pet Shop Boys, Depeche Mode, Joy Division, New Order, Yaz, Goldfrapp, BT, Moby, Aphex Twin and Slayer, I told Owen how Grayson had such an eclectic taste in music like I did. I said how he'd loved the song "Walking on Sunshine," by Katrina and the Waves and every time it was on the radio, we'd have to listen to it, many times to my annoyance, even if I didn't want that much peppiness at the time. Just as I'd finished saying that, we heard, "Here's another one picked out just for you by 104.1 Jack FM," then the beginning cords of "Walking on Sunshine," began to play out of my little transistor radio that was sitting by us. We looked at each other in sheer amazement, knowing Grayson was there with us. We got teary, then leaned over the CDs for a quick hug before continuing with our project.

The next day I went to church to go over the plans for the memorial service, and what I wanted to include within it. I was very fortunate that it only cost $450 for the service, the pastor, the luncheon reception afterwards and the bulletins. I didn't have to pay for a casket, or transportation for it, or cremation because Grayson's body was at the U for research for the next year or so and would return to me cremated.

I calmly walked into the church, sat on the brown sofa in the pastor's office and began talking about my husband's memorial service. Oh, man. This was really happening. I was a W-I-D-O-W. Holy cats. I looked around, thinking of how many other people must have sat where I was, doing the same thing, but probably at much older ages than I. I told the pastor I had specific music to be played before, during and after the service, as well as a photo slide show near the end. After I gave my wishes, I thought we were done, not even thinking that there was a traditional Lutheran service that would be part of the memorial, as well. Grayson and I had never identified with one denomination, instead choosing a church based on how well we felt it fit for us. I knew that our pastor would honor Grayson well, as he'd gotten to know him over the last two-plus years. I walked home in a slight daze, thinking about how I knew I'd be giving my husband the best send-off possible, while also trying to come to terms with wrapping my mind around all that was happening. It all felt like a graduation of sorts, finishing or closing a book of my life, ending the 11.5 years of my life with Grayson. I had to move on to whatever my future held for me.

On Thursday Felicity and I put together the gift bags of sweaters and CDs for a few of Grayson's friends and family to receive in the next few days. I felt a rush of relief in sharing pieces of Grayson with those he loved who loved him right back. I looked in my closet and found I had nothing to wear to the service. I'd gained weight from the combination of endometriosis, hospital food and lack of energy or time to exercise. To boot, I was in extreme pelvic pain at the worst time possible. Felicity let me know that Poppy, her lifelong friend, who was like a sister to me, was flying in the next day, and they'd go shopping for dress choices for me, to my relief.

I felt overwhelmed, as if it was my wedding all over again. Friends asked what they could do to help, thank God, and I graciously accepted the offer, asking Angela if she could bring flowers for the sanctuary, to add to the arrangements I'd already received at home. The rest of the day I attempted to chill by napping and waiting for family to arrive. My dad, brother and his family arrived that night, providing me with a growing sense of security and comfort.

On Friday Poppy, Grayson's aunt Anna and his cousins Dean and Jason flew in. I went to the church to approve the bulletin, this time with lighter footsteps. This was going to happen and I had to keep on trucking no matter what. The second round of "Team Grayson" bracelets

I had made when Grayson got sick again had a truck on them and said, "Keep on Trucking," and it was time for me to follow the motto that was for our joint team, for myself. In the afternoon Felicity and Poppy had dresses for me to try on, along with Spanx to suck in my belly. I thought why not as far as the Spanx went, and settled on a white and pink striped dress with a matching white belt, panty hose and white shoes. My sister Diana was not able to fly in until later that night and Victoria, Bernard and Natasha had decided to stay in St. Cloud to do their own thing that evening.

My parents, Felicity, Owen, Aunt Anna, Jason, Dean and I had dinner from El Loro that night, spending time together in the living and dining rooms in a big group. At one point Jason came into the kitchen, raising an eyebrow at me as he found me chugging Pepto-Bismol straight from the bottle. My stomach was so nervous and there was nothing I could do to change that. I gave Jason some sweaters and the neat Fossil watch I'd given Grayson several years ago, and to Dean, I gave sweaters and the folder of the six CDs that Grayson had made specifically to be played during his radiation. They shared a love of music and being DJs. Grayson had been "DJ Spun-G" back in the day at some parties, which made me giggle. Other than the radiation techs and physicists, they were the only people to ever know what was on those CDs. I thanked everyone for being there, gave many hugs and then stayed up way too late with a type of nervousness I cannot describe.

Felicity and I lay in bed that night and giggled as we read Grayson's Health Care Directive. My now late husband was so silly. I knew in the next months and years I'd experience a world of hurt and pain, but I'd also be able to hold tight to the memories I'd made with him.

Below are the actual answers on Grayson's Health Care Directive he wrote in February 2011.

1. *The things that make life most worth living to me are*: "My beautiful, compassionate and intelligent wife Rachel. My entire family, especially my mother Victoria. Music, art; namely photography, enjoying a good pint of beer and dinner with my friend Owen; going to see a favorite band in concert; traveling and being witness to historical places, nature in its pure form; God's love and blessings."

2. *My beliefs about when life would no longer be worth living:* "When all my friends and family are gone: if hostel aliens from outer space have taken over the Earth and if I am bitter and have turned into the walking dead: aka: a zombie."

3. *If I am nearing death I would want my loved ones to know that I would like*: "Prayers, positivity, celebration of my life, my love for my wife, friends and family and to play the song "Ceremony" by Joy Division."

Grayson was certainly something else. Even his requests about his death and dying could make me laugh. Felicity and I laughed, hugged, then went to sleep.

Chapter 22:
Bright Colors and Memories

Saturday, May 4th: The Memorial Service

That morning flew by in a blur of slight chaos as my parents, sister and I prepared for the service. I stuffed myself into the Spanx my sister had bought me, then put on my pink and white striped dress with the matching white belt and shoes. Felicity curled my hair and I opted to skip my usual mascara, only doing eyeshadow; I didn't want to look like an Alice Cooper wannabe if the mascara ran. Poppy hugged me that morning as she cried and said, "I am so sorry, I have no idea how you're going to move on, there will never be another man as great as Grayson!" I thanked her and didn't really know what to say. I had to move forward and wasn't able to think beyond that day.

We piled into my parents' van filled with flowers and mementos and drove down the block. We walked into the empty church, prepping for the service by setting up photos on the tables that had been set up, and putting the pretty, brightly-colored plants and flowers up front in the sanctuary when Angela arrived. I was so nervous, I felt like I was going to throw-up. I took a Xanax to calm me down so I could focus and be in the moment, to do what had to be done. I gave the sound tech the flash drive with the slide show and music to play and the appointed times to do so.

Jack and his family soon arrived, as well as Diana. Jack had dyed his hair pinkish red in response to my request for everyone to dress brightly. Victoria wore a bright yellow jacket with a red skirt. I asked her how she was feeling when she arrived with Bernard, Anna, Jason and Dean, to which she replied, "Oh terrible! I don't know how I am going to get everything done for tomorrow!"

My eight-year-old niece Emma came up to me and handed me a red and white angel that she'd sewn with "Grayson" at the bottom, causing me to briefly cry in awe and envelope her in a hug. I gave Natasha and Ken hugs when they arrived, then brought Natasha down the hall to a private quiet place where I sat on the steps as I handed her a box. I gave her Grayson's first wedding ring, a plain gold band that hung from a gold chain. I'd later replaced that ring with one I'd had made from his late dad's rings, along with the "bling" of a couple little diamonds he requested, when I surprised him with it at the Statue of Liberty, when we were on vacation in NYC. She was surprised and thankful at the gesture, then handed me a box that contained a neat pink rope necklace that had a "G" hanging from it, along with a little pink crystal and a silver tablet with a Bible verse. She was wearing the same necklace, but in black.

The next thirty minutes was a carnival of hugs and welcoming friends and family I hadn't seen in so long, as they came through the door. My boss and supervisor gave me hugs and told me that my clients missed me, and how valuable I was to the company. I was thrilled when my best friends Wyatt, Sandy, Bella, Vera, Hazel and Sage all arrived. Cassie walked in with a man I knew only from a Facebook photo to be the kind widower Tony, who had been so generous when Grayson was in the ICU both times. We'd talked late at night on the phone when I'd been scared, and he gave me questions to ask the medical team. I continued to meet and greet in the blur and bizarreness that was my life, feeling a little loopy from the Vicodin I'd had to take an hour before for the severe endometriosis pain, until I heard the Coldplay song that signaled the service would start in ten minutes.

For nearly a decade I'd had Moby's "Porcelain" on my own funeral playlist, and had recently added Bruce Springsteen's "Jesus Was An Only Son," both of which I'd decided to play that day. The foyer was jam-packed with loved ones and looked more like a concert venue, and less like a memorial service for my husband. This was the best kind of celebration I could have hoped for.

The pastor requested that immediate family join him in the library for a prayer before the service started. I held one hand with Felicity and the other with Owen, as the pastor said a blessing, asking the Lord to be with us all in this place to honor Grayson's life, then instructed us to line up outside the sanctuary. The calm and collected voice of my beloved Springsteen started to fill the sanctuary, as I prepared myself to walk down another aisle for Grayson, the love of my life, this time without him.

Grayson's parents, sister, my soon to be brother-in-law, aunt and cousins all filed into the church, followed by my siblings, then parents. Owen and I walked in together. We both had lost our best friend and it was time to face the literal music. I linked my arm through his, quickly stood up on my tippy toes and gave him a quick "we're in this together buddy" peck on the cheek and said, "Ok, ready or not, let's do this." I kissed my Grayson tattoo on my wrist as I took my first step forward into the sanctuary. Everyone turned to look at us as we walked in, which was such an odd and bizarre thing to experience. Grayson should have been walking down the aisle with me as we renewed our wedding vows, instead of us all honoring his life. It was amazing to see the sanctuary filled with so many bright colors and liveliness per my request. We filed into the front pew and I sat between Owen on the end and my mom on my other side. I quickly turned around and saw my siblings behind me, and my dad next to my mom, and felt comfort in their presence.

The pastor began to talk about celebrating Grayson's life and thanked everyone for attending, then called my dad forward to deliver the following eulogy:

"Good morning: Thank you for being here today. Grayson wanted a colorful and happy time to remember his life. The music and pictures you hear and see are things he wanted. I see Jack has colorful red hair; Grayson would laugh. When Rachel asked me to say a few words about Grayson, as we all celebrate his life, I wondered what he would have liked me to say. It has been a real honor and privilege for Marie and I to have been a part of "Team Grayson" over the past twenty-seven months or so. We were privileged to spend many days with Grayson and with Rachel since he was first diagnosed with leukemia in mid-January 2011. I believe "Team Grayson" was formed that very first week, when Jack dropped everything in his world and helped them begin to plan for the difficult future they would experience. Grayson would want you to know how grateful he and Rachel are for you; and for each and every one of you here today that have been a part of "Team Grayson." Each of you have been so important in sustaining both of them: your prayers and assistance has been so helpful throughout this most difficult process. Whatever part you have played in "Team Grayson", please know they are both forever grateful to you."

"From the time they first began to understand the realities of Grayson having Acute Lymphoblastic Leukemia-known as "ALL," until today and into the future, Grayson was "ALL in" in trying to overcome this type of cancer: not only for himself but for others as well. He told me a number of times that he prayed that others could benefit from his struggle with this illness. As most all of you know after three attempts in the fall and winter of last year, standard chemotherapy treatments were unsuccessful in preparing him for a stem cell transplant procedure. Grayson understood that there was a need for more extensive chemotherapy and radiation if he were to have a chance to beat ALL."

"We were all hopeful when he was admitted to the hospital on January 21st of this year to begin treatments leading to the stem cell transplants that occurred on January 31st. Grayson always remained continuously hopeful as well, even when things got very tough for him. There were some very difficult days. More than once he told me, "If things don't work out for me…I want my body to be donated to the University of Minnesota Medical School and I want to be cremated and my ashes to be buried beside my dad." But there were also many very positive days as well."

"Imagine with me a newborn baby Grayson. There are probably only two people here today who actually remember the newborn Grayson. What joy there must have been on that last day of October in 1975: Halloween. Time and time again during Grayson's treatments or his hospitalization periods, he was asked to give his name and birthdate. Most often followed by a discussion of Halloween. Grayson really enjoyed the fall season, especially Halloween."

"Maybe a few more of you remember Grayson as a toddler learning to sit up; to walk; to talk. Or maybe elementary or junior or high school child Grayson. We have seen wonderful pictures of Grayson and his sister Natasha as they grew up. What beautiful children they were. What fine adults they became. Maybe more of you remember a teenage Grayson making his way through high school, discovering the world around him, who he was and how he might fit in. The loss of his father after a long illness was a great setback for Grayson and all of his family. He loved music and attended the McNally School of Music in St. Paul."

"As an adult he was a loyal and hard worker, working many long overtime hours, many days and weeks. All for the same company for nearly twelve years. Somewhere in those years Grayson and Rachel met and in August, August 20th, 2004 they were married at the Wabasha Street Caves. I would kid Grayson and Rachel now and then by saying, 'What did you expect? You got married in a cave!'"

"Throughout his illness Grayson was a model patient. He did everything he was asked to do and often more. No matter what function an employee of the University of Minnesota Medical Center Fairview had in helping Grayson, he treated them all with respect and sincere interest. They were pleased to be assigned to him and to help him in any way they could. It was a Joy to witness his interaction with each one. Through the weeks and months they too became his friends."

"Throughout the very tough process he found himself in, Grayson consistently demonstrated all of the fruits of his True Christian Spirit."

"Grayson Loved: He loved all of his family-each and every one. He especially loved his mother Victoria who has been supportive of Grayson and Rachel. He loved his sister Natasha. Natasha, I don't know how many times he explained to someone how you found abandoned puppies, picked out Greta for him and how you and Ken drove from Louisiana to bring her to him. He had a special love for Greta and for his cats Puddin' and Rufus. Grayson loved his "special" Aunt Anna. Anna, I'm so glad Grayson and Rachel were able to use your place in Colorado at times. They talked about it often, how beautiful it was there and how much they enjoyed that time. Anna's son's Jason and Dean, younger than Grayson, were special as well. He enjoyed the times they could be together. Grayson talked about how much he enjoyed the trip to South Florida, that Bernard and Victoria took him on a number of years back."

"Grayson had a very special love for and bond with Rachel. Marie and I and our entire family will forever be grateful to Grayson for the love he shared with our Rachel. Grayson also cherished his long-time friendship with Owen, who he loved like a brother. He had a number of close friends as well. Each one meant so much to him."

"Grayson was a Loving Man: There was True Joy in Grayson's Life: his family, his wife, his friends. He enjoyed learning on the internet, looking up almost anything he could think of; playing games, he was interested in cars, Sci-Fi movies, and funny shows. Grayson could be a very funny person himself, he liked to make people laugh. Grayson enjoyed the outdoors. Recently he talked about fishing with his grandfather as a youngster and how he would like to go back to Louisiana to see how it has changed. Grayson had a gladness not based on his circumstances, but in his heart- He was Joyful."

"Grayson truly enjoyed Peaceful Times: Calmness, quietness. In the early mornings in his hospital room we often had long periods of silence. He so enjoyed times when there was unity and caring with those he cared so much for. The Bible's book of Romans 14:19 (New International Version) states: Let us therefore make every effort to do what leads to peace and to mutual edification.' Grayson was a Peaceful person."

"Grayson was usually a very patient person: For those of you here today who helped him get to an appointment or brought things to Grayson and Rachel-we thank you so much for your gift of time and effort to Grayson. And if you did take him to an appointment, I know Grayson helped you to learn to be a patient person as well. The book of Proverbs 14:29 (New International Version) states, 'A patient man has great understanding, but a quick tempered man displays folly.' Grayson was a patient man."

"Grayson was a Very Kind Person: He was eager to put others at ease and to let them know that he really did care for them. From Proverbs 11:16-17(New International Version): 'A kind hearted woman gains respect, but ruthless men only gain wealth, a kind man benefits himself, but a cruel man brings trouble on himself.' We all know Grayson was a very kind man."

"Grayson displayed Goodness through his Life: He was an open hearted person: from (New International Version) Psalm 23:6: 'Surely goodness and love will follow me all the days of my life and I will dwell in the house of the Lord forever.' Grayson was a good person."

"Grayson was faithful: He was a loyal person, full of trust: (New International Version) Proverbs 3:3 states, 'Let love and faithfulness never leave you: bind them around your neck, write them on the tablet of your heart.' Love and faithfulness never left Grayson."
"Grayson was a gentle person: He was humble and had a non-threatening manner about him. Proverbs 15:1 (New International Version) "A gentle answer turns away wrath, a harsh word stirs up anger." He was a gentle man."

"Grayson nearly always exhibited self-control: He was slow to anger-again from Proverbs 29:11 (New International Version) 'A fool gives full vent to his anger, but a wise man keeps himself under control.' Grayson was that wise man."

"Grayson's spirit is described in Galatians 5:22-23: (New International Version) 'But the fruit of the spirit is Love, Joy, Peace, Patience, Kindness, Goodness, Faithfulness, Gentleness and Self Control, against such things there can be no law.'"

"Grayson would want you to leave this service knowing how he loved each of you-how grateful he was for his entire family, for Rachel, for my family, for the First Congregational Church where he grew up, his mother's church whose members have been so supportive of his parents, for this church and Pastors who have been so helpful to Grayson and Rachel, for his many friends, his wonderful neighbors, for all those on the medical teams and hospital employees who helped him and helped Rachel. He knew people in Minnesota, Wisconsin, Michigan, Illinois, Georgia, North Dakota, Massachusetts, New York and so many other places were part of "Team Grayson," praying for him and assisting him in so many different ways.

"I hope when you think of Grayson you will think of his smile as he looked in your eyes."

"I hope you remember the fruits of Grayson's spirit."

"What a true gift each of us has been given!"

"How grateful we are for the life of GRAYSON."

Throughout the eulogy, I held Owen's hand in my left and my mom's in my right. It was difficult to hear my dad's voice shake as he talked about Grayson. At one point I burst out sobbing, glad that my mom was next to me, prepared with tissues. It was so unreal to be in a church full of people who were all grieving the loss of my husband, my other half. He was gone and never coming back.

The pastor gave a wonderful sermon that fit Grayson to a "T." After that, my slideshow began to play, showing photos of Grayson from birth up until his transplant, while Joy Division's "Ceremony," his favorite song, then New Order's "Bizarre Love Triangle," a favorite of ours played. It was wonderful to see so many photos of life and happiness to reflect upon that had come before the ugly illness and death I'd just seen. I sat there in sheer agony and pain at losing my beloved, while also feeling such weightlessness and relief that he wasn't in pain anymore. The pastor gave the benediction before "Heartbeats," by Jose Gonzalez was played, a treasured song of Grayson's. The grand finale to the service was the playing of George Michael's "Freedom 90," that Grayson had adored as a teen, especially with Linda Evangelista in the music video. I joyfully headed back down the aisle and out of the sanctuary with Owen, celebrating that Grayson was free of cancer and pain, despite the heartbreak I also felt at the same time.

I went up to Victoria as she exited the sanctuary to ask her what she'd thought of the service, only to get a dry-eyed and grimaced response as she spat, "Why weren't my flowers on the front alter table in the sanctuary? They were supposed to be up front so everyone would know they were from me!," she said as she pointed to the giant display of flowers with a big white sash that said "SON" in large gold lettering, sitting on the table that held the bulletins. I told her I hadn't known she had wanted that, to which she backfired, "I spent all that money and no one saw them during the service!" then she huffed and walked away. I just let it go, and moved on.

I was pleasantly surprised to see so many people there including my former boss and a coworker, our realtor from years ago, and several medical professionals from the U. His psychologist, three nurses, a medical assistant, the hospital chaplain, and his lead PA Tessa and clinical trial research nurse Nadia were all there. I gave Tessa and Nadia big hugs and thanked them for coming. They told me how sorry they were for my loss. I replied, "I should thank you for taking such excellent care of Grayson these past two-plus years, and giving me that time I would not have had if he didn't survive after the first hospitalization. Thank you so much for your care and support," to their shock. They told me that it had been their pleasure to work with Grayson and me, then hugged me and left.

One of Grayson's best friends from high school was Bella, who I'd been talking to almost daily the last few weeks. She had graciously created a little boat-shaped sign that said, "Off on Adventures," along with hand painted and decorated rocks in a flower box for attendees to take as parting gifts. Grayson was no longer here on earth, but off on adventures, free of sickness and most certainly exploring the treasures above. Bella, who is of Native American heritage, had also brought me an eagle feather she'd found on the ground in the woods near her house that she said would protect me and bring peace. I still have that feather and it most certainly has done what it was supposed to do.

I retrieved the music and flash drive from the sound engineer, thanked him for his help, and was surprised to be handed a recording of the service. I found my sister-in-law Maddie sitting in the second pew up front still, holding my sleeping niece Samantha. When she saw me she started to softly cry, saying she wished she'd been there more for us, and that she had really loved Grayson. I hugged her and told her she had been a busy mom of three little girls, and Grayson had known and felt her love and loved her very much as well.

As I made my way into the reception hall, I was delighted to see so many loved ones eating the luncheon of deli meats, cheeses, breads, salads, chips, desserts and beverages while listening to the playlist I created for the occasion. I'd had to cut out some of Grayson's favorite songs like the Beastie Boys' "Fight for Your Right," as it wasn't church or parent-appropriate, but did play the Pet Shop Boys, Interpol, New Order, the Cure, Depeche Mode, Peter Gabriel, the Police, the Postal Service, Feist, Pete Yorn, Stevie Wonder, 80's and 90's songs and an eclectic mix that Grayson would have quite enjoyed.

I went table to table, thanking people for coming, just like I had all those years ago at the Wabasha Street Caves when I'd first married Grayson. But this time, instead of happy smiles and well wishes, I got half smiles and condolences that were very much appreciated but also felt so odd. So much attention was on me in that moment. I went up onto the little stage in the front of the room and said, "Thank you for being here. It means a lot to me that you're here today to honor Grayson. He was such a great person and human being. I spent 11.5 years with him, 8.5 married, and am so thankful for that time God gifted him to me. He was so silly, funny, and the kindest person I've ever met. I feel grateful that I was able to be in this fight with him to the end, and know he'd want me to thank you all for supporting us through the two years and three months of his battle. He fought harder than most of us could or ever would, and I'm so, so proud of him. He will miss each and every one of you. Again, thank you for coming. This is going to be really hard without him, but somehow I know I will be okay." I stood there in my new dress, feeling so out of place, but also calm. It struck me that no longer would Grayson ever be a phone call away, in another room, at home or in the hospital. He was gone and I was literally talking about it, so it had to be true. After I finished, Bernard got up to say a few words. He somberly said that he would miss Grayson, and that he wished he'd taken more time to spend with his step-son, to know the real Grayson.

Afterwards a few of my close friends suggested we have an "after-party" at my house to sit, relax and just be together to honor Grayson just among friends, which I thought was a great idea. When I walked into my house I was welcomed with hugs and smiles by my close friends as well as Greta who came up to me with a dog smile and her tail wagging. We sat around and drank mimosas, ate chocolates and just chilled. It was an odd feeling to have closure. The memorial service was now over. I had given Grayson the send-off he would have wanted and deserved, and in the coming days, weeks and months, I would somehow move forward. That night I had a potluck dinner with my parents, siblings and Owen, then went to bed in a dazed mess.

Afterlife Preparations: Although you can never truly plan for the death of your spouse/significant other, it is helpful to have a game plan in place. Funerals and memorial services can be costly, stressful and tiresome for anyone, then double that if it's your other half. You may have already done some of the things on the checklist before your loved one died, or maybe you were like me and were optimistic- thinking it would never happen to you. Either way a plan is necessary to honor what your loved one would want.

- Planning: Have a family member or friend sit down to help you plan the service by drafting ideas and making a checklist of what needs to get done.
- Obituary: I ran Grayson's on a Sunday in the big obit section as more people generally read the paper that day. You can write whatever you want, or just give details and let the obit writer create it. I had them do mine pretty much verbatim, and it turned out great.
o The average obituary costs between $200-$500.
- Ask for help: Delegate tasks to family members and friends. Simply ask them to help.
o This is not the time to be prideful, to try to take it all on yourself. If you do try to do it all alone, you may crash and burn, later wishing you'd spent more time on the details that you couldn't see to clearly, when you were in the haze of the shock of the death.
- Financing the service: Actual costs of a service for a casket with transportation and a cemetery plot can cost between a minimum of $7,000-$9,000 these days.

o   Consider what you can really afford and of course what your loved one wanted. You do not want to use your life savings or all your reserve/emergency savings -or have gone into credit card debt with these new expenses, then be so tight on money you cannot afford regular life expenses because you paid for a fancier service and burial than your means allowed. The added stress of financial strain is bound to happen if you were a two-income home. You don't want to add more to your plate after your loved one's death when you are in the thick of grief and loss by having debts for the after death services, if possible.

- Casket vs. cremation:
  - Caskets, casket transportation, funeral home/church expenses, burial plots and headstones can be a very expensive, but a more traditional way for some.
  - Cremation including the actual cremation itself: $1500-$3000, then adding in the costs for the urn and the funeral home/church hosting or at home hosting is quite a bit cheaper financially. With this route you can also of course have a burial plot, headstone, etc., which will add to the costs. Do what is most comfortable and within your budget.
  - There is nothing wrong with cremation, an urn and a gathering for friends and family at a park pavilion or living room if that's what needs to happen. (For me, Grayson's body was used for research for year, then I received his remains. My total costs were under $700. I was very lucky, even though it was unconventional.)

Do what you need to do, make the smartest decision that you can at the time in your heart and mind and then move forward -- no regrets.

- Flowers and food: If people ask what they can do to help…can a friend or friends do the flowers for the service? Is someone good at making desserts or appetizers that could provide food for the gathering? Use people's talents to your advantage. Many people want to help but don't know how, and you can save a lot of money by utilizing their gifts and talents.
- Eulogy: If you aren't sure who should do the eulogy…ask yourself who really knew your person, inside and out, and will reflect the most accurate picture of your loved one.
- Music: Choose the music or songs that you know your person liked/loved or even songs you have thought you'd want at your own after-death service.
- Your image: Do not care what others think about you during this time…do what you have to do to survive and make the best choices possible. It's not a beauty contest at

177

the service and you want to be stylish yet comfortable and not worry about fashion malfunctions, whether you are a woman or a man.

- o Let someone help you pick out what to wear to the service, you may want a second pair of eyes to help. Trust me…you're going to be in a surreal cloud and not know up from down during the first couple weeks.
  - People will undoubtedly look at you just like they did at your wedding, and everyone wants to see how you are reacting.
    - o Do not let it bother you! Be yourself, cry, wail, fall apart on a trusted loved one. It's probably going to happen…it's not a big deal. God gave us the ability to have emotions and feelings for a reason. Your other half died and real feelings reflect that.
- Bulletin/program: If you are able, have the church or funeral home, or even a friend create a program with your loved one's favorite song lyrics, poem or other writing. Personalizing this is key.
- The day of the service- have a little bag with tissues, Chapstick, Tylenol, antacids, bottles of water, and whatever else you may need. Take deep breaths.
- Here are some websites with some useful tips:
- o http://www.forcremation.com/how-to-plan-a-memorial-service/
- o https://tomorrow.me/trust-worthy/planning-ahead/how-to-plan-a-funeral-for-under-1000/
- o https://www.creative-funeral-ideas.com/planning-a-memorial-service.html
- o https://www.brownmem.com/memorial-service-ideas-on-a-budget

- I will say it again- in my humble opinion-do not go all-out if you cannot afford it. If you do not have a big support network or those who can pitch in, do the best you can, and do not break the bank paying for these services. Make the smartest decisions you can, get comfortable with them and move forward. You are now the widow or widower, and the survivor of your other half. You will need to be able to move forward with as much confidence and gusto as you can…despite how you may feel inside. You CAN do this. I did, and think you can, too!

Sunday May 5th: Felicity flew home that day, which was really difficult, but I was forever grateful for the handholding over the course of the past two weeks.

This was the day of Victoria's memorial service in St. Cloud with "her own people and those that knew Grayson best," as well as the Mall of America fundraiser that Cassie had organized for me. I opted to stay home from both. I was toast. Despite Victoria's pleas for me to attend, I knew I didn't need the extra fatigue or drama. I decided to stay home alone, while Jack and his family, Diana and my mom went to the fundraiser, and my dad went to the other memorial service to represent me.

I napped for an hour then dragged my tired body to the living room where I watched the nine-minute slideshow that Victoria had had someone create for her service. I was shocked to only see images of Grayson from infancy to age twenty-five, the year he met me. The photos were set to an odd arrangement of music that ranged from a cherub-sounding child, to a salsa version of "Awesome God," that happened to dance its way in, on a photo of Grayson at probably age eleven dressed up as the grim reaper for Halloween, scythe and all. Only the last three photos of the slide show had me in them, one at our wedding, and the last two were from past Christmas cards. So yes, ladies and gentleman, it was almost like the last eleven and a half years we'd had together, along with me, never existed.

When my dad returned, he told me he'd worn his "Team Grayson" fleece along with Bella, and had been asked to sit in the front of the church, in one of the two rows that held family. He said the church was full of nearly three hundred people. The pastor started out the service stating he hadn't personally known Grayson, and proceeded to perform a service that would have been more appropriate for the death of a young child, scriptures and all. Bernard, who had gotten up the day before and stated he wished he'd known Grayson more, got up and talked about how close they were. After the service my dad stood in a line with the family, shaking hands with nearly one hundred people that all told him, they too, had never known Grayson. I still greatly do appreciate every person that prayed and thought of Grayson and I during the illness, but it was just ridiculous how many people were there that had never met him.

Dad said after that many people, he decided to step out of the line, and talked to Bella for a while before heading home. She'd made cream puffs for Victoria, which had been Grayson's favorite treat in high school. Bella and my dad talked about how the service offered little reflection of the Grayson they knew. They also both noticed the slide show was void of photos of Grayson's life with his wife.

Later my siblings and mom came back from the fundraiser with big smiles and stories of how cool it had been, a bowling and arcade pizza party with a silent auction of neat things to bid on, and a great sharing of love and stories of Grayson. I felt so enveloped in comfort from that. I didn't care about the money, but knew Cassie had done that for me and that so many people had come out to honor Grayson and I.

Chapter 23:
Time to Get Real with Widow Logistics

My boss called to tell me I had to either come back to work or I'd be let go. I knew from head to toe I could not go back yet, so I thanked her for her kindness and quit. I thanked God for the ability to take time off, and knew that it was a rare gift.

Diana and I went through the cards from the memorial service, reading the kind and comforting words, then deposited the checks I'd been given. I cried in grief at the ATM when I saw on the screen "Rachel and Grayson Checking," and my sister attempted to make me laugh by doing a funny skit like act to distract me. That afternoon I got out my budget sheet and went to town organizing my finances. The life insurance company sent me a form that I had to have Grayson's doctor sign to prove that when we'd taken out the policy, Grayson had been able to do the basics of bathing, toileting, etc.

Over the next few days Diana dug countless holes in the flowerbed in front of my house for my mom to plant flowers in that would, and did, spring up in Grayson's memory every year around the anniversary of his death. I was stationed on the couch most of the time, too tired to move. I still felt like I was responsible for Grayson and his medical care. I'd been on caregiver auto-pilot for so long; now my mind was like a hamster running in circles on its wheel, but the wheel had been taken out of the cage.

My dad went back home, which was really hard. I thanked him for the gazillionth time for everything he'd done for us, and cried saying that I would not have been able to do it without him. He told me he really didn't think that Grayson was going to die and it would take us all a long time to recover and heal from this. He was very somber yet talked about how glad he was that Grayson wasn't hooked up to machines and in pain in the hospital, like he'd endured the last two and a half years, that he was now free of those confines and living with God. I nodded in agreement and looked around my living room where Grayson would never sit again, not sure of my future.

I was becoming surer every day that I'd be okay, even though I had no idea how.

~

Party of 1:

Finances: Now that it is just you, you may need to do another finance evaluation. You're most likely going to have to make some difficult decisions, even though all you probably want to do is hide from the world. It's time to decide what you can realistically afford in this new life without your spouse/significant other.

- o If your loved one had income coming in, prior to their death, from work, disability or Social Security, you are probably used to having that money to pay for part of your living expenses. Without that, you are going to need to figure out what you can and cannot afford now:

o   How long can you pay for things as they are with the money you have in your checking and savings?

o   Was there a trust or life insurance plan in place to help you for any period of time?

 o   For wills: there may have been stipulations or gifts to other family members. Despite any reservations you may have for whatever reason, dole out the money or items to those your loved one wanted things to go to, even if you may not have the best relationship with them. Some families get along great, and some very much do not.

o   Your spouse/significant other's debt: Anything with only their name on it and not yours, such as a credit card is not your responsibility to pay, at least that's the way it was when Grayson died in 2013. I took money from Grayson's stocks and paid off one of his credit cards only to find out they would have written it off, as they did another credit card. Check to see what other debts your loved one had just in their name, to see if you are legally responsible to pay them. Most times you are not, but I cannot guarantee that!

o   Mortgage/rent: Can you realistically afford where you are living on just your income now? You may need to downsize. This can be discouraging, disheartening, frustrating, and just sad to have to leave your home that you shared with your spouse/significant other. But…you have to really look at the numbers and see if you can now afford to live there with just your income.

- What is the cost analysis and benefit of moving?
    - o   If you do need to downsize, you will not have to worry about making ends meet monthly if you realistically cannot afford things as they are.
    - o   Live within your means, not beyond them. Now is not a time to get in over your head financially when you will most likely be on a grief rollercoaster for some time.

o   Cars/automobiles: If you were a two-car household, you may need to sell your loved one's car. Factor in their monthly car payment and insurance in addition to yours. Is that feasible? You can always sell it outright yourself, or trade it in with your car as well and get one car just for you. Either way, do what works best for your budget.

o   Utilities: Electric, gas, (trash, recycling/water, sewage -if you are a home owner) will always be there, and those are usually not adjustable.

o   Student loans: If you have student loans, contact the loan company and if necessary, request a forbearance. Forbearance allows you to skip monthly payments for the available/agreed upon 3, 6, 9 or 12 months. Interest will still accrue, but this will allow you a short-term reprieve. (Contact the vendor directly to find out what needs to be done if your loved one has their own student loans).

o Internet: I was able to negotiate a lower rate and lock it in for a year at a time. Call your internet provider to see what they can do.

o Credit cards: Call the companies, tell them your spouse/significant other died, and see if you can lower the interest rate. It can't hurt to try! I was able to get one of mine lowered by doing this.

o Food: Unless you're a robot, most likely when you are hungry, and do eat during the first few weeks and months post death, you may not feel like cooking. Watch your budget, splurge and treat yourself with a pizza every now and then, but try to stick within your means. You will need a chocolate and comfort food fund for a little bit! I did: Sometimes a girl or guy just needs a good dessert and some time to heal. Try to only buy groceries you know you will realistically use; don't let perishables go to waste.

o TV/movies: I think a lot of people still do have cable/satellite TV, but this can get pricy. For years I have had Netflix, Amazon Prime and Hulu which totals around $36/month. This has been the most affordable route for me. It provides hundreds of shows and movies to choose from. I wasn't that choosy about what to watch after Grayson died. Anything to distract me was great when I came home from work and crashed. I found that watching old friends like Frasier, Friends, Roseanne, Cheers, the Office and other classics were what I turned to most often.

*You will need to get several copies of the death certificate to send into creditors and vendors to take your loved ones off of the bills. You can get copies at the DMV.

☐ You don't have to be a pro at everything right away. You will learn how to balance it all in this new life, in time. Breathe, regroup and work on planning things out the best you can.

Facebook: May 7, 2013: 2 weeks and 2 days: It's hard to fathom life without the real deal, most incredible human being by my side. I am numb and feel like an empty shell. Cancer is the devil. I would take away his pain, suffering, etc., but this love and cancer journey has forever made me a better human being, who I hope to reclaim to be, once I can breathe again.

- You are such a sweet, kind girl. As your hubby struggled, you reached out to me over and over again. Just remember to breathe, one breath at a time. It's all we can do as we feel like half a person. The loss is too huge. Call me whenever. We can be wise witty wonderful widows.
- I have great confidence in you!
- Praying for you.
- Rachel, you are extraordinary...lots of love to you
- Keep breathing and writing it out, Rachel. May the world be gentle with you as you move through this.

- Hang in there Rachel, can't imagine how hard this is on you. We're all here for you when you need support and encouragement.
- Rachel, I've continuously been thinking about you and praying for you. I am so so sorry for your loss.
- Oh Rachel, I am so sorry from the core for your loss. The love you shared was palpable. Cancer is an evil teacher who takes so many wonderful people before their time, and yet in a twisted way teaches us so much about life. Lots of hugs for you Rachel and all of those who loved Grayson.

Diana left on Thursday the 9th after lots of hugs, laughs and telling me she was only a phone call away. It was so hard to see her go, but I was so thankful for the time we had. Felicity called me shortly thereafter, telling me she was going to add me to her family cellphone plan, buying me a new phone as I'd switch to her carrier, and also would pay for my largest student loan. I couldn't believe my ears. I was so grateful and blessed. I called the Social Security Office to officially report his death and to ask about collecting the $250 one-time payment as the deceased's spouse. I was immediately asked "What was the date of expiration?" I was floored. Grayson was not a can of beans or a box of cereal, he was my husband! Sigh.

~

Widowhood Here We A Go-Go

CaringBridge/Facebook: May 10, 2013: My mom is leaving later today. Am looking forward to some quiet time, oddly all I have is quiet time. It's still strange to not only lose Grayson, but the entire ecosystem of the medical system too. Watching lots of Cheers reruns and napping.

My mom told me she could stay longer if I wanted her to, that she had no idea how to leave me after what we'd been through. I told her I'd be okay as we attempted to say goodbye outside by her car. A woman drove up and down the street trying to find where the scent she was adoring came from. This chick in an old brown Buick, with big hair and sunglasses kept turning around and asking, "Where is that wonderful smell coming from?" in a smoky voice. My mom threw up her hands in defeat and face palmed, as we looked at each other and busted out laughing. I pointed to the cherry tree across the street and the woman smiled, waved and took off. Mom and I hugged, cried, hugged again and she left.

Later that afternoon I came up with the idea to make a place where I could write, cry, vent and emotionally bleed while asking for support. The Lord shoved me in this direction of putting it down in Facebook posts in the private group I created, where I'd later learn how much I truly flourished as I wrote it all down. Even if it was just a simple statement or what I was watching or listening to, I felt less alone and heard.

Healing Blog: May 10, 2013: This is a private group, where I can/will post honestly and blog, ask for support, etc. I need to write, but don't want to make it seem like I am whining on the Team Grayson group page. I need so much support, and plan to journal this post-Grayson journey. Thanks

- I love that you're doing this!
- Wonderful idea. Much love, support, and props for doing this!
- Thanks for including me in your support network. The grieving process is long and we are here for you.
- You are a rock star.

Facebook: May 10, 2013: Books: What I am reading: "Widows Wear Stilettos: A Practical and Emotional Guide for the Young Widow," and "Happily Even After: A Guide to Getting Through (and Beyond) The Grief of Widowhood," both by Carole Brody Fleet.

I got the idea to look up books on widowhood the week Grayson died. I wanted a touchstone to help me when I was swimming in this ocean with no lifejacket. I began to read these books at bedtime a few pages at a time before I fell asleep. I felt so comforted and less alone. I was the first person I knew to have a cancer spouse, and now was the first young widow I knew as well. I felt thrilled to find kinship in these books.

Facebook: May 10, 2013: Hour 2 of being alone, alone, alone. Mom left. Sad but looking forward to time off. Am here with our lovies Rufus, Puddin' and Greta. Am a very independent person, but this is going to suck big time.

I was on an emotional rollercoaster by the hour, if not the minute.

Facebook: May 11, 2013: Day 1 Widowhood: On the docket, possible gardening. For now, finally watching Silver Linings Playbook in fleece pjs and eating beloved green beans and mashed potatoes. Slept in too!

CaringBridge: May 12, 2013: Grayson died 3 weeks ago today. I went to Menards, then put together a dog house for Greta and a finch feeder. I fenced in the pretty yet toxic Lily of the Valley flowers, so Greta wouldn't eat them, filled in a giant hole by the fence that the dog had dug, fenced in the back garden, watered the flowers and filled the bird feeder. I feel numb, but my yard is ready for summer. With the help of a neighbor I put Grayson's dad's old brown leather chair and ottoman onto the three season porch with a rug, for my cozy new hangout.

I tried to carry and boost the heavy and wide chair up the narrow stairway from the basement. I literally got it stuck between the slanted wooden ceiling above the steps and the railings. I had to acquiesce to sanity, and go get help after many sweaty failed attempts to lug it up the stairs myself. It was a learning experience for sure.

Facebook: May 12, 2013: Went to Walgreens to fuel up on junk and comfort snacks. Can't even make a decision, everything is a blur. I hate this.

I was in a daze of napping, eating, animal care, reading, sleeping, rinse and repeat. I could not believe how tired I was. The last couple years of the go-go-go had really kicked my butt and drained every ounce of energy that I had. I had been in deep survival mode at the time, and God had given me natural energy drinks into my soul with His faithfulness, grace and guidance. I'd been carried through work, running around to and from medical facilities, and balancing family, friends and pets. My time was split between being a wife, best friend, cheerleader, medical and pharmacy coordinator, independent living skills worker, daughter, friend and pet mom. I was toast.

I have told many people this in the years following Grayson's death- when your spouse dies, you don't eat salad. You eat comfort food and fill yourself with what is delicious and satisfying, not necessarily what is healthy and good for you. I knew it might make me gain more weight but didn't care right then. Root beer, BBQ chips, and chocolate were in my Walgreens run. I would eat and snack, watch TV until sleepiness dragged me down, then take a nap. I always apologized to my two cats and one dog, telling them, "Mama needs to go sleep, she is so tired from her life, running around with Papa when he was sick."At times I would feel so guilty for sleeping again, that I would go hug them before I lay down for a nap.

Facebook: May 12, 2013: Last night I had a panic attack. I didn't cry much, but completely freaked. His clothes are hanging up, his big shoes are in the closet, all waiting to be put on, and there is a car ready to be jumped in for a Rachel and Grayson road trip never to be had. Am tired from yard work, depressed and watching the remake of an '80s classic, which is sure to be awful. I am blessed though. Thank You God, for my love and life with Grayson.

Each time I woke up, either in the morning or from a nap, I would forget for milliseconds that I was a widow. I'd look at the walls as the light streamed in the windows, or I would stare into the darkness and just lay there taking it all in. He was gone, gone, gone. God had a plan for me and I didn't have any blueprints to guide me in what that would entail. Many times I was just living hour by hour, numb and too tired to cry. I'd shower every other day or sometimes in the middle of the night. I didn't have a regular sleep schedule; my mind, body and heart were all competing for different things. The peace within my soul was there, but locked deep inside a chest and thrown off the end of a boat, deep into the bottom of the ocean. I was calm and relaxed, but lost in a sea that I had no idea how long I'd be swimming in, despite positive people, places and things I would experience.

Healing Blog: May 13, 2013: Numb, tired, bored. I have 185 Facebook friends, and only put 71 people in this. If you are in here it is because I trust you, and feel like I can be myself with you. I quit my job. I can't get through this, driving around all day helping physically disabled and mentally ill adults, when I can barely drive myself, and eating and showering is a chore. I am taking a few months off to breathe. For the past 5 yrs I've worked in direct client services and half of that as a cancer wife=grab a knife and some butter....this girl is toast! (Grayson always rolled his eyes when I would say that last line).

- You deserve to have time off to do whatever you feel like doing. I spoke to a few people at a retreat last January who had been both cancer patient and caregiver. They agreed that being a caregiver was way harder than being a patient. This time is for you. Do absolutely nothing for a while if that is what you want to do.
- You definitely need some wallow time. I'm glad you are still reaching out to us through it.

Healing Blog: May 13, 2013: Last night I took off my wedding ring, and Grayson's as well, that I had been wearing since 2 days before he died. I thought it would be a huge, monumental loss. I consulted the widow books and the Facebook young widow group I am in. Today I kept moving my finger to adjust it, as I had for 9.5 years, but it was not there. It was just a symbol, making me sad. It took me a whole 24 hours to look and realize he is forever with me, on my wedding ring hand/arm...tattooed on my wrist. On January 21st, 2011 he started chemo, 6 days after diagnosis.....and a few days later, cried, and asked me to never leave him. The next day I got my first tattoo, and never left him. I am shredded please pray for me.

Healing Blog: May 14, 2013: Extreme exhaustion and sadness. Last night I unraveled to my mom on the phone. This was not supposed to happen with this incredible human I planned a lifetime with. We won't ever have kids, travel, grow old together, etc. We wanted to move to the country in our 60's and have a hobby farm with llamas, goats and chickens. Now Grayson is gone and my body is in so much endo pain, I don't think anything but adoption someday is for me. In this time off I plan to get a hysterectomy. Am grieving the life I will never have.

- I'm thinking of you and holding you close to my heart, keep writing. I don't have any words for you except I'm here and I know....call me whenever you need to or want to. Hugging you with prayers dear sweet Rachel.

Healing Blog: May 14, 2013: I cannot stop crying. I want my Grayson.
- Let yourself cry, it's a good day to cry, my eyes burn from crying. God bottles our tears and saves them in heaven. I think all the salt water in the oceans are from our tears. I get to the point where I get all cried out at times and then I start again. It happens.
- I wish I had some amazing words of wisdom to bring you comfort right now. But I don't. All I can say is that my heart aches for you. You are an incredible woman. It is always OK to cry when you feel you need to. Please know that I am thinking of you and hoping you find a little peace tonight so you can rest.
- Oh honey, my heart aches for you. I'm so sorry. I'm always here if you want to cry to someone.
- I have no words that will take away your pain. Just know that you have so many people who love and care about you. You are never alone. Hugs to u Rach. Love you girl.
- I'm so sorry Rachel. Big hug for you.

Facebook: May 14, 2013: It's apparently hot today. Am sad, but comfy in my pjs, in a cool home with no AC running, watching TV. I talk to Grayson sometimes, know he is here. One of my sisters said she thinks he'll fulfill his promise to always be with me. In the meantime

Greta is happily heaving and chewing on a Kong toy filled with peanut butter. Am sure Grayson is giggling up there.

I decided that I had to get out of Dodge. I had been in the world of cancer and slowly losing Grayson one day at a time, engulfed in survival. Now I needed a release, to leave our home and just breathe. Grayson and I had planned to travel abroad exploring Europe, and now that plan was in the dust, like the kind of dust a real Dodge pickup would kick up. I researched online for several hours, weighing my options. I wanted to go somewhere totally new, but didn't think I'd have it in me to stand in long lines at the Louvre and certainly not to learn a new language. I wanted the ability to emerge myself in a solo healing adventure, while also not having to forage too much for comfort. My body had so many aches and pains with endometriosis, my brain was mush with grief, and I didn't want to worry about where my next meal or bed would be.

I settled on an Alaskan cruise from June 24th to July 10th. I'd always wanted to go there and felt a sense of peace and wonder in my choice. After I booked the trip, I called my parents and told them. They were thrilled and understood my need to clear my head.

When I called Diana, she said, "What?! Did you ask Mom and Dad if you could go? You've never talked about wanting to go to Alaska before!" I told her that I was excited, and no, I didn't need permission from our parents, I was thirty-one, my husband had just died and I needed a break. And lastly, why would I talk about Alaska when my life had been hospitals, clinics and a juggling act?

Facebook: May 16, 2013: A month ago today was the last time I had a conversation with my husband. I skipped visiting him on the last day he was alive, not on life support. I was tired and needed to rest after being there for days on end. I regret not seeing him, but can't coulda, woulda, shoulda, as I know I was there all the time, even tho it hurts now. We had 2 phone conversations, and the following morning were able to say I love you, speaking to each other one last time, on the phone before they intubated him. This was the last time he ever said I love you verbally. This is horrible and I wouldn't wish it on my worst enemy.

- Can't imagine but you are so right in what you said. Praying for you every day!
- Hugs Rachel.

The Victoria Lunch: Victoria had texted me two days prior, asking me to call her. She told me she was coming for the day, that she would take me out to lunch, and listed several items that she wanted back now that Grayson was no longer alive. I was not surprised by this and also shocked at her agenda.

I had to give it to her, she was always the gladiator, ready to come into the arena, hold an audience and let it be known what was going to happen. Now that Grayson was gone, I really did feel like I was just something she had to deal with, despite the sweet-talking tone in her voice. Grayson, her only son and pride and joy, was always the focus and I was the wife/partner/sidekick that she had to acknowledge whether she liked it or not. She told me she wanted the silver flatware set that had been her mother's that she had given Grayson and I for our 7th wedding anniversary that she had polished, and put in a special case with her parent's anniversary date on the top, as well as ours. We had never even taken it out of the box it had been wrapped in. She also wanted a large framed pheasant art print that was in our basement that Grayson's late dad had given Victoria's parents years ago. I was fine with returning both.

I went through the house leading up to her arrival and gathered all of the silver picture frames she had given us of herself, her and Bernard, youth family photos and other non-Rachel and Grayson-esque items that I no longer had to keep in my house. I didn't have to keep the façade up, or keep the fancy little trinkets that I'm sure she thought were lavish gifts that we'd adore. This lady didn't like me, had never liked me, and now that her son had died, she seemed ready to grab her crap and get going onto greener pastures. I put all of it in a giant storage tub and set it by the front door. I made sure to hide the one thing that Grayson treasured most that had become a treasure to me as well, praying she would not ask for it.

When her car pulled up, I said a quick prayer to the man upstairs, asking Him to give me patience, strength and courage and to hold a hand over my mouth when I was challenged. As history could attest, I'd hear odd or cruel things, which I knew would happen in no time. She came in, asked me if I had her things, then asked where I'd like to eat, suggesting my favorite Thai place that Grayson and I had taken her and Bernard to in the past. As we rode in her car, she filled me in on the events, committees and things she had been busy doing, and the friends who had come over and continued to give her gifts, flowers, food, etc. I sat in silence, adding verbal 'oks' and nods in the appropriate places. Don't get me wrong, I was not heartless. I just had had way too much time with this woman who had almost always seemed to make things about herself, especially in the midst of her child being sick, then dying. I was proud of myself in each age of my life, we all figure out who we are, make mistakes and learn, and are carried by God's grace and will, but this lady was very conditional, based on praises, love and niceties. If it worked for her, or she thought it was pleasing to her, then I was great. But if I had my own opinions, or had made life choices as a young growing adult and had created a life with her son, then that was not okay in her eyes. A few times I'd had to sit in the back of their van as they drove around St. Cloud as they pointed out houses for sale that they wanted us to live in, not even a thought to factor in that we loved and enjoyed the life we'd created in the Cities. What she wanted was the crème de la crème and everything else was just so-so, as she'd wrinkle up her nose and tell me. She came over onetime on November 1st, the morning after I'd had a Halloween birthday party for Grayson, years ago at our old apartment. I'd moved around lights and furniture for the party. She looked at a light and said to me, "With this light on, it actually looks civilized in here."

We sat down at a table in the middle of the restaurant amongst the pleasantly painted jade green walls, Buddha statues and other Thai art. I ordered my beloved Szechuan green beans and carrots over white rice. As we waited for our food to come, I nervously played with my white straw wrapper. Victoria asked me what I was going to do now. I told her that I had quit my job and was going to take a few months off to breathe, rest and regroup.

She immediately told me several things. One: that she was only willing to help me with a mortgage payment for June and July, then she wouldn't help me anymore. This was totally not what Grayson's sister had told me right before he died. I was chilled by the air-conditioning and so uncomfortable in my seat, but remained clear and calm on the outside. The first thing I thought was "Well crap, Lord, what am I going to do now?" Followed by, I know I will be fine, God will provide, I had a financial plan. Most importantly, Grayson would be horrified and infuriated that his mom had lied to him as he literally was a week away from his deathbed at that time.

Two: she told me that I was going to lose my house and have to go on welfare. This was interesting to me on many levels. As an ILS worker I helped disabled individuals who literally could not work due to physical and mental disabilities apply for county and government assistance, and I knew I was eons away from needing that kind of help. Also this was the lady that told me one time when I was going to have a garage sale, "Have it on the first of the month, that is when the poor people get their welfare checks and go to thrift sales," as she herself apparently would never peruse a garage sale. I calmly told her that I knew what I was doing and she kept shaking her head over the course of our meal, telling me I had no idea what I was doing. She told me that she had several friends that had given her cards and large checks for me, and that she would mail them to me later (I never ever saw these cards or money. Victoria either lied about them, threw them away or kept them for herself).

Shortly thereafter, we left the restaurant, she dropped me off at home, handed me a check and loaded the things she wanted back into her car, gave me a hug and said we would talk soon, then left.

I let out a huge sigh of relief, waited until her car had pulled out and away from the driveway and let out a big whoop of excitement and stated, "Thank You, Jesus!" My treasured item was safe and the meeting was over. Time would tell, but I had a feeling she just metaphorically "washed her hands" of me. God certainly had a sneaky way of putting people in my life that could teach me lessons of who I did and didn't want to be like, and Victoria was a prime example of what I did not want to be like. I wanted to treat people with unconditional kindness, respect, compassion, love and authenticity.

~

Facebook: May 17, 2013: Thanks Jasper for fixing my outdoor hose plumbing issues! Am out for dinner and a 12 a.m. viewing of the new Star Trek movie in 3D with Grayson's buds. Grayson would be proud. Honey, I am geekin' it up!

Facebook: May 17, 2013: I am ready to share a piece of my history I will never forget: This is the playlist of the songs I played him as he died. Grayson, I love you forever. I still can't believe you are gone, my love.

1.   "Fade into you" Mazzy Star

2. "The Luckiest" Ben Folds
3. "La Cienga Just Smiled" Ryan Adams
4. "Heartbeats" Jose Gonzalez
5. "To Make You Feel My Love" Billy Joel
6. "Northern Sky" Nick Drake
7. "On Your Side" Pete Yorn
8. "Standing Outside a Broken Phone Booth with Money in My Pocket"   Primitive Radio Gods
9. "Answer" Sarah McLachlan
10. "Pride (In the Name of Love)" U2
11. "When the Stars Go Blue" Ryan Adams
12. "Love Will Tear Us Apart" Joy Division

~The love I had with him, and have for him will forever drive me to appreciate the world. Healing though, is going to be excruciating, but I have God, family, and all of you. ☐

I can remember clear as day sitting on the plush tan couch in the living room with my animals around me, my iPod in my left hand and my eyes staring straight ahead. I looked down at the music player as I heard the hum of quiet ringing in my ears. As it got louder and louder in the deafening silence, I felt a little nauseated at the thought of playing it. I took a deep breath, hit play and waited for the tears to fall and/or the vomit to rise. Nothing happened. I just sat there numb... feeling the rug below my bare feet and gravity holding my body to the couch....looking around my living room that was now mine and only mine. I sat in the same position and listened to every song, not moving an inch or crying. Ten or fifteen minutes after the music ended I got up, let the dog out one last time, then went to bed. Tomorrow was a new day.

~

I began to see my friends Jenna and Josh at least once a week during this time. They lived only five minutes away and had a really cute, energetic and fun son, Caleb, who was five. Jenna and I would sit outside and drink lemonade as she gardened or puttered around on whatever project they were working on. Josh had met Grayson in an LLS support group a year previously, as they both had blood cancer. Josh had had two bone marrow transplants and had been fighting the cancer for a total of eleven years. They were very sweet and fun to be around, and as fellow believers, always had healing words of encouragement that were a balm to my heart.

CaringBridge: May 18, 2013: I am working on healing; it's been nearly 4 weeks. As I cry and grieve, I am comforted by our years of love, honesty, silliness, calmness, craziness, and sincere, soul mate love. There are few people in life who are this lucky, and I was, which means I am going to be okay!

191

My church had been so sweet, supportive and encouraging during Grayson's illness and beyond. They'd graciously helped us pay a mortgage payment during the illness. Daisy who helped plan it on the other hand, was a handful. She was on the board of the Christian financial organization Thrivent Financial that decided to hold an ice cream social fundraiser for me at church, and would match 100 percent of what was raised. I was floored by the ongoing generosity of cards, calls and kindness. It felt amazing to be supported, yet I was very aware of the smiles with hints of pity, sadness and not quite knowing what to say to this young widow. Daisy had stopped by my house once a week or so in the last month to see how I was doing.

The church had an ice cream social following the 11 a.m. service. I stood behind a table serving chocolate and vanilla ice cream into little Styrofoam bowls, with assorted toppings of maraschino cherries, sprinkles, chocolate and caramel syrups to be put atop the frozen treat. I'd invited friends to attend via Facebook invite, but did not expect any to attend as I'd just had a gigantic fundraiser weeks before. Owen showed up minutes before it started to help me scoop. There was a little woven basket with a napkin inside that held the money that was donated by each person as they came to get their ice cream. I was so humbled and surprised by the parishioners who would drop in five, ten, and even twenty-dollar bills as they would tell me, "I am so sorry for your loss," "We've been praying for you, and will keep praying," and "We are so sorry we didn't get to meet Grayson, he sounded like a really nice man."

I felt so at peace standing there, while also feeling like I was floating outside of my body, seeing myself and Owen scooping ice cream for these kind people. I saw older couples walk away hand in hand, arm in arm and knew that would never be Grayson and I again. I stood there for over an hour totally alert but also in a fog. I'd had to take a Vicodin pill for severe pelvic pain in order to be able to stand there for that long. At thirty-one, I felt like an old lady, but had to do what I had to do in order to function, and be there for this event. I thanked Daisy for setting this up, gave her a hug, helped clean up and then walked home.

That afternoon Owen and I sat and listened to music on our local indie station 89.3 The Current. We drank local craft beer and talked about everything and anything. I showed him the old high school notebooks I'd found of Grayson's, and we laughed and thought of happier times with Grayson. I worked on ignoring the endometriosis pain I felt, glad that it was only moderate, not the extreme amount I'd had in past days.

That same afternoon Owen and I briefly kissed. Was it the beer or the vulnerability I felt in that literal painful and awful space? Grayson had only died a month before, and I kissed someone else. I didn't feel the shame and horror so many people would think that I would have. The names of what someone would call me, or "Her husband's body isn't even cold yet, and she kissed his best friend," rolled through my head over the coming days and weeks, yet I knew that that was not me. I had given Grayson one thousand percent of my heart, my life, my love and I was in a weird and odd place, as was Owen. His wife had had issues and they'd divorced, leaving him a single dad of two small children, when he'd planned on being married forever, just as I had. We were both in an ugly place of grief, and had gravitated towards each other. Not romantically, but this would forge a friendship that was nearly unshakable for the next couple years.

Right after the death of your spouse or significant other, you feel invincible. No one can touch you. You're absolutely invincible and no one can understand what you're going through. Owen was like an old hoodie or comfy pair of jeans. Old and familiar. What I would come to learn and reflect on, was that he and I had both lost our best friend when Grayson died and my late husband had gifted Owen and I, each other. We began to hang out regularly, nearly every week and kissed one other time beyond this first time, a week later, and after that we never kissed again. Later, I'd feel confused, thinking I loved him, and much later than that, learn it was the grief talking.

The day of the first kiss, he said as odd as it was and felt, he'd realized he'd had some feelings for me in his time of grief as well. It was all so confusing. I was on a sinking ship of grief and loss that I had no idea I would be riding on, that at times would plummet to the bottom of the ocean, and other times nearly drag the entire ship onto dry land and wellness. Owen and I held onto each other metaphorically, as it was easier at times than facing the current desperation and unknown future. I trusted Owen and he was and would be a representation of security during this time.

I'd been used to physical contact and being a part of a little family of two. I would later learn that the support I'd had during the cancer journey would begin to lessen then nearly cease altogether, as people went back to their normal lives after the crisis of death was over. I would get confused and hurt along the way, but God had me, and man, oh man, would I, and did I, learn a lot about myself.

Chapter 24:
Complacency and Calm

Facebook: May 20, 2013: Tomorrow will be a month since Grayson died. Am dreading it. A whole month. I miss him so much, but I've grabbed the life raft, and am holding on! I know he would be really proud of me. Thanks for all the love and support.

Facebook: May 20, 2013: I miss my best friend. Am beginning to laugh again and enjoy things, despite my broken heart, which is amazing. I know it's because I was so loved.

Healing Blog: May 20, 2013: Just went through some tubs in the basement storage area and found negatives of pics Grayson took when I was 19 and 20 that I have never seen before. I was just a baby! Also found a whole folder of old girlfriend letters. So funny

Facebook: May 20, 2013: Found this online, made me smile. "And I learned something from that experience: grief is a hairy twisted monster. Death is something we all have to face, and in a lot of ways it's beyond our normal modes of comprehension. The effects it has on us are varied, and it's not our place to judge anyone's grieving process, unless their grieving process is to hurl typewriters at laughing children or something." (Author unknown)

- That's fantastic.
- I hate grief.

Facebook: May 21, 2013: Today has been a month. I feel okay. I feel like I should be more upset, but these are the facts.

1) Grayson was my true love. The great shebang, the real deal. I expected us to hold hands on the porch in rocking chairs as we peed our pants in old age.

2) Grayson fought with such bravery, courage and grace.

3) Pre-transplant the statistic of 2+ yrs out for the space age radiation +chemo+transplant, was only a 19% survival rate. I heard it, digested it, and put on my armor and we carried on, started the process and I was there through and through.

4) I had an amazing life with him, and believe the combination of my Faith, and the medical actuality and biological reasons he had to die, plus his adoration and love he had for me (of course I for him) and the time at home to get used to this, is helping me heal. In the meantime, I nap a lot, hang out with friends, and cherish the life I had, as I face an unplanned future.

Facebook: May 23, 2013: Today it is beautiful out. Lilacs are blooming, sun is shining. Still don't feel the best, but have plans with friends the next few days, and a summer of sunshine and awesome music planned. And 4 seasons of Rhoda on DVD.

Healing Blog: May 23, 2013: I feel very at peace emotionally. I know it's the time off and the space to breathe, but also the circumstance. Friends and my therapist have said, subconsciously I have been grieving Grayson since the day of his diagnosis. What I know to be true, is that the way he died was beautiful, compared to a lot of widow stories I am encountering. Some women have lost their husbands to post-war suicides, war, murder, sudden, unexplained aneurisms and illnesses, freak work or car accidents. I got to be with my guy, since day 1, and was in the trenches with him until the end. This was a gift. He was taken away from me way too soon, but good Lord, am I blessed and lucky compared to the heartbreaking stories I have recently encountered in the helpful widow groups I am a part of online. We were all blessed to have had Grayson, and will all be better people because of it.

I began going to Owen's house weekly during this time, hanging out with him and his little two- and five-year-old daughters. I found spending time playing My Little Ponies when I'd brought over my original ponies in their barn carrying cases and ice cream parlor-shaped Mary Jane shoe, was a great way to clear my mind and focus on just having fun. It was freeing to be silly and watch the imaginations of these little beings at work.

Over the next couple years Owen and I would attend concerts, watch movies and share new music over pizza, Thai and Chinese food and craft beer. We began to know each other outside of the roles we'd had as Grayson's wife and Grayson's best friend, different from the almost 12 years we'd known each other before. Owen was a lot wittier and snarkier than I'd ever known. It was fun to see him let loose and have fun the way my husband had. We'd talk on the phone every few days about work, music, family, or whatever came up, as best friends do. God gifted us each other when we'd lost our spouses and best friend to the harsh realities of the world. I loved how'd he roll his eyes and tell me, "Oh Grayson was just out of this world in love and enamored with you. He'd talk about you all the time!" It was fun to hear stories and things like that, to hold deep in my heart, after my husband's passing.

Facebook: May 27, 2013: Just read C.S. Lewis's philosophical novella "A Grief Observed," while listening to Jack Johnson. It chronicles the author's wife dying of cancer and how he processed grief and moved on. I thought I'd be a complete mess about now, but I am amazed at the strength God is giving me. I felt Grayson's presence the first couple weeks after he died, he must have known that. He's gone now though, off on adventures, where he is not sick or in pain. I'd often tell him over the years when he'd think I was kooky or out of my gourd, "You signed up for this field trip!" I am at peace that our field trip has ended. Grayson was my other half as I was ushered into my adulthood and made me who I am today. I am blessed! Thanks Grayson!

Facebook: May 28, 2013: Laughter is the ultimate medicine that is healing my soul. Thanks to those of you who are making me giggle, you all know who you are!

I met up with my best friend Wyatt at least once every week or so for lunch or just to hang outside during the spring and summer months. We'd often eat brunch at the Seward Café among the hippies and grungers at one of our favorite places. It catered to the veggie crowd and was an accessible place that Wyatt's power wheelchair could navigate easily. It was nice to sit out on their back brick patio, in black metal chairs eating omelets and kale at tables, with the sun shining on our faces as we ate and talked about music. I was able to lose myself and not focus on grief. To this day I still treasure those times so much with Wyatt, when I was in the beginning of my grief. He's such an amazing friend and I love him dearly.

Healing Blog: May 29, 2013: This blog is quite therapeutic for me. I am unable to sleep and started journaling at 1:15 a.m., which I haven't done in years. Am trying to use it to bide my impatience about a few things, but also am finding it's fun to do. I write poems, general journaling and doodle little pictures. After an hour of writing in bed, I kept looking at the closet which held mostly Grayson's clothes. I got out of bed and spent 25 minutes deciding what to keep, donate and how to make the empty closet just mine now. I guess I thought I needed to keep more of his things, but he's got a whole new wardrobe with God for his adventures up there!

As I listened to 104.1 Jack FM, I opened the armoire and began working toward reformatting the hard drive of my brain and life. I kept the warm tan wool cardigan sweater that I got all sweaty running around in my winter gear in Macy's to find as a Christmas gift one year, as well as a pair of jeans and a few other items. I tried to smell Grayson on the clothes but there was nothing there, I found to my disappointment. Tears sprang to my eyes. I was in a sea of clothes, knowing he would never come back, yet still had the whisper of a hope that he'd somehow miraculously walk through the front door someday.

The only other person I knew in real life in the same predicament was Sheila, eighteen years my senior, a cancer survivor Grayson met in the LLS group. During his BMT process, Sheila's husband was fighting for his life in the cardiac ICU. I found her and introduced myself, and spent a lot of time sitting with her around her husband's bed for the last days and hours of his life. However, she had seven children and many grandchildren.

I was alone and spent hour after hour either being super productive or a sloth. It was an odd mix and I never knew what would happen when, with no one to check in with.

Healing Blog: May 29, 2013: Feeling quite positive today. Fatigued, but positive.

Healing Blog: May 29, 2013: AM BLESSED!

~

Into the Heat of Summer

Facebook: June 5, 2013: Have been awake for hours.

CaringBridge: June 5, 2013: This past weekend I went to San Diego, thanks to my amazing friend Angela- to the San Diego Rock and Roll Marathon with 23 TNT participants/friends. The MN team raised $85,000 for the Leukemia and Lymphoma Society, and the 1,500 LLS/TNT total marathon participants raised a whopping $4.5 million. I enjoyed the weather and palm trees and was able to grieve and cry while being surrounded by understanding athletes fighting blood cancer. I felt so blessed and honored that they had Grayson's name on the TNT jersey this year. I also was party to seeing the fastest 1/2 marathon =13.1 mile record broken in the United States ever! A Kenyan man ran a 4.4 minute mile, so 13.1 miles in only 58 minutes!

My friend and TNT mentor Angela surprised me with a trip to San Diego to get me out of the house and around supportive TNT people in sunny California. I was thrilled to have this space and time to regroup. From the time Angela picked me up, to the welcoming TNT team at the airport, to each and every meal and event, I felt more whole, welcomed, and at peace. Even in a month, I felt such solace and inner health. It was like seeing a spotted deer drink from a fresh stream of water in a lush green forest. I was slowly beginning to feel natural, refreshed, and like a real human again. Not a cancer wife, not a widow, not a shut-in, but like a real person out in public eating and being among the living.

Angela and I went to a nice restaurant for dinner the first night there. It seemed so exotic to be out doing something so simple like sharing a meal, as I'd become so used to sterile medical environments. We spent time walking around downtown. I smiled to myself being so out and about when I'd been confined to my couch and bed for the past month.

The night before the marathon the "Inspiration Dinner" was held in a large ballroom with huge banquet tables. As the host went over the statistics of increases in blood cancer survival rates and advances in medicine, I began to bawl my eyes out because my cancer patient had died. I threw my arms around Angela and let the tears fall for a couple minutes as the others at the table looked at me in sympathy. Gus, a larger fellow with a beard who was sitting next to me, patted my arm, said he was sorry and cracked a joke in attempts to make me smile.

Later that night as the coaches met with the team to give their night-before motivational pep talks, I came up with a mission for the team. I told them with a shaking voice through a few tears, "I want to thank you all for your hard work to get here. Tomorrow when you're tired and you hit the wall and feel like you cannot go on, I want you to push harder in memory of Grayson. He was so geeked to know that TNT existed and wonderful people like you raised money for patients like himself. Just keep going and kick cancer in the teeth the way he did. Thank you all so much!" I was given several hugs and high-fives then went to our room and watched Angela prepare for her race, as I had done so myself the year before, but with Grayson watching.

The next day I woke around 8 a.m. to sunshine and God's grace. I got ready, then wandered around the post-race area. I reveled in the fanfare, as I happily ate snacks and enjoyed the weather. I followed Angela's race progress from an app on my phone. When I saw that she was halfway through, I headed to the stadium to take in the main act of the event, The Psychedelic Furs. I took a seat. Minutes later as I sat in a sea of green plastic empty seats, I was rewarded with the opening beats of "Pretty in Pink," that caused me to dance in my seat. I reminisced about the first time I watched the movie in my friend Kristen's basement on a Friday night at age fourteen, for one of our sleepovers. I immediately fell in love with Andie, Duckie and Blaine. I smiled and looked up to the sky, as if Grayson were there listening to it…he could have been, who knows? God is quite wonderful.

Thirty minutes later I received a call from Angela from a medical tent, where she was getting checked out. She had to stop running, as her heart was beating irregularly and she didn't feel well. I met up with her at the Minnesota TNT tent and gave her a hug, telling her I was sorry that she had to cut the race short.

As we sat there, Cameron, a big guy on the team, came and told me, "I hit that wall and thought of exactly what you said. I pushed on kicking cancer in the teeth for Grayson! Thanks for saying all that last night." I jumped up and gave him a high-five and hug. Angela and I went to the hotel for naps before lunch. She decided she wanted seafood and beer for lunch, and I was game as I'd find a salad or something to eat. In the fifteen minutes that we waited for a table, I had an internal war with myself as I drooled, looking at the banner with a picture of their fish and chips on it. It had been ten years since I'd eaten any form of meat. I wondered if I ate the fish if I'd get sick, as the body can become intolerant to foods it hasn't processed in a long time. I ended up giving in and trying the fish and chips. I enjoyed it very much along with a Stella Artois beer. For the next couple hours I couldn't stop exclaiming out loud, "I cannot believe I just ate fish!" as if I'd just eaten a monkey brain, to anyone who didn't know my story.

That night I was excited to learn that mahi-mahi was being served at the post-race congratulatory dinner. As I sat with Angela, Gus and other TNTers sharing in their accomplishments of the day, I reveled in feeling so special to be included in this experience. Angela was my angel of a friend, to pay the pretty penny it cost to include me in her trip. That night I cried a little at bedtime, telling her how grateful I was to her for getting me to a literal new place of peace, to be part of something bigger. When I arrived home the next day I thanked Angela profusely and returned to my bubble with my pets, wondering what was next.

199

The next day I called the cryogenics clinic to request to have Grayson's sperm destroyed. There was no point in keeping it if I didn't have Grayson with me to raise our mini-Graysons and Rachels. I received the paperwork in the mail, numbly signed it and sent it back. So many wishes and dreams died with Grayson, and having children naturally would be one door I would have to close as well. I reached to God for comfort in knowing what was done was done, and I had to move forward the best I could.

Facebook: June 5, 2013: Today I am suffering severely with a migraine and allergy face pain due to the merry-go-round that is Minnesota weather. I went to my fabulous therapist today, bought yummins' at Trader Joe's, and am going to nap this headache away hopefully.

Facebook: June 7, 2013: I need prayers please. Day 3 of monumental migraine with pain. Eye swells, teeth hurt, cannot sleep.

- Praying right now for you. Lord, please give Rachel relief from this horrible pain, ease her mind, bring her your peace as she trusts in you. Grant her sleep. Amen.

CaringBridge: June 8, 2013: Please pray for a little 3yr. old boy named Danny who is having the same kind of transplant Grayson did. Cancer makes me so angry. I vow to dedicate my life to working in social services, to help people and to honor Grayson. Tears won't stop falling. It's hard when people say they understand, but if they haven't been through it, they do not. We need a world with more survivors and less widows, widowers, and empty armed parents. Please hug your significant other and children tight tonight, life is so unpredictable, and I never thought I'd be where I am now.

~

Owen and I went to the Fine Line in Minneapolis to see the band Chvrches perform. It was a great show, and it felt so nice to be out and about, among people my age at a public place where I'd attended so many concerts in the past. I stood there listening to the songs "Recover" and "Mother We Share," that I loved while drinking a beer and letting myself get lost in the music and the moment.

Facebook: June 9, 2013: I feel really good. I painted for the first time in years which was very therapeutic. I am pleased with how I am doing so far. Eight weeks ago I wouldn't believe I'd feel this okay, probably instead thinking I'd be hiding in the bottom of a closet crying. I'm so thankful to my friends for their support as I go through all of this. Upcoming is my Alaskan trip, then rest, then my big surgery. Deep breaths and prayers.

- Proud of you babe, you are amazing
- Enjoy the fresh air tonight, proud of you
- Your strength and positivity is amazing! You're awesome.

That week I went to see my gynecological surgeon to request a hysterectomy. When I told him Grayson had died, he said, "Oh no, Rachel, I am so sorry." I told him my pain level had been unbearable, I took painkillers nearly daily and couldn't take it anymore. He agreed to perform the surgery but warned, "Once I take everything out, I cannot put it back in…" I told him I understood, I wasn't able to function well and wanted a better quality of life.

I'd dreamed of being a mother, had twenty years of childcare experience including raising babies as a nanny, and always thought I'd have my own biological children, yet my body was at war with itself. I knew many people had reproductive issues like my own, but didn't think it would ever come to this. I scheduled the surgery for early September and drove home subdued to yet another hard reality in my young life. Sigh. "God give me strength," I said to myself as I drove and reflected on how the last time I was in that same medical office, Grayson was there with me, was alive and we had such hope that he'd get better after the transplant. Life is not fair and a slap in the face, a kick in the teeth and sometimes so darn unjust.

Facebook: June 9, 2013. Rachel's late night chill-out, calming, waiting for sleep meds to kick in music: "Banana Pancakes" and "Better Together" Jack Johnson, "Waiting on an Angel" Ben Harper, "Crash into Me" Dave Matthews Band, "Tranatlanticism" Death Cab for Cutie, "Paper Bag" Fiona Apple, "Molly: 16 Candles" Sponge.
Facebook: June 9, 2013: Am very loved by the 3 pets, especially Greta who randomly runs up to me, with adoring doe eyes and wants pets, fully believing she is a 2 yr. old real girl.

Healing Blog: June 10, 2013: Am happy girl today. Ran errands around in weird weather, on the phone on hold- dealing with post-Grayson provider issues, and the lovely Jenna is coming over soon, then I shall get crafty around my house.

Healing Blog: June 10, 2013: I just took down in my bedroom the quote "Every Love Story is Beautiful, But Ours is My Favorite." It was depressing. I always said there was no Grayson and Rachel without Grayson. I left up the word "Love." I have a lot of living to do and loving in my young heart.

- Good idea to leave up LOVE. I like that you changed it but did not remove it. It's very symbolic

Facebook: June 10, 2013: Lots to post to you, my supportive peeps. Today: major laugh-doorbell rings, young guy tries to tell me about his home remodeling business and Greta goes all Cujo on him behind the door, meanwhile, said young guy asks if the homeowner is around. Apparently the little chickadee in a Twins tee and bright green and pink Hello Kitty pants doesn't look like the homeowner.

Healing Blog: June 10, 2013: In the past week, I have reconciled with my heart and mind that I began slowly watching Grayson die before my eyes, and grieved the whole time he was ill even when I didn't know it. Despite the laughter and fun he and I shared, I didn't let myself

201

realize the severity. His illness and cancer life was our norm. I am choosing to be grateful for what I had and to try to be positive each day.

Facebook: June 11, 2013: Creaky from climbing all over my house like a monkey, stencil painting. Now time for cocktails and my beloved Hubbell Gardner and Ka-Ka-Katie in "The Way We Were."

I learned during this period that sleep would come only when it wanted to, causing me to stay up late at night and nap during the day. One night I went online and got ideas on stenciling my walls to change up my new house, to reflect my new place in life. The next day I bought wall stencils and a variety of Martha Stewart acrylic paint sets at Michael's. When I returned home with my art tools, I was devoid of energy, so I put off the project 'til later. After being unable to sleep that night, I popped out of bed at 2 a.m. and stood on my couches stenciling for hours as I sang along to Fiona Apple's "Tidal" and Nelly Furtado's "Whoa, Nelly!," albums of my youth.

It felt like coming home, holding the stencil frames on the light cream walls, as I painted pink swirled intricate designs onto the walls and I sang the lyrics I knew from heart about wanting to be a bird that flies away and being a shadow-boxer. It was just me now and if I was going to make this house mine; might as well make it girly. As I painted, I shut my eyes a couple times and prayed, thanking God for carrying me this far. I'd later come to learn how much grief was like a Ferris wheel that let other passengers get on and off, like when I'd spend time with friends and loved ones, but ultimately I was stuck on the ride, and had to learn how to live with the constant changing and movements. What I didn't know at the time is how many tools in my tool belt of life I would acquire, and how valuable each experience would be, as it all contributed to who I am today. I finished painting at 4 a.m. and collapsed in bed, happy with my creations.

Facebook: June 12, 2013: In the process of negotiating selling Grayson's car...big monkey off my back!

I had a red PT Cruiser that had stopped working; it needed new brakes and a new alternator. I knew I couldn't keep it. I was able to sell it for $1,800 on Craigslist, and was grateful it made it out of the driveway in one piece! I had to sell Grayson's car and decided that I would trade it in for a bright orange KIA Soul that I found online not too far from my house.

I felt calm driving his car to the large dealership; however I began to feel a bit nervous as two salesmen exchanged looks before one walked over to greet me. I test-drove the car and although it was not a manual transmission like my last several cars, as I preferred, I could not pass up the look of it and its low mileage. I sat at the salesman's desk and looked at the paperwork in front of me, with the large fluorescent lights shining above me. This was the first major purchase I'd make without Grayson. I began to feel nervous as I negotiated a monthly payment. The kind salesman told me, "If you say yes to this amount and it gets approved, this is what it will be, it cannot be changed." I knew it was just me now and I would be solely responsible for the car, house and all the bills, but would return to work in time and have an income coming in. I agreed to the monthly payment we negotiated and within forty-five minutes I was able to drive off the lot in my new sweet little orange boxcar. Huge life purchase as a widow-check!

Healing Blog: June 14, 2013: 6 a.m. cleaning, organizing and watching Breaking Bad.

Healing Blog: June 14, 2013: Insomnia...again. I had a late night painting party again, this time listening to the local country music station K102, as I climbed on top of my kitchen counters to paint little red circle like flowers with the stencils on the cream colored walls. On the red accent wall I stenciled green twisty vine like designs, as I listened to the music letting myself get lost in the moment. Painting those stencils, listening to that music and having my dog lay on the kitchen floor with me, brought me such peace that night in ways that nothing else could or would. The living room stencils turned out great, and I hung up my Frida Kahlo print of "The Wounded Deer," that up until then had hung in the basement as it creeped out Grayson. No boys lived here now and I am making it mine!

In those days and moments God gave me such grace that I needed in ways I did not know. The ability to move forward, one foot in front of the other, whether it be redecorating my house in small ways, or being able to go a chunk of minutes or even hours without thinking of myself as a widow or what my new widowhood would entail, was such a gift of grace. It was something I would feel and know, but not completely comprehend until I could look back on it years later.

Healing Blog: June 14, 2013: Yard-work day and housework: to my mother's horror, I climbed on a tall ladder in the garage to change garage door opener lights (and didn't call someone to tell them I was up, then down the ladder and not broken, alone, laying on my garage floor). And used a weed whacker for the first time and still have all of my appendages! Single girl, taking the home/garden world on her own! Bell bottom jeans and yellow tank top, hair pinned up, Rosie the Riveter I may be...

Healing Blog: June 15, 2013: Super busy week. Lots of hangouts, reconnecting with friends, and house/garden work done, as well as new hobbies struck. Am bummed I only have 1 episode of the Catherine Tate series left, as I adore it. Now if I could keep healthy and pain free, I'd be set! Busy week ahead with close friends and whoever else participates in my shenanigans!

Healing Blog: June 17, 2013: Happy girl, happy heart.

I unfortunately had to stop seeing my therapist; as my COBRA insurance premiums were too high, and I could not afford the expensive deductible. I began to process some things through friends and knew that the coming months would be harsh and nothing I could prepare for, but that I'd make it. I had studied anthropology in college and now I was learning about the culture of widowhood. There were things I couldn't help and wouldn't be able to fix...like how I'd feel nauseated every time I went down highway 94 and passed the U's Fairview Hospital where I'd left Grayson's body. I always looked back at it, even though it made me uneasy, knowing they were working on his body in some building, somewhere.

Facebook: June 17, 2013: 8 weeks/2 months and am doing worlds better than I'd ever imagined possible. Grayson will always be a big part of me, and Thanks Be to God! For my Strength, Faith, and Courage!

Healing Blog: June 18, 2013: Awake way too early. 450 a.m.! It's for the birds! Ahhh, will nap later. More sleep now, then 9 a.m. revolutionizing a friend Jenna's upstairs attic room with my mad, nerdy organizational skills, girly gossip, cancer support, grocery store, then yard work, bathe Greta (smelly girl), then nap, then grilling dinner! Tuesday, Blue Light Special, Aisle 9.

Healing Blog: June 18, 2013: I hope my late night philosophical thoughts don't come out or come across like Jack Handy's fireside musings from Saturday Night Live. I think it's not about seeing the silver lining in the clouds, it's about knowing the clouds are permeable, ever changing, can cause rain, and ugly storms, but are also beautiful, shade, comfort, and are a constant in life, no matter where you are, or how old you become. Understanding that life gives no guarantees, but that you have the ability or choice to still want to strive for happiness and fulfillment despite hardships. -Late night Rachel hippie happiness for the fortitude I have.
- I see a book in the near future.... Rachel's Musings

Facebook: June 19, 2013: Shocking evening. Wowsa.

Four days before I was to head to Alaska, I had the worst migraine and my power went out. It was blazing hot, getting to the low nineties during the day and only dropping a few degrees at night. I spent as much time as possible in the cooler basement, but could not even open the windows as everyone decided to mow their lawns or run loud generators. My pounding head could not take it anymore. I called Bella and asked if I could stay with her to have a girl's night and share her AC. She immediately agreed, and we invited Hazel to come over for drinks and hang out later as well. I quickly packed up some clothes, covered up my standing freezer with a blanket in an attempt to save any food as instructed by my dad, and loaded Greta into the car. I drove all the way to St. Cloud with the air conditioning blasting its sweet coolness onto my face and body.

Bella and I caught up on life, love and her twelve- and fifteen-year old kids. She was remarried to a nice guy, and reluctantly shared custody with her abusive and manipulative ex-husband. Bella used to run a bed and breakfast with her current husband until she fell one day and hit her head that resulted in a traumatic brain injury. She was receiving Social Security for herself, as well as payments for her children. She'd recently found out that the kids' payments were somehow sent to her ex, who was keeping the money for himself. That day he'd been served with contempt papers for this violation and was not too happy with Bella.

Hazel came over that night and had wine with Bella, while I drank strawberry Boone's Farm, a cheap, candy- tasting malt wine. As we sat there, Bella began to talk about how it was so awful the way Victoria treated me. She joked that we should paint Victoria's windows black and egg her house. We laughed. Of course, it was something we would never ever do, as we were nice to the core and not spiteful or revengeful girls. Having overheard her, Bella's fifteen-year-old son laughed and then went to his father's house for the night.

Bella chugged down her second glass of wine, which is like double that to someone with a TBI, and suggested we call Victoria. Bella refused to take payment for the desserts she'd made for Grayson's St. Cloud service, and suggested they share a bottle of wine sometime instead. Bella called her that night under the guise of getting together to share the wine. I had no idea what to expect as I sat there quietly.

Bella put the phone on speaker in the middle of her glass coffee table, as she sat on the couch with Hazel, and I sat on the adjacent sofa holding my glass of strawberry malt wine.

"Hey, Victoria, it's Bella. How are you doing?"

"Oh hey, Bella, I am ok, how are you doing?"

"I am well, I just wanted to call to check in to see how you are doing with everything. It's been several weeks since we last talked. I wanted to see if you wanted to share that bottle of wine sometime, and how you think Rachel is doing."

"Things are going ok, I have my good days and my bad days. Yes, we will have to get together sometime to have that bottle of wine. I am not sure about Rachel. There is a lot going on with her."

"Yeah? What have you heard about her?"

"Well," (sigh and low throaty chuckle) "you know Rachel has always been a bit odd and just does what she wants, ya know?"

"No, not really, what do you mean?"

"Well she told me that she is going to quit her job and take time off. I have no idea what she is thinking. She doesn't know about the realities of life. She is going to lose her house and will have to go on welfare."

My eyes nearly fell out, my mouth dropped open, and I slapped my hand on top of my mouth, as Hazel looked at me and mouthed "What!?," and threw her hands up in the air. Bella held her finger up to her mouth in a shush motion, then continued to talk.

"Um, I don't think that will happen. Rachel is really smart and needs to take some time to heal and have a break from everything going on. I know she will not lose her house, she is just taking some time for herself."

"Yeah, well' (small snort chuckle noise). "I don't know what is going on, she is going to have a hysterectomy and will be sorry one day that she cannot have babies. She is making so many mistakes right now."

"I think that she is taking good care of herself, she needs to do what is right for her body. I had to have a hysterectomy years ago myself. I know Grayson would want her to be healthy and happy. I know it was hard for all of us, when Grayson left here when he was in his early twenties and started his new life in the Cities without us."

"Yes, he did. He had so much he could have done for work and school, but now there is nothing else that can be done, he is gone now."

"Victoria, he had a good life, he loved and adored Rachel and had a great life with her and was happy."

"She is not who I would have picked out for him, but yes, he did love and adore her. She has just made so many choices that I don't approve of. The way she has looked, acted, jobs she has had. She's just so different from what I know. That took Grayson away from me."

"I know it can be hard as a mom when your kids don't make choices we agree with, but Rachel was the best wife in the world for Grayson, and she did everything she could for him up until the very end."

"Well I don't know, I just know she is making rash choices and won't be able to keep up her standard of living and who knows what will happen. I have to go now, but I will talk to you soon. Nice talking to you, bye."

"Bye, Victoria."

Bella, Hazel and I sat and looked at each other in shocked silence. "What in the world?" I said aloud.

I knew that Victoria didn't like me and I was definitely not who she would have chosen to marry her baby, but to hear the things she said was just almost otherworldly. I said it before and I will say it again...when you're someone like me who is really nice, you don't necessarily expect the best in everyone, but you are surprised each and every time that someone bashes you. This level of her annoyance and weigh-in of thinking I'd pretty much end up in a cardboard box, was just too much.

The three of us detoxed and rehashed the phone call, before taking a breather from the drama to play a board game. An hour later after more wine Bella decided to call Victoria again, and when Bernard answered, Bella said, "Hey Bernard, I just wanted to call Victoria again to check to see if she wanted to share that bottle of wine tonight, she sounded pretty upset when we talked earlier." He told her that Victoria was in the shower and that tonight would not be a good time for a visit. Victoria lived only blocks away from Bella, and Hazel and I had to use all of our might to convince our beloved friend with a TBI to not walk over and drop by for a visit.

We chatted and giggled late into the night. I decided that night that the next day I was going to get a large tattoo on my leg of a peacock feather and was very excited. After Hazel went home, I crawled into Bella's daughter's empty bed with Greta lying right below me, and fell fast asleep after listening to a Ryan Adams song on my phone.

The next morning I sat in Bella's living room, lounging on her couch with Greta at my feet on the floor. I happily ate a blueberry muffin that Bella had made the day before and discussed the day's plans with my good friend. All of a sudden there was a loud bang on the door. "Coming," Bella yelled as she hobbled to the door on her crutches. I heard some talking and then Bella leaned around the corner and said "Uh, Rach, there is a police officer outside asking for you."

"What?" I said. I looked down at what I was wearing…a light brown shirt with a dark brown peace sign on it that said "Dirty Hippie" across the top, on the back it said, "Flower Pickin', Baby Kissin', Puppy Pettin', Tree Huggin, Bleeding Heart Liberal" along with my white Hello Kitty pajama pants with a print of her riding on hearts down rainbows. I grimaced to myself at my attire, and went outside barefoot.

The police officer took off his sunglasses and told me that they'd received a tip that Bella and I were going to cause property damage to Victoria's house. I told him that Bella's son heard his mom joking and must have told his dad. I could tell the kid thought it was funny, and her ex had reason to be mad for being caught stealing the disability benefits. The cop said that Victoria and Bernard had received a call from a police officer warning them of some possible pranks by their daughter-in-law Rachel. They had stayed up the entire night, worried that I was going to come to their house with Bella and cause property damage. Lovely, I thought to myself. What a mess!

I told the police officer that we were sitting around as girlfriends, chatting and having a cocktail and had no intent to harm Victoria or her home. I filled him in on Victoria's history of dislike for me as her son's wife, and the recent conversations we'd had regarding her being upset with me about money and my life choices. He smiled and said he knew friends get together and vent, but next time not to make any phone calls. I thanked him for his understanding and went back inside. When I told Bella what happened, she quipped, "You have pelvic pain and can barely walk, I am on crutches and have a sprained wrist and a TBI; we are barely one whole healthy person put together. Why would anyone really think we would do property damage to Victoria?" We laughed so hard we cried for a few minutes, then went on to plan the rest of our day.

An hour later I got a phone call from the same police officer. He told me, "I just got a phone call from Victoria and after telling her I had talked to you, she wanted me to tell you that she will no longer talk to you, or have any contact with you unless a third party is present, and that any money she has is for the living, not the dead, and that you are connected to the dead, i.e. her son, therefore she will no longer help you with any finances." He asked me if I understood and I confirmed that I did.

The powers of the St. Cloud reigning couple had gotten to even the police. Bernard and Victoria both held city volunteer roles they'd been voted into by many fans. I was apparently seen now as some sort of deviant in the eyes of my in-laws, and the local police department, too. Dear Lord, what has the world come to? When the call ended I set my cell phone on the table and told Bella everything that had just happened.

Her mouth dropped open as she, too, could not believe it. "I am so sorry! My dumb mouth and my kid who went and blabbed to his dad. Now you won't have help paying for your house!" I told her it was fine, it would all be okay and that my ties were for sure severed with Victoria now, as she never wanted to talk to me again without a third party present, which was fine with me. She really didn't like me and I had to start my life all over again. I needed only positive, non-toxic supportive people in my life. I called Hazel and Owen to tell them each what just happened, as the sheer bizarreness of it all blew my socks off and around the room.

An hour later we parked on a side street and walked to the brick building that held the tattoo shop. As I waited for my turn, I took in the walls and photo books of past artwork done there. When my name was called, I followed the artist to a private room with a bench for Bella to sit on near me. I told the artist I wanted a giant peacock feather with the word "Serendipity" scrawled around it, in the same font as my other tattoos. I said he had freedom with the artwork and colors, just to make sure it was colorful with several pink feathers.

For the next three and a half hours I endured some of the sharpest pain of my life. I had Bella take pictures of the progress to let me see how much was done so far, as I lay on my side with my right leg out as the ink was seared into my flesh bit by bit. As I lay there, I thought about Grayson getting poked and prodded with needles in his spine for his lumbar punctures, his bone marrow biopsies and hundreds of blood draws via ports or IVs. If he could go through that hell, I could get this done easily.

I also thought about Jesus on the cross and how he suffered for all of us to be able to have rights and liberties and unconditional love and life in the name of God. The inking on my leg was not even 1/1000th of a fraction of what happened when the nails went through Jesus's hands, as he was nailed to the cross. I bit on bobby-pins to keep from squealing in pain, and the artist had to shush me a few times, so I didn't scare other patrons. Bella sat by my head part of the time, as I kept exclaiming, "Victoria sent the Po-Po to get me!"

I lay there listening to music and reflected on the wonder of how I got from point A to B in the cancer journey and how the "Serendipity" on my leg reflected that despite so, so many bad things that had happened to me, and happened in my life, I continued to have surprising wonderful things happen as well. I was supported and loved by family and friends, and was moving forward with God's grace and devotion. I wanted to mark that on my leg, to never forget that even when things get really bad, good things can still come…there really is light at the end of the tunnel, you just have to bring your own flashlight sometimes. That night I went to sleep in Bella's daughter's bed again, this time icing my sore and throbbing, newly-inked leg, and chuckled to myself in the dark at the oddness of the day. In two days I would be leaving for Alaska!

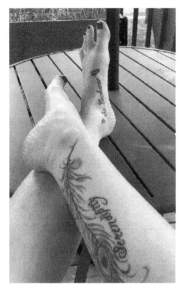

Serendipity and "The Luckiest"

Chapter 25:
Alaska, Here I Come!

The next day I packed my suitcase with nervous excitement for the seventeen days I would be in Alaska. I packed warm and colder weather clothes, tennis shoes and sandals. I packed my "Jesus Calling," devotional, a new non-fiction travel book I'd found online called, "Walk in a Relaxed Manner: Life Lessons from the Camino," and a small journal. I took a deep breath in as I folded all of my clothes and set them carefully into my suitcases. My cats lounged in and out of the doorway, Greta lay on the hallway rug and hot winds blew in the windows that were still my only source of light, as the power was still out. I threw out all of the food I knew would spoil while I was gone, listened to music on my little transistor radio, and sang along to Run DMC, Def Leppard and AC/DC while I ran in circles making sure I had everything I needed. I brought one large suitcase with clothes, another large one that was empty to bring treasures home in and a small carry-on bag and purse. I had two small pouches that opened up into bigger bags for my day trips, one into a backpack, and the other into a duffel bag. I had wanted to go to Alaska for eons and could not believe I was going on my own! I felt like a warrior princess about to stake my claim on a new frontier.

Owen came over around 4 p.m. the next day to help me take Greta to my friend who would watch her while I was gone, and to bring me to the airport early the next morning. Jenna was going to come over to feed the cats and water plants as well, which was a huge blessing. I bought Pizza Luce for everyone as a thank you for helping me before I left. I slept on Owen's couch in the cool air-conditioning with his dog Ella laying near me. I took a Benadryl, reached my phone to make sure I'd get up to make my 8 a.m. flight, watched a rerun of "Friends" and fell asleep.

Healing Blog: June 23, 2013: Serendipity defines the fortunate circumstances I have had lately, which is scripted above my peacock feather tattoo=my free spirit and willingness to fly forward. Tomorrow am going to Alaska for 17 days, so no Facebooking. Am excited for this solo adventure after years of exhaustion and heartbreak.

I woke up to the alarm on my phone at 5:30 a.m., took a quick shower in the kid's bathroom, with ducks and toys at my feet, dressed, regrouped my bags, and was ready to get out the door in record time. Holy cats! I felt like such a little adventurer. No one had any idea that I was a widow, my husband had died, and I was going on a trip to take some time to heal myself. It was really neat and special that this was mine, and only mine, and no one would know what I'd just came from unless I told them.

I flew straight from the Minneapolis/St. Paul airport on Alaskan Airlines to Anchorage on a six-hour flight. I was wedged in the middle seat and alternated between sleeping, snacking and listening to music. I arrived in Anchorage at 12 p.m. local time, excitedly walked off the jet way, through the terminal, gathered my luggage, then called my friend Sylvie's husband Greg to come pick me up. Sylvie and I had been in the same social work graduate program at the U. I hadn't seen her for years and was really excited to catch up, but Greg came to get me, as she had to work. We gave each other a quick hug, loaded my luggage into the car then settled in for the two-and-a-half-hour drive to the small town of Whittier where the cruise ship docked.

I was in such shock at actually being in the real Alaska. I was in awe of Alaska the entire time I was there, but right at that moment, I felt like pinching myself to make sure it was all real. We headed down the highway with the top down on their Jeep and caught up on recent events.

After we'd been driving for an hour, Greg pulled over on the side of the two lane road where we got out, crossed to the other side and looked down over the railing at a small waterfall and beautiful moss-covered mountains, to see if we'd find any brown bears like he had seen there many times before. After ten minutes of not seeing anything, we got back on the road to ensure we'd make it through the one-way tunnel on time, or we'd have to wait on our side for an hour. We made it, careening through a darkly and barely lit ancient tunnel that was so small, cramped and a bit spooky, but also very cool. First super interesting thing to experience that I'd never seen before-check!

We got to the boat around 2:45 p.m., I gave Greg another hug before I slung on my purse and backpack and began dragging my two suitcases to the large metal airplane hangar with signs directing me where to check in. I couldn't get over the massive size of the ship, my home for the next two weeks. I'd always said in the past, "I will never go on a cruise or big boat, tell me what you will, I've seen the Titanic!" That was then and this was now. I didn't think I'd be a widow at thirty-one, either.

I made my way through the rope lines, checked in with an agent and received my keycards and maps, then made my way up the ramp to the entrance of the Norwegian Sun. Once I'd been scanned in, I made my way to the main level where I took in the marble floors and glistening dark wood staircases as soft music played overhead. All around me were floor-to-ceiling windows that displayed Alaska's beauty, which I knew at that point was only a glimpse of what was to come. I found the elevators and navigated my way to my room. Everywhere I looked inside was beautiful polished cherry wood. I had a queen sized bed and end table, a large closet and shelves, a desk with a bookshelf and TV above it, a small sofa and a spaceship-looking bathroom with a cylindrical shower.

For the next fourteen days this would be my safe haven that I'd come to know and trust when I was happy, sad, distraught and so very lost. The trip I chose went from Seward down to Vancouver along the Inside Passage. The small port towns that I would disembark in and venture around were accessible only by boat or plane, along hundreds of miles of coastline and glaciers that would leave me speechless and awestruck. I chose to take time going down then up the coast because I had the time, space and freedom to rest, reflect and recharge.

I took the next few hours to explore the levels of the boat and familiarize myself with places where I might want to spend time during my stay. I found a great little seated area that looked like a good place to read and watch the sights go by on a top deck, a library with nautical décor and several piano bars that hosted music and dance nights. The casino, tiki bars, hot tubs, pool and volleyball and game areas might not be something I'd utilize, but were entertaining to see.

I attended a jewelry show out of curiosity, and was rewarded with vouchers for a free piece of jewelry in each port. I ventured to the dining area where I was not prepared to find so many offerings. The gigantic salad bar was brimming with more fruits and vegetables than I could eat in a month. Anyone's tastes could be met by all of the meats, cheeses, sandwiches, ethnic and cultural offerings, desserts and even a crepe station. Holy cats! That was just lunch and dinner! I took my plate of veggies, salmon, bread and cheese to the outside deck where I'd eat most future meals, and then went to the bar. I took in the drink menu as I waited my turn. I engaged in small talk with the bartender and ordered the featured drink of vodka, cranberry and orange juices topped with cherries, telling him I was there as a widow to take time to heal and rest. He thought I was kidding when I said I was a widow and laughed, thinking I was joking as spouses joke at being so frustrated with their spouse they could kill them. I told him yes, I was serious, paid for my drink and as I walked away, gave him the friendly tip to take someone's word next time, as you never know if they are kidding or not.

I took in the mountains as far as I could see, along with the very small port town that mainly consisted of remnants of the railroading business from a century ago. As I ate my meal, excitement pulsed through my veins as I sat on the nearly empty deck. A loud announcement said the boat would set sail in ten minutes. I finished eating, stood up and headed to the dark wooden railing where I asked God to protect me. As I closed my eyes, tears sprung forward and I said, "Grayson, show me that you're here with me, show me a sign!" I looked up and within seconds, a bald eagle swooped down in front of me, no more than twenty feet away, turned its head and looked at me for a split second then took off out of sight. I sniffled, laughed and said, "Ok, I know you're here," then returned to my room. I started to go through the itineraries and maps while sitting on my bed, as the boat began moving, only to launch myself into the teeny bathroom to empty the contents of my stomach for the next ten minutes as the activity director loudly announced that night's entertainment. I thought to myself as I cursed that featured drink I'd consumed not long ago, "If my parents could only see me now!"

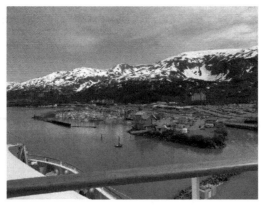

Whittier: Waiting for the ship to take off.

I napped for an hour, chugged water, then forced myself to go explore. There was no way I'd miss out on the sights, as it was the sole reason I was there. I armed myself with my room key, phone, trusty little bright red point-and-shoot camera that would take National Geographic-worthy photographs, and a jacket. I found a brown wicker lounger on the exercise and viewing level to sink into, as I took in the landscapes of richer blues, greens and browns than I'd ever seen in my life as we went around the Gulf of Alaska, passing Prince William Sound and the Columbia Glacier.

This forty-foot-long glacier was the first one I'd ever seen, and as I stared at it in pure glee I learned about the magnificence in front of me. As I attempted to comprehend its massiveness, I learned how falling snow on glaciers compresses and becomes part of the glacier where air bubbles are squeezed out, causing ice crystals to enlarge, which results in the ice becoming blue. I heard a churning sound in front of me, in the water that caused me to rise from my seat to see these "calves" that broke off of the glacier in sizes ranging from a basketball to a car. The baby cows had chunks of beautiful blue that was visible as they churned in the water. This all fascinated me, causing me to desire to learn more about Alaskan nature, topography and geography. I called it quits as I'd gotten up so early for my flight, and went back to my room, despite the bright daylight that I'd have to ignore as there were twenty-one hours of daylight at that time of year. I learned to rely on the alarms I preset in the coming days.

I woke up the next day at 7:30 a.m., showered, dressed and walked downstairs for a breakfast of fruit, toast, and tea that I ate while looking at the passing scenery outside. As I took in God's beauty, I thanked Him for getting me thus far since Grayson's death, and reflected on how I could have been a balled-up mess still at home. Instead, I trusted in the greater plan despite not yet knowing what it was. I decided to read and explore the ship; that day was a full day at sea. I enjoyed the fact that I didn't care what anyone thought I looked like. I was alone, resting in the comfort of hoodies, jeans and flip flops. Despite the fact that it was June 25th, I was often chilly from the cooler outside temperatures or continual flow of the

AC inside the ship. I was accustomed to the swampy humid temperatures of Minnesota, but was happy as a clam as I loved the cooler temps much more.

I spent several hours outside listening to the rolling winds and water, breathing in the sea air and resting my sore leg that still smarted from my tattooing just days before. It felt freeing to not think about much, to tune out the ship's announcements and conversations of those around me as if they were shadows on the sidelines. Every now and then I'd turn to see a small child running around enjoying themselves. I'd smile to myself, but for the most part I was in my own little bubble, despite being on a ship housing nearly two thousand people.

I'd always been an avid reader, and on this trip, after such a long and painful loss, I found a connection to another text, to my delight. As I read "Walk in a Relaxed Manner," the story of a sixty-year-old woman who spent thirty-seven days walking across the Camino del Santiago in Spain with her retired pastor friend, Tom, I felt such kinship. It allowed me to walk through the ups and downs of the journey I'd just been on with Grayson. The book filled some holes in my soul I didn't even know were there, as I reflected on my past at a comfortable pace while not triggering the cancer wife, then cancer widow PTSD I'd later learn would be a part of my future. I think God gives each of us gifts to share and connect with others, and Joyce Rupp, the author, gave me that platform to process and discover parts of myself I'd locked inside while balancing the world of my late husband's illness and death.

At some time that afternoon when I allowed myself to put the book down, I filled a plate with veggies, fish and fruit again and headed to my same spot on the deck to watch the serene landscapes before me. I went to the lounge and watched "The Guilt Trip" movie that stars Barbara Streisand and Seth Rogan among the older ladies in track suits, fancy nails and big hair. That night I watched "Who Wants to Be a Millionaire," on stage, then bought a Coke and sat outside to watch the beautiful landscape go by. I quickly learned that the shows every night were at 7 p.m. and again at 9 p.m., as the theater was directly below my room. Whether or not I wanted to hear round 2, I would! I read my Jesus Calling book, watched one of the sitcom repeats that was on a loop, and went to sleep.

The next day I showered, dressed and ate while excitedly listening to the overhead announcements describing the stop at Icy Strait Point. The ship docked an eighth of a mile from the actual shore, where then those who disembarked rode in dinghies to the port. I took the little red boat with twenty others to land, took a guide from a greeter and mapped out what I'd do in the five and a half hours I had to explore. I wore my Nike tennis shoes that I'd used for my half-marathon, jeans, a long sleeved shirt over a tee and my maroon and pink Columbia windbreaker jacket that would be such a trusty part of my Alaskan uniform.

Icy Strait Point is a unique village that is owned and operated by Alaskan Natives which directly supports the Hoonah community, the state's largest Native Tlingit village. Just reading about the indigenous culture made me more excited to explore and experience the museums, restaurants, tribal entertainment and gift stores. The wooden buildings before me were painted in a sharp red that housed the Historic Canning Line and Historic Museum that told me the stories of the lives of those who lived and worked there decades before. From 1912 to the

1950s the world had been enjoying King Bird and Real Red salmon that had been caught, cleaned and canned by hard-working men straight from Icy Point Strait. I enjoyed walking through the museum seeing the mock pieces of fish on the canning line, colorful diagrams and vintage advertisements and cool artifacts hanging on the walls. As I looked at the photographs and artifacts of the Salmon House People, I thought about what it must have been like to use the oars and boats so long ago. I watched Natives singing and dancing for ten minutes then went to The Cookhouse Restaurant where I had the most amazing fish and chips of my life. The halibut and fries that I ate with lemon wedges and tartar sauce from the little cardboard box along with my root beer was pure heaven. That was the kind of food angels must eat up in the clouds. I learned at that moment that any fish I'd eaten until then had never stacked up to Alaskan fish, especially the halibut that had been caught that morning.

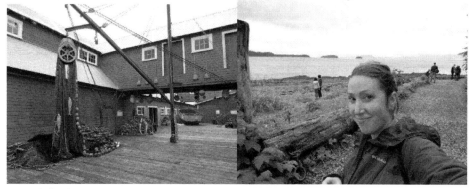

Icy Straight Point

After lunch I walked down the gravel path to the forest, looking at my map so I wouldn't get lost and not make it back to the ship in time. Within minutes I could no longer hear my feet crunching on the gravel; in its place I could hear the whispering winds in the trees which sent a calm yet electric bolt up my spine. I was in awe that I was walking in the Alaskan rainforest! I was surrounded by such sweet-smelling and bright, lush green trees, plants, grasses, mosses, and winding paths. What I saw and did during this excursion, as cliché as it sounds, are the things you imagine in dreams. I walked up and down trails just reveling in the massiveness of the forest around me, as I heard and felt the air rolling off the sea behind me. The flora and fauna surrounded me with scents of new life and growth. It was invigorating to be enveloped in new life and thriving wilderness when I'd been living in environments of sickness, dying and death. I'd been robbed of so much and this Alaskan rainforest was just the cup of tea I needed on that day. I passed a bus that looked exactly like the one that had been in the movie "Into the Wild," thanking God that I was on a positive and protected path during my journey. I just could not get over how good everything smelled. I wanted to stop and live there forever, sending for my animals and a few essentials.

I walked over to the zip line and watched people career sixty miles an hour down the fifteen-hundred-foot drop down Hoonah Mountain as they were dropped three hundred feet above the rainforest. I thought it looked fun but knew I'd either puke or poop my pants or both if I did that. I began chatting with the guy on the bench next to me who was waiting for his husband to come down the line. Once his husband arrived, we all chatted and made plans to meet for dinner at one of the restaurants on the boat that evening.

I continued walking, saw moose burgers on the menu of a restaurant, and found a small fire pit that I made a wish on. A little basket next to the burning pit held small envelopes with flat, three-inch by one-inch pieces of wood inside a little paper that said the Tlingit people had gathered with friends and family to pass down stories and traditions over time, and to feel free to add the fire chip to help keep the tradition alive. I said a little prayer, quietly asking God to continue to protect me, to help me heal from my loss and to have a great life going forward, then threw the wood in the fire.

I spent my last hour wandering around the gift shops looking at the native jewelry and wares while talking to the Native workers. I felt a strong interest and connection to Native culture. Like the book, "God is Red," that I read in one of my Native American classes in undergrad, I believe that God is in the dirt (red), trees, plants, and everything that is living. He created it all and it is all His masterwork and that we are only here borrowing the space and land that He made, for a short amount of time, therefore we need to take care of it and respect it for future generations. I am nothing without God and the world is nothing without His creation. The cyclical ying and yang of Rachel's philosophy. I purchased a small silver pendant with teal, black and red Tlingit totem animals on it and some postcards.

I sat on the sand near the shore, took off my shoes and socks, despite the chill in the air, as it was only fifty-five degrees, and sank my feet into the sand. I collected shells and rocks all around me, then arranged them next to me and took a photo. I closed my eyes for a minute, taking in the sea air and smiled at the new wonders around me. Twenty minutes later I was back on the boat, took a nap, then met my new acquaintances for a sushi dinner. I went to Sam Fedele's engaging comedy show that night and laughed quite hard for the entire hour, feeling happy at my spirits lifting. That night I slept well. I was excited for the next day in Juneau. God kept blessing me and holding me together, despite my body pains and grieving heart.

The next day when I woke up I turned on the TV to the ship's camera channel, to watch the view from outside above the boat only to see the fog covering most of the screen, above the rich green and blue water. I got ready for the day, grabbed breakfast and headed outside to watch the scenery. I went inside to the auditorium to get my passes for my whale-watching excursion, and made a quick call to my parents before we docked. They were ecstatic to hear from me, "The Alaskan Traveler," as my dad had said.

Once the boat docked, I scanned out again, took the dinghy to the shore, then waited in a misty rain in line to board the giant white tour bus that would take me to the whale-watching cruise. It was quite chilly on this June 28th day, compared to the humid summer I knew at home. I bundled up and found my seat, then stared in awe at the several bald eagles that were sitting on top of telephone poles nearby.

On the thirty-minute ride along the Gastineau Channel to Allen Marine by Auke Bay, I learned neat little tidbits such as a gallon of milk was $5 and a loaf of bread was $4, because the land was reachable only by boat or plane. Residents had to pay high prices for everything in exchange for their chosen hideaways. I easily pictured myself hidden in a little cabin with just my animals, a long-distance job, books to fill my house with a roaring fireplace in the winter, and a sea to look out upon in the spring and summer.

That dream was quickly shaken from my head as I walked on the cool and wet metal ramp that led me to the small boat I'd take for the three-hour trip. I took a bench seat, settling in among the couples and families. While we careened up and around the North Pass, I learned about its history, weather and native animals, including the otters I saw floating on their backs. As we passed little islands along the way I was able to see a Dall's porpoise bobbing up and down as well as many sea lions that were sunbathing.

One of the tour guides carried around a large black curved thing that I had never seen before, as he told us it was a nine-foot long baleen plate, the filter-like feeding system inside a whale's mouth. It filters out water through the toothbrush bristle-like hairs to catch krill and small fish. It was humbling to see and touch something from one of the world's largest creatures. Once we'd been on the water for a bit, I went upstairs to check out the view from up there, only to find wet seats and even colder winds whipping across my body. That was secondary to my comfort as soon as I saw nearby ripples in the water of what I was told was a male whale that weighed close to twenty-five tons and averaged a length of forty-six feet! All I could think about was how amazing God was, to have created such a creature.

We traveled another fifteen minutes without stopping, giving me an opportunity to warm up below with cider and a donut. Just as I finished my snack, the driver cut the boat engine, requesting over the speaker that we remain silent as a mother and two babies were nearby. I went to the back of the boat, shivering in the rainy winds as I trained my eyes on the water in front of me. I gripped the railing as I held my breath and waited. Within seconds several small ripples appeared in front of me, followed by a large black nose peeking out of the water for seconds before it disappeared below. For the next twenty minutes I stood as the cold rain pelted my jacket, watching these magnificent beasts take turns coming up to the surface, then crashing into a deep dive with their tails lingering up above the water. It was by far one of the coolest things I'd ever seen and still is to this day. On the way back I warmed up inside and watched a father explain to his small son in another language how the whales breached the surface. He used hand movements and noises that were understood by anyone without a language barrier. I smiled and reveled in what I'd just seen. On the bus ride back I nodded in and out of sleep in sheer exhaustion from being so cold and attempting to keep myself warm, while I watched the beautiful homes and cabins go by.

Back at the Juneau port, I went to the jeweler with my voucher to receive a silver whale tail pendant, then explored the area. I spent time going from store to store, many of them art galleries or boutiques that sold handmade artisan items from locals that spent the winter months creating items for the May to October tourist season. I saw incredible photograph after photograph of the rich greens, yellows, blues and purples of the Northern Lights stream across dark black skies that were taken there, instead of what I'd only seen up until then in pictures online or books. I lost myself in the photographs and paintings of snow-covered houses, villages and animals in winter scenery, wishing I could purchase it all and fill a giant home with it all somewhere deep in the wilderness that would become my new safe haven. I purchased a hoodie, some small art prints and trinkets before boarding the dinghy and heading back to my room to change into warm clothes. I had a late lunch and smiled to myself thinking, "I am really doing this!" as I looked out the window at the sea. I felt so at home, that I could do this the rest of my life. I chuckled a bit to myself. I could imagine someone asking my parents, "How is Rachel doing?" "Fine!" my dad would say. "She took a cruise to Alaska and decided to never come back. Yea, it was crazy. We shipped out all of her things and her animals to her and she has lived there happily ever since!"

That evening I sent a few emails to family and friends. I'd purchased an internet plan with a very slow connection. I opted to skip that night's entertainment, as I was not a fan of musicals and went to the piano bar instead. I sat there in so much pelvic pain, sipping my Coca Cola as I listened to the pianist sing Billy Joel, Elton John and James Taylor covers. When he started to play "You Are So Beautiful," by Joe Cocker, I shifted uncomfortably in the black suede-chair, uncrossing and crossing my legs. By the time he got to the chorus I was in tears and bolted to the lobby. I heard only my flip flops smacking the marble floor and the beating of my racing heart as I stalked to the elevators.

Everywhere around me I saw people together and in love. My person was dead. I sunk into the empty elevator and said "Oh Grayson, where are you?" out loud between sniffles. I made it to my room, picked up the love doves made out of towels, chucked them onto the sofa and collapsed into a blubbering mess on the bed for the next hour. The injustice, the tragedy, the pain and loss of all of it blew up in my face right then. I was a seven-layer dip right then of sadness on top of anger, on top of pain, on top of fear of the future without him, on top of being okay and knowing God was there, on top of the joy of the years I had with my Grayson, on top of being there and healing in Alaska, all layered up in that space and time. I fell asleep that night with tears streaming down my face with the musical roaring loudly below me.

The next day I woke up feeling refreshed, frowned at the memory of the night before and said aloud, "Lord, let today be better," as I got ready for the day. I headed to the coffee bar to grab a Coke to try to help ward off the headache I had from all the crying the night before and sat down at the counter to chat with Lourdes. I met her on my first morning there and had come to visit her daily for a morning cup of tea. We quickly bonded over being the same age and chatted about our lives and the things I had done or would do that day. She lived in a small room with another employee and sent as much money as she could home to her mom in Ecuador who was raising her four-year-old son while she worked. She was short, kind and became my best friend the duration of the trip. That day my head luckily got better within an hour, just in time to explore Skagway.

Skagway was my favorite port city on my trip, one that I would spend time in twice, as I came back up the Inside Passage as well. It was the "Gateway to the Klondike," the historic center of the 1897 Gold Rush boom.

The town revolved around its historical portrayal of the actual events of the time through costume dress, train rides along the Yukon Pass, stores and buildings set up as they'd been long ago and restaurants and plays based on true events. I'd purchased a day excursion pass for the Alaska 360 Experience which included an Iditarod Dog Sled Racing Musher camp, gold panning, and themed restaurants and stores.

I spent the next four hours in an area that was situated between mountains that had been used for mining in the Gold Rush days, feeling like I'd been taken back in time. The staff was dressed in the clothing of the late 1800s and used Yukon accents and all, which made me smile. I watched a re-enactment of what gold panning had been like before I took a try at it myself. I climbed on one of the only remaining dredges from that era and learned about the mining process and what it would have been like to live and work back then, before I toured a small soda factory and tried the sugary liquid goodness.

I excitedly participated in "The Chilkoot Chill: 40 Below Experience," where I learned about what temperatures that cold did to the lungs and bodies of humans and animals, before putting on a parka and venturing into the frozen ice block enclosure. I only lasted seven of the allotted fifteen minutes, until my nose hair froze and my lungs began to hurt.

From there I went to the musher camp, which was my favorite part of the day. I listened to an actual Iditarod musher tell our group about the 1,100-mile race over the course of seven to eighteen days that participants from all over the world came to attend, as I pet the beautiful dogs before me. The sled dogs were an array of black, black, white and tan, and tan and white. My favorite had sea-blue eyes. I stood in amazement as the musher told his tale of racing in negative fifty degrees for four or five hours, before stopping to feed his sixteen dogs and rubbing salve into each of their paws before making his own food, resting for a couple hours, then starting to travel again. It was an epic tale that I could never imagine myself doing. I watched the adult dogs race around the gravel rink in their harnesses to demonstrate how they run together, before petting and holding four-month-old puppies that would one day be Iditarod dogs themselves. I held these sweet, little wiggly pups while having my photo taken amongst the green trees and blue skies and felt so free and at peace.

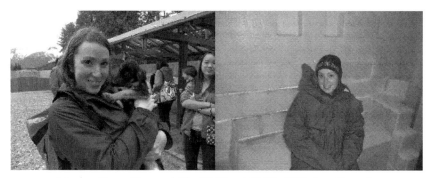

Musher Camp Pup and The Chilkoot Chill: 40 Below Experience

Back in Skagway proper, I spent an hour exploring the local shops and taking in the gorgeous pottery and art. I collected my free purple gem stud earrings, purchased a couple art prints, made a few phone calls then headed back to the boat.

That night I went to the casino, bought a Heineken beer, lost $20 on slots, then went to my cabin to read for the rest of the evening. I had to work hard that evening to block out the images in my mind of such an ill Grayson, willing my mind to think of the healthy and happier times. It was hard; the healthier times had happened so long ago.

I spent June 29th in Ketchikan, my second favorite Alaskan port. When I was there I spent more time talking to locals, like the kind Native American waitress at the crab shack as I ate amazing-angels-can-only-eat-this-good halibut tacos with an Alaskan White Ale. She told me how her permanent home was sixty miles away, reachable only by boat or plane, and that she stayed in a bunkhouse with roommates for the tourist months. She shared some recent community tragedies, and discussed the community resiliency and teamwork that helped make bad things better.

I spent time walking along the waterfront and through the town, before perusing the local shops and boutiques. Everywhere I looked I saw various sizes of totem poles, carvings of animals in glass, marble and wood, and a few large stuffed bears in doorways. I went to the Christmas in Alaska store and found very cute little felt and fake fur hooded Eskimo doll ornaments I purchased for myself and as presents. The store was full of reds, greens, golds, cheer and a dressed-up live Santa.

Lastly I went to the Southeast Alaska Discovery Center where I walked through their neat exhibits on forestry, fishing and wildlife, that made me really miss my brother Jack. When I exited the building I called him and told him I'd wished he was there to experience this with me. I hefted my duffel bag full of treasures onto my back, smiled feeling fulfilled and enriched, and returned to the ship.

I spent the next day relaxing, visiting Lourdes and reading as it was another entire day at sea. I took my book and journal onto the pool deck and settled at a table until I was too tempted to get in the pool for a bit. I'd only been in there ten minutes before rain began to fall which made me laugh. I wanted to freeze in that moment and to have an aerial photo taken of me in the pool inside the ship atop the sea, all in the falling rain. I had no idea what was in store for me and all I could do was take it day by day and trust in God and the greater plan, rain falling on me and all.

The next morning, July 1st, was the last day of the cruise heading south. We docked in Vancouver. At 8 a.m. I took my birth certificate with me and set off to explore for the next eight hours. I was without a plan. Of course, I hoped to magically run into my favorite singer Sarah McLachlan who lived there.

I looked at a map and headed toward Stanley Park. By 8:45 a.m. I was walking toward a dozen-plus homeless people waking up in front of a series of broken down buildings. As I took in the giant mural of the Simpsons cartoon characters and got closer to the individuals, I realized I was in a Skid Row-esque area that was littered with needles, condoms and broken bottles on the ground. As a mental health professional I knew these people most likely were harmless, but I started to walk faster nonetheless, silently asking God to protect me. I declined to engage with them or give them money and kept my eyes to the ground. Once I'd gone down a couple more blocks, I turned the corner and took out my map to only realize I'd been walking in the wrong direction for the past hour.

I backtracked, going over a block to avoid where I'd just been and in time was on a bus and headed to Stanley Park. I found out that it was Canada Day, or as I'd refer to it from then on, "Oh Canada Day," thus why I'd been the only person I'd seen in quite some time on the deserted streets, as everything was closed for the national holiday.

At Stanley Park I purchased breakfast, bought a cool little green wallet with orange and red maple leaves on it, and some maple sugar candy for my parents. I passed several artists who were painting and had other artworks for sale leaning against their easels, as I walked among the tall trees and explored the war monuments and statues. Around 10 a.m. I stumbled across the Vancouver Aquarium that was just opening for the day, which was a pleasant surprise. As I walked along the featured exhibits of jellyfish in colors of reds, pinks, oranges, yellows, greens, blues, purples and multicolored in baby, medium, large and gigantic sizes, I stood in wonder at God's creations. I learned incredible and amazing facts about the animals and people of the British Columbia and Pacific Canadian areas, the Amazon Rainforest and Canada's Arctic regions. It was then that I came face to face with a beluga whale. I stood there in awe watching two white whales happily swim in front of me, until I had to sit down. I was absolutely floored in how I'd gone from walking past the drug addicts in the sketchy area I had been in only two hours ago to seeing the wonder in front of me now. I knew it was only by the sheer grace of God. I wanted to tell my parents that right then and there so badly. I laughed at my luck and circumstance.

In the afternoon I explored the beautiful gardens, walking around display after display of gorgeous tulips, roses, rhododendrons, and other beautiful perennials and annuals in every color imaginable. I wished that my mom was there with me to see them all. I explored the Japanese garden with its intricate paths and perfectly manicured plants, then looked at my map to decide what to do next as the blazing sun and heat beat down on me.

I walked along the seawall, passing many walkers, rollerbladers and people on bikes, until I came to the Brockton Point Totem Poles where I sat in the grass and just stared at their magnitude in size and artistry. I wished that I had water and Tylenol as my head began to pound. I felt so unprepared; I'd usually had a purse stocked with every pain reliever or first aid item should I one day need it.

I walked across the street, passing the tall West Coast Rainforest trees that weren't even the largest in the park. They reminded me of the trees in the opening sequence of the "X-Files." I perched on the seawall. I sat there with my feet dangling over the wall, with sand below me and water to my left, breathing in the sea air and saying a prayer. I called my sisters and parents for a quick hello, then made my way along the paths, passing Canada Day parades and gatherings to find the exit to the park. The farther I walked, the louder the bands and fanfare were to me as I kept walking, willing myself aloud with a pep talk to get to the bus stop. I ran to the stop when I saw the bus approaching, then sank into the vinyl seat and closed my eyes in the cool blasts of air conditioning.

When I reached the pier I was able to find a pharmacy to purchase a Canadian version of Excedrin, then lined up in customs. The agent didn't want to let me back on the boat without a passport, but after several minutes of adult whining and telling him that the woman who helped me book the cruise said my birth certificate would be enough, he gave in and let me through. I practically ran to my room after boarding the ship, had a snack, napped and rested the remainder of the day. Thank you Lord for the USA!

On July 2nd with the second voyage starting its first official first day, I took t time to rest and relax my body as it was sore from all the walking in Vancouver. It was interesting to see so many people dressed for warmer weather who thought this would be a summer voyage, not the chillier days I knew were ahead. I slept in, went to get tea and catch up with Lourdes, checked my email, and rotated between reading on the deck, napping and eating. I went to another jewelry show which allowed me to get vouchers for each of the ports again. That evening I went to another game show in the auditorium and went to bed early. I know, I know, I was such a party girl!

July 3rd: I enjoyed my time in Ketchikan again, this time doing more walking and hiking around the town. The boat docked at 9 a.m., which gave me time to burn before many places opened. I grabbed a newspaper, hot tea and mini donuts from the store near the wharf and sat by the historic piece of art, "The Rock," along the water. I loosely followed the walking tour on the map I'd found on this overcast morning, first perusing the Soho Coho Art Gallery where I fell in love with the sarcastic and witty art of the local artist Ray Troll. I spent an hour or more just looking at the beautiful artistry of the local artists in the forms of pottery, masks, totem poles, jewelry, blankets and carvings as I went from shop to shop. I then made my way around the town around Eagle Park, Harbor View Park, and the Waterfront Promenade up to the Eagle View Area, where I saw five bald eagles all just hanging out. I felt such grace and solace in that moment, being on my solo adventure when going through the hardest thing possible in my young life.

The sun came out in the afternoon over the little village as I made my way to the Salmon Market, a large steel shed with red, white and blue stars around the name on the awning. They had the best smoked fish I would ever eat. I tried the garlic flavor atop crackers and wasn't sure if I'd like it, but feel in love instantly. I took photos of some of the neat-looking buildings like the Arctic Bar and Totem Bars, both of which looked like they'd be in the show Northern Exposure. I had fish and chips at the Fish House, along with an Alaskan Amber Ale

On the 4th of July I spent nine hours tromping around and exploring Juneau. I disembarked the ship at 7 a.m., going straight to the Tramway to take me up to Mount Roberts. I felt so free and weightless as I rode 1,800 feet up to the summit, yet sad and pensive at the same time. Grayson should have been there with me, and was not. I kept seeing places and things we would have loved to have experienced together and he was not there. I wanted to tell him about these things, and he was not there. He would never be by my side again in this earthly life. People would tell me I would see him again someday in heaven, but that, my friends, was a very long time away.

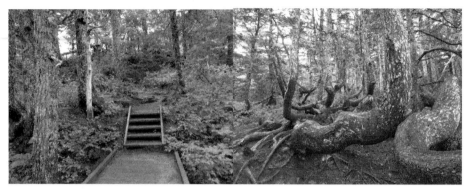
Juneau Alaska, Atop Mount Roberts

I really liked the fact that Alaskan Natives owned and operated the Tramway as well as the mountain's nature center and gift shops. I watched a really neat film at the Chilkat Theater on the history and culture of the Tlingit people, then went to watch women bead and sew in Raven Eagle Gifts. At the nature center I compared my wingspan to that of many birds, saw an eagle's nest, put my hand in the paw print of a bear, then a wolf, and made my way around the trails in the forest. I came across several Living Tree Carvings, one of a little tribal man and another of a raven that were the replicas of the ancient custom of putting one's clan crest into a tree to signify owning an area or trail. I climbed up countless flights of wooden stairs dug into the earth as I crossed over little creeks. I came across some of the most twisted trees and green plants, flora and fauna that I had ever seen in my life. I occasionally met other people on my hike, but was alone out there most of the time. I climbed until I reached the observation point where I looked out over the wharf below me and the main tourist drag.

I took a deep breath and looked at all of the blues and greens as far as the eye could see and felt like I'd been holding an empty bucket while also holding my breath. In this moment my bucket had been filled and I could breathe again. I felt close to God and to Grayson in heaven, just above me. I lifted my hand and yelled, "Hi Grayson!" as I sat down on a nearby rock to thank God for bringing me there and keeping me safe. To this day, that was the closest I've ever felt to God's actual presence, as I looked at the nearby mountains, sea and trees.

I felt great, while also so alone as a fresh widow who was forced to reboot my life like a computer that wasn't working. My life literally depended on my ability to adapt and accept things as they were to move forward. This healing journey was giving me the respite in ways that I still cannot quite articulate. When you have seen what I have, and had to do the unthinkable things I have done, and then are able to experience what I was seeing right then, there are no words.

While still on top of the mountains, I made quick calls to my parents and siblings, telling them where I was and thanking them for always supporting me. According to my parents, some close family members had a hard time understanding how I could go on such a big trip after friends had had a fundraiser for me. My parents said they told them that they had no idea what my life had been like and this was something I needed to do for myself to heal. My experience was one I wouldn't wish on my worst enemy. I was proud that by the grace of God I had been able to do everything I had done for my husband.

Back inside the main building, I had the most amazing salmon burger of my life with an Alaskan Amber Ale as I studied my Juneau brochures and looked at the bearskins and animal heads on the walls around me. For the next couple hours I was completely loopy after the one beer, I believe from the altitude. I bought a few treasures in the gift shop, then headed down on the Tramway, a bit regretful to leave the beauty I'd been in for the last few hours. I claimed my free fake pearl pendant at a jeweler, then went in search of Ammolite stud earrings, the rainbow-looking gem I'd never heard of before this trip. I spent the afternoon alternating between walking and sitting, enjoying seeing the local art in shops as well as the downtown 4th of July parade.

At the Mt. Juneau Trading Post I saw hundreds of amazing wooden carvings of Tlingit art in rich aqua, black, red, green and light blue colors that transfixed me as I looked at them and acknowledged the skill, time and effort it must have taken to create each one. I was especially taken with the canoe paddles that hung on the walls. I wished I could afford them and had a home they'd fit in. I went to the Alaskan Brewing Co. store where I bought coasters and took note of the pint glasses I'd later purchase online when I returned home. I bought a few other little items for my friends, then hit up the Taku Store near the ship launch where I purchased bottles of Alaskan fish oil vitamins, salmon jerky, Moostard's roasted garlic and blueberry mustard and Taku brown sugar and maple salmon rub. Oh yes, I was loaded up with delicacies to keep this little chicky happy for quite some time. I exited the store then took one last look around and boarded the ship.

That night I sat in the hot tub, loaded up on curry and salad then went to the auditorium where I saw a European husband and wife team that balanced, twisted and contorted in hoops and fabrics that hung from the ceiling while music filled every corner of the auditorium. I slept well that night after all of the walking I'd done.

On July 5th, my last day with a stop, I wanted to soak up as much as possible while in Skagway. I started the day with an egg, spinach and cheese sandwich and a hot tea while I sat on a park bench and watched the city wake up. I attended a play called "The Days of '98 Show" about the legendary reign of Jefferson Randolph Smith aka "Soapy Smith" who, although he'd portrayed himself as an honest philanthropist in the town, had been a conman. I bought a map and took the self-tour around town comparing the businesses of long ago to those now, and walked around the cemetery of Skagway's well-known citizens of the past. I had the best fish and chips of my life at the Skagway Brewing Company, where I enjoyed the peppered fish and local ale. I walked several miles around the small town, going back into its neighborhoods passing homes, churches and small businesses, imagining what it would be like to live there. I spent an hour in the Skagway News Depot looking at maps, books and newspapers before purchasing a few books about local history as well as some Alaskan-themed children's books. I was armed and ready to sink into Alaskan culture and history when I got home. That night I went to another one of Sam Fedele's comedy shows then watched TV, read my devotional and fell fast asleep.

I awoke after a restless sleep, rising early to see Glacier Bay as it came into view, only to find it was not viewable due to fog. After looking outside for thirty minutes and not seeing anything, I went to sleep for an hour, then woke up to see the beauty of Glacier Bay National Park. I attended an hour-long presentation by an Alaska Geographic naturalist where I learned about the native animals and climate. I was able to see and touch animal skins, fossils and other neat artifacts. After that, I spent the afternoon on one of the higher quiet decks reading and watching the beautiful scenery. I saw a giant brown bear along the far away shores as well as otters floating by on their backs. That afternoon I met and talked with the comic Sam Fedele, whose shows I'd enjoyed each week, making a friend I am still connected with online all these years later. By then I was beginning to miss my pets and the comfort of my home.

On July 7th, my last full day at sea, I spent the day bundled up outside looking at the Hubbard Glacier, taking in its beauty and thanking God for the wonderful time I'd had to rest, reboot and reflect. I packed up my clothes and treasures as I smiled at the wonders I'd seen and neat things I'd done over the past two weeks, wondering what life held for me when I returned to Minnesota. I went to say bye to Lourdes, and hugged her as she frowned and said she'd miss me so much. She took the tiny silver and faux pearl clip out of her hair and gave it to me, telling me not to forget her. I still have that clip in my jewelry box, all these years later.

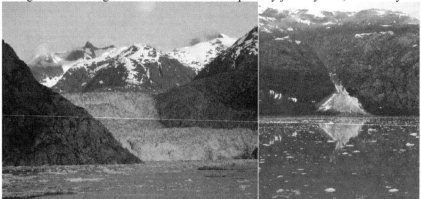

Glacier Views from the Ship

On the morning of the 8th I disembarked at 8:30 a.m. after having Nutella crepes on the outside deck one last time. I sat waiting in the grass for my friend Sylvie. I pulled up a picture of Grayson on my phone and held it up in front of me and took a photo with my camera. I wanted to remember at that moment, him in heaven and me in this heavenly place after my healing journey on the water. Sylvie and I gabbed the whole drive back to Anchorage, before she showed me around her city.

Facebook: July 8, 2013: I feel very healed due to my time in Alaska. Luckily, I still have a couple days! God's beauty in nature is very authentically, spiritually healing. You cannot help but feel like a tiny morsel in the world, amongst the gigantic mountains, ocean, seas and large mammals. I am so proud of myself that I took the leap of faith to do this big expedition by myself. Thank you so much to my family and friends that donated after Grayson's death to help me stay afloat-(literally, now) this beauty is hopefully preparing me for hard times to come, including my upcoming surgery. I have a summer planned with lovies- of music, fun, hangouts and joy. I cannot imagine how hard my life would be now, if I hadn't quickly chosen the route I did- to be happy for what I had, grateful, and carried it with me to move on to a new life. I didn't plan any of this, as you all know. I am a planner- I like to know things in advance. I had to give up so much control this year, and especially in past months. I gave my heart, soul and destiny to God and the universe, and I believe it has given me back tenfold the strength I thought I had lost 3 months ago. Thank you all for continuing to hear me, support me, and love me. R.

- You are inspiring!
- I'm so glad you did this!!

That night Sylvie, her husband Greg and I feasted on fish and chips and local beer at the Sleeping Lady Brewing Company. I ate the three pieces of beer-battered fish, one halibut, one salmon, and one cod as I filled them in on the events of my voyage as we sat outside in the warm, inviting sun. From there we went to the Marble Slab Creamery for ice cream before driving to Chugach State Park, where I was in awe at the green rolling hills and plateaus. It reminded me a little of Ireland or Scotland that I'd seen in photographs with the overcast skies above the water as far as the eye could see in the distance. We took several pictures together then went to their home where I attempted to sleep when it was stark daylight outside at 11 p.m.!

The next morning on the 9th, on my last full day in my beloved Alaska, I walked the mile and a half into town and enjoyed walking from store to store and around downtown Anchorage. I took photos of the reindeer hotdog stands, and neat oddities around the main drag, then headed to the Anchorage Museum. I spent several hours walking through awe-inspiring exhibits of Native American clothing, instruments and tools from the early 1900's that had been made with such intricate detail from every part of the animal they'd hunted. I enjoyed seeing the exhibit on the history of flight in Alaska, then headed to the planetarium to watch a film on the Northern Lights.

As I sat there watching the documentary of the hundreds of hours a Scotsman took of the night sky at the Arctic Circle, I began to cry. With tears dripping down my face while I watched the swirling colors dance across the sky, I felt like God had wrapped me in his arms and that I'd be ok. I had this epiphany as I saw this masterpiece of His work above me, that I would be okay somehow as a thirty-one year old widow. I'd been so unsure of myself, and still was, but knew in that moment, God had me cradled and that no matter what, I'd been healed on this journey in Alaska and was stronger and would be okay. I reflected on how God had carried me through the hell of Grayson's illness and death and that, yes ma'am, I, Rachel, was going to be okay.

That afternoon I met Sylvie for a delicious lunch of halibut tacos surrounded by the Alaskan art of Ray Troll that I had adored back in Ketchikan. I spent that afternoon walking around town and finishing up my shopping, before taking a longer walk home around the back of town along the water. That night we had dinner at the Glacier Brewhouse where I had my "last meal...or death row meal," as I called it, which was halibut that had been caught that day atop sautéed spinach with garlic mashed potatoes, with freshly brewed ale and their root beer. After dinner we dropped off Greg, then had girl time driving to Kincaid Park to look for moose. I was out of my mind thrilled to see a mother and baby across the road, taking photos out of Sylvie's window, thinking how cool it was to see them. As we drove farther down the road, right as we came across the bright yellow moose crossing sign on the side of the road, a mother and two babies came out of the woods and walked right in front of us. I snapped several photos with my mouth agape, hardly believing that I'd just had the Northern Exposure moment I'd been dreaming of this whole time! I read the last of my book, texted Owen to confirm my flight details and happily went to sleep.

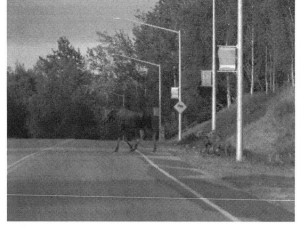

The next morning was bittersweet. I really wanted to stay in Alaska, but was also excited to get home to my animals, and back to my real life, despite the grief and loss I knew I'd have to face head on. I hugged Sylvie, dragged my heavier luggage filled with treasures into the airport and got ready to go home. On the plane I sat next to a nice older Scotsman who had just taken a cruise at the urging of his wife's Alzheimer's assisted living staff. He hadn't been able to see many animals and took photos with his camera of my photos off of my camera "to trick my lads," as we shared our life stories. He had been in the services early in his life, and took my address to send me a copy of his book. Sure enough, two months later I received "The Carin Line of Steamships and Nautical Tales Beyond Leith," by Gilbert T. Wallace that had been sent through the Royal Mail.

That evening, after Owen and I had caught up for a little bit, and I'd spent time with my animals, I went to bed and slept for the next fourteen hours.

Chapter 26:

Home Again and Buckling Up on Grief Bumper Cars

Healing Blog: July 12, 2013: Yes, yes! Serendipity has brought me courage and blessings.

Healing Blog: July 12, 2013: No Doubt's "Just a Girl," feels like my theme song right now.

Healing Blog: July 14, 2013: This weekend marks 3 months since I held Grayson as he bravely died, after being such a fighter. It feels like it's been more like 6-8 months. My healing journey helped me more than words can ever say, I am so grateful. I thought I'd be a mess for a very long time, but am moving on with gratefulness and happiness for the life of Grayson and Rachel, opening my eyes, ears and heart to the possibilities of the future. I know God has great plans for me and serendipitously some of them have already popped up in a garden of positivity I have chosen to grow and see.

- Your post is beautiful and sad. Yet hopeful and inspiring. Thinking about you and praying for more peace and joy to enter your life. We will keep kicking cancers butt together!

That week I decided it was the day to clear out my house of any negativity that was in it, feelings of death, illness or whatever, and to move forward. As I listened to Tom Petty's "Learning to Fly," with tears in my eyes, I lit the sage stick that I'd purchased in St. Cloud with Bella before my trip to Alaska, and began to go to work. I ran the sage around every doorway and window in my entire house, as I listened to Tom Petty croon about moving on and starting over. I got rid of the negativity that Victoria had brought into my home so many times, the face of illness that was in my mind when I thought of Grayson, and through a dripping nose, prayed to be as positive as possible to move forward as a young widow.

Healing Blog: July 15, 2013: A few weeks ago I belonged to 5 widow groups online, now only 2. I am past a lot of the tough things widows young and old are processing. I am amazed at where I am at, adapting to being alone, and navigating this new life. Today was very uplifted at church and feel very blessed. Quitting my job and being on hiatus has given me time to grieve, heal, breathe, read, travel, relax, learn, sleep, and spend time with my lovies- human and animal. Happy girl □. Thanks Grayson! You make me smile for the life we had and the joy I have in life now, due to it. Am going to schedule surgery this week, nervous but good thing.

~

That summer I quickly learned how fortunate I was to have had the time I did with Grayson. Through the widow groups I was a part of, I'd heard horror stories of women losing their husbands with no ability to have closure. Veterans took their lives after returning from war; one very short woman had to have her eleven-year-old son cut down her husband in their garage, after he'd found his dad hanging there. Another had her husband tell her to come lay down with him for a nap, after it was already too late -- he'd taken a handful of pills unbeknownst to her. I felt so lucky. Although it would never make sense why my husband had to die, I knew his body just couldn't go on after so many medical issues.

Facebook: July 17, 2013: Happy Girl. Also nothing like driving home on a hot summer night with the windows down and awesome tunes: Men in Hats' "Safety Dance," Foo Fighters' "Learn to Fly" and Bruce Hornsby's "The Way It Is."

Facebook: July 18, 2013: Bad endo pain today. Zero energy and pain is keeping me down and out, had to cancel friend date I was excited about.

Facebook: July 19, 2013: Please pray for me. Pain is so disabling I can barely walk. Bah!
- Prayers going up now for you
- Oh honey, hopefully it will be over soon!

Healing Blog: July 20, 2013: Can't sleep. Due to endo/migraine pain/issues as earlier described, am a little more sad than normal. It's been 3 months/13.5 weeks. Today I had to tell the Schwan's man that I couldn't afford the service anymore that Grayson had died. He was surprised and sad as they'd been chatty friends every month. My sister and her family came to visit today. I got out a My Little Pony cup for my three year old niece, and it made me sad as Grayson called me "Pony," and it dawned on me that I'd never again hear him say that, or any other word. We'd never have our Wham or New Order dance parties or fun times again. Sigh. My angel, was too awesome for this world, he burst into stars, and left us all heavy hearted in losing him.
- I'm so sorry and I know how you feel. I miss my husband so badly, our life, our inside special funny things that were ours alone. My heart hurts for you. I'm praying for you dear sweet girl.
- The whole thing sucks. I really wanted to get to know him better and talk music. I'm sorry you have had to go through this; it shouldn't have happened. We are here if you need us for anything.
- Hang in there. Let me know what you need.

Felicity, her husband and daughter came to visit for a few days. I'd been sitting on my front porch waiting for them to arrive, and as they pulled into the driveway, my sister popped out and exclaimed, "Oh my gosh! Rachel! You look like a totally different person since I was here last! You look so rested and less tired!" She told me that several times over those days. I had finally begun to rest after the twenty-seven months of cancer wife running, and I guess it was showing.

Facebook: July 21, 2013: I have been homebound since last Wednesday. I am grateful for my blessings; I have money for food, bills, and am healthy for the most part and had an amazing life with Grayson. Yet, I sit alone in this house I'd planned to have babies running around in with my husband, in so much endo pain. I will never have that. I got robbed and it just sucks. I am ok 90% of the time so far, but that other 10% is pretty hard. Hug your family tonight. I cry for my monumental loss.

- I am sorry Rachel, if there was something I could do to make all the pain go away I would.
- Oh hon I'm feeling for you right now. I wish so much that you didn't have physical pain - especially while you have emotional pain to handle. Hugs and love to you. Try to call it a day for now if you can.....
- o Rachel: Thank you both. It's so hard to be so tired, I can barely shower or get out of bed. Jenna, I know you know. If I was better physically it wouldn't be so bad.
- o Rachel: It's July 21st, I have Lollapalooza Aug 1-5, then a full week last week of August. Otherwise, chilling with friends, then big surgery in September, then will look for oncology social service work in the fall once I heal. It's managing the pain now that is hard. I see my surgeon on Tues to set date.
- I hate that life messed with you so badly.
- I am so sorry. Chronic physical pain is a monumental challenge on its own. Losing the love of your life in the prime of your life must be the worst and most difficult experience. Combining the two of them and trying to cope with both must be unbearable.
  - Rachel: Thanks. I know it could be worse. I had so many different plans.
- The pain is unreal. Vicodin doesn't work
- o Thanks. I feel so crappy... This is temporary. When pain is less, mind is better. I miss Grayson today more than I have in a while. It probably sounds awful, but it feels as if he's been gone 8+ months or more. I am surprisingly well adjusted and usually fine. Being this ill makes it all so much worse.

Healing Blog: July 22, 2013: In the midst of a breakdown due to lack of emotional control due to horrific endometriosis pain, God brought me Jenna for a late night chat. I have had pain so badly am thinking cysts are rupturing. Imagine whacking your ovaries or nuts with a hammer. It's where I am at.

- Hugs, Rachel. Why are they making you wait until September for surgery?
  - Rachel: It is my choice. Have some fun concerts and things to do first. Plus when I requested one in May, my doc wants to make sure I have enough time to process and grieve this loss too.

Healing Blog: July 26, 2013: I thank the Lord that my positivity and attitude has carried me thus far so successfully, weathering this storm.

Healing Blog: July 27, 2013: Had a bad dream about watching Grayson walk away and knowing he was going to die. Woke up with a migraine then cried for a bit about the realness of the dream. It's so surreal sometimes that my husband is gone forever.

I wanted to pick up the phone and call him at work. I wanted to hear the clinking and running noises of the machines in the background. To see his hair long on his sweaty blue shirt collar, as he'd not taken the time to go get it cut, the ink on his pants, under his fingernails and the smell of his hair and sweat, when that had normally always smelled not so fresh to me in the past.

Around this time my best friend Hazel starting calling me a "unicorn" for my uniqueness, and the way I "was handling things with grace and strength, when you could have a really crappy attitude and just be bitter all the time." She'd knitted me two rainbow scarves, gave me a unicorn Funko Pop, and sent me countless gifs and pictures of unicorn sayings and jokes, years before the unicorn boom of popularity was in full swing again.

Healing Blog: July 28, 2013: A frequent mp3 of mine: Ben Harper's "Waiting on an Angel."

Healing Blog: July 28, 2013: K. Am going to widow whine and vent. I am alone, alone, alone. Yes, I have support, but outside my house. No one is here to hug me or hold me, like now when I am crying. All I want is to be held, nothing else. I am healing emotionally and mentally yes, but am here alone, in daily chronic pain, waiting to have surgery, waiting for the day I can actually exercise, waiting for the day I am healed and can go back to work. I chose this time off which was/is one of the smartest things I have ever done, and have some fun things planned in coming weeks pre-op, but still am waiting for so many things, in pain and alone in a house and space in life that I didn't plan, and am hurt.

- Oh Rachel, I am sooo sorry. It is moments like you are having that truly suck. I have been there, just not in the same way, but I do know that you are stronger than you think. I know how it feels to feel like you are going to be crushed by the silence.
- If I could afford the gas to get there I'd show up on your doorstep right now.
    - Rachel: Hazel, that made me smile!
  o Good! And I mean it!!

Healing Blog: July 28, 2013: Feel quite shredded inside and out. Was reading old Team Grayson posts from February til recently. It's so surreal and awful. May you never know this pain til you are old and gray. I told Grayson a week or so before he died, he was my plans, my future. Little did I know, I'd soon lose him forever. Cannot stop crying

- I'm so sorry Rachel. I don't know what you are going through, but know I'm always thinking of you.
- Love and prayers for your continued healing. I know Grayson is proud of you. I have no idea what it feels like to be you--I think my worst heartbreak x infinity. It doesn't help that you feel unwell as well

- I'm so sorry, lovie
- I'm so sorry... you are always in my thoughts and prayers. Wish I was there to give you a hug!!
- Don't know what to say other than we all love you!!
- I'm glad you're able to share, Rachel. I'm sure you're getting plenty of "things will get better" etc. advice. Sometimes it's just okay to take your time & be real with what you're feeling.
- I'm so sorry sweetie. Big hugs next time I see you. Wish there was more I could do.
- My heart Loves your heart
- Thinking of you. Hugs.

Lollapalooza: The first weekend in August Owen and I went to Lollapalooza, the giant music festival held in Grant Park in downtown Chicago. I'd asked him if he wanted to go when I'd found tickets on a lark the month before, knowing it was worth ponying up the money to see New Order and the Cure that I'd been listening to since I was little, and as they were some of my joint favorites with Grayson. We drove there in my little orange Kia, listening to some of our favorite bands and talking about anything and everything. On the first night there we had dinner at an outside Greek café as we poured over the schedule for the following three days. We had to pick and choose the bands we wanted to see amongst the seven stages that continually showcased musical acts all day long. Luckily we had likes in common for most of the bands and would be together a majority of the time, so we wouldn't get lost among the thousands of attendees.

On the first day we grabbed a quick breakfast then walked through the front gates, to find that we hadn't gotten the memo that little flower child hippie attire was in. I was surrounded by young men wearing little tank tops and shorts and girls wearing cut off jean shorts -- Daisy Dukes, with tiny tops and flowers in their hair. I felt dorky in my modest but cute dresses and sneakers so my feet would survive walking and standing for days.

On the first day we saw The Neighbourhood, San Cisco, Icona Pop, Smith Westerns, Monsta, the Crystal Castles, Imagine Dragons, New Order, Hot Chip and the Killers, between walking around and checking out the massiveness of Grant Park, and finding food. We'd brought water bottles that we filled up at stations all around the festival, which was a welcome relief as it was blazing hot most of the time. I had to take painkillers most of the time, as I was in intolerable pain, which made me feel like a granny with my purse of pills, but had to do what I had to do to get through the day.

That first evening we staked our spots for New Order among the crowd, standing in the mud after a brief fifteen-minute rainfall. We'd luckily been able to hide under a nearby awning, so we were not drenched. As I stood there, off to my left on a large black metal camera crane I felt Grayson's presence, as if he were sitting up there for a front row seat. I told Owen, and he agreed that he could feel Grayson there as well.

When New Order's lead singer Bernard Sumner began to sing, I had a rush of excitement mixed with sadness. This was the band and voice I'd loved nearly my whole life, then along with Grayson and he should have been standing next to me. I danced and sang along until they started playing a few Joy Division songs, the band before New Order until the lead singer had taken his life in the early '80s.

When they played, "Ceremony," Grayson's favorite song, the one I played at his memorial service just months ago, I began to cry. Owen briefly put his arm around me, said he was sorry, then took it back and danced along, as I stood there locked with my feet in the mud below me, filled with joy at being there and despair at the loss of my husband. I danced and had a good time the rest of the concert, and looked up at the crane to my left again, quietly said bye to Grayson, before kissing his name tattooed on my wrist and walking on to the next act.

An hour later I found a dry grassy spot and enjoyed a performance by the Killers, as Owen went to see the Nine Inch Nails. I sang along to the songs I knew and felt more joy rise within me. That night I lay in my bed crying in the dark, telling Owen when he asked from his bed across the room, that I was so sad that Grayson was gone and should have been there with us. I fell asleep with wet tears stinging my face, praying that tomorrow would be better.

The next day was filled with sunshine, laughter and more familiarity as we'd gotten our bearings by then of the festival grounds. Over the course of the day we saw the Wheeler Brothers, Shovels and Rope, Cole Plante, Ben Howard, Court Yard Hounds, Local Natives, Eric Church, the National, the Lumineers and the Postal Service. We sat in shady spots as we listened to the music flow in front and around us. I delightedly danced and sang along to one of my favorite singers, Eric Church, in the blazing sunlight that afternoon while Owen opted to stand and hold his spot for the National, as he hated country music.

When we perused the artisan booths between shows, I found a really cool pair of wooden tribal-looking earrings, and thanked the young man and woman who manned the booth for DKMS Bone Marrow Matching Org. "We Delete Blood Cancer" for being there. I told them that my late husband had benefited from donated stem cells and that I knew how important their mission was, to their shock and surprise.

After sunset, we sat on the ground waiting for the Postal Service, one of my favorite bands of the last decade, to play, as we smoked the cigars I'd purchased on the way there. When the band began to play I got up and danced while Owen remained seated on the ground. Within thirty minutes it was completely dark. Tons of people in front of us had put together glow sticks that they wore and twirled in front of them, turning our experience into a colorful dance party. Owen got up and danced with me as we heard, "Such Great Heights," and I smiled to think of how Grayson had put this on a mixed tape for me so many years ago. That night we discussed the day's events over some of the salmon jerky I'd brought back from Alaska before falling asleep. No tears for me that time.

On Sunday, the last day, we walked along the trampled park to see Makeshift Prodigy, Jake Bugg, Wild Nothing, Leanne La Havas, Tegan and Sara, Grizzly Bear, Beach House and The Cure. The day was a blur as we dragged our tired bodies from stage to stage, attempting not to run into people and sitting in the grass and shade every chance we got. My thirty-one years to Owen's almost thirty-seven years were not holding up like the late teens and early twenties of most of the crowd we were amongst. I needed a lawn chair and someone to fan me with palm leaves, a real fan or I would have even taken flapping me with a magazine. I was hot, tired, and in old lady pains again with that darn endometriosis. I had fun nonetheless, and danced and sang that night in awe at seeing the Cure live, and in front of me, with Robert Smith's crazy hair and bright red lipstick like I'd seen for decades in music videos at home. It was amazing and something I'll never forget.

The next day we drove back in the rain as we talked about music, life and what my future might hold. It was so uncertain at that point.

Healing Blog: Aug. 8, 2013
Tree branches sway back and forth
Winds that have been howling quiet down
Darkness gives to light
Starting over
Sleeplessness bites like a bee sting
Calm
Quiet
Loud
Desperation
Laughter
Exhaustion
Smiles
Numbness
Memories
Uncertainty
Starting over
The tree dries out in the sun and the buds wait to grow, for the seasons to change and the cycle of life to continue
- Painful and beautiful

Healing Blog: Aug. 9, 2013: If I could fast forward time I would. Healing would be easier, the gaping obviousness that Grayson should be here and isn't in this empty house, would be less/smaller. I look forward to the day when I am healthier physically, more healed of heart and life is a little easier. I am really proud of my progress, I know I am strong, but I wouldn't wish these harsh experiences on anyone. I still have a tough road ahead, especially with the surgery, but here I am, starting over at 31.

Healing Blog: Aug. 10, 2013: Death Cab for Cutie "Transatlanticism" is on repeat for me.

CaringBridge: Aug. 11, 2013: 16 weeks/4 months today. I count every couple weeks, and find comfort in the stretches of time getting longer. Time heals. I tell people it makes 100% sense biologically why he had to die, his body gave out. It will always 0% make sense why my Grayson had to leave me, us all, in the big picture of life.

Healing Blog: Aug. 13, 2013: I feel very alone in this banana boat of mine. Only time will do the trick.

Healing Blog: Aug. 13, 2013: Alright, here goes. From the depths of my losses: 4 months ago, my future crashed, I lost my best friend, partner in crime, the funniest person I have ever known, the person that could make my face light up like a firecracker, my travel buddy, my roommate, my person who made up jokes and stories with me, about how if we were so poor and had to, we'd put hats on the cats and have them tap dance in downtown Minneapolis on Hennepin Avenue for spare change. Since then I've had to adjust in ways I never imagined. I've gotten closer and farther away to friends which I hadn't anticipated. I've gotten closer to my church, and found more love and acceptance in my heart. I had to have my cryogenic "kids" destroyed, and now I am choosing a better quality of life, so I'm having a hysterectomy. I will never count my own babies' fingers and toes, the baby that was half me, and half Grayson. I know I can still adopt or foster, but it won't be with him. I feel overwhelmed and depleted. Sigh. Thanks for listening.

- At least the surgical pain will end and in the end be "healing" pain. It may not be as bad as what you are dealing with day to day! Love you always and you were a beautiful child! You will still be a beaut without a ut! Love you!
- Love-Rachel! Inbox me your address again I can send you post cards from Africa
- Here for you.
- Hugs and prayers to you, Rachel.
- Love, hugs and many many prayers Rachel!
- Virtual hugs your way! Cuddle with those animals and take care of yourself!
- Wow, you are so brave and open. I think the openness is what makes you so beautiful! I would never be able to handle this with as much grace and dignity as you!
o Rachel: Thanks!
- Love, you know I am here if you need anything. Now I've got your number and I might be a bit of a pest-- but you can tell me to stop. I've had so much pain/sickness and it really surprised me who my friends were.
- Rachel: Thanks everyone.
- You are always in my thoughts dear Rachel. You are very brave and a true testament to strength, courage, and fortitude. I have a care package ready to send your way after your surgery.
- All my love, friend.
- I had my hysterectomy at age 28, and I can honestly say it gave me my life back. I did so much good work in the area of helping children that would have been impossible without the surgery. Now that I can't do much, I'm so grateful to be able to look back and feel I did all I could do when I could do it!

236

- Best wishes, I'll stay in touch.

Facebook: Aug. 13, 2013: God brings people into our lives. God takes people out of our lives. God puts the right people in our lives. God purposely puts us in other people's lives. Only God knows what will happen, what the plan is. Grayson always told me, God put us together. I'd like to believe this-I know I was able to be his devoted angel, as he was mine. Now this girl is chilling and waiting, to see what God has planned next.
- Love your attitude of gratitude!

Healing Blog: Aug. 14, 2013: Was in a new widow/widower insomnia sleep blog on Facebook and just had to delete it. Some gross guy was trying to find women to have sex with. Nice, take advantage of sad, sleepless widows. Ick!
- Rachel: Eww. Creepy guy just applied to be my friend!
- Gross.
- Tell him off!
- Block him
- Creepy

Healing Blog: Aug. 17, 2013: Had some odd and not so great things happen this week, however the weekend has been much sunnier. Was able to spend time Friday with Jenna, Mike and Wyatt. Today had fun with Gus at a beer fest, dinner at Sawatdee (his first Thai experience!). Tomorrow: church, then Gasthof's fundraiser: catching up with good friends and TNT peeps. Am blessed.

On Sunday, August 18th, Gasthof zur Gemutlichkeit's German restaurant allowed me to have a fundraiser to benefit the Leukemia and Lymphoma Society in honor of Grayson. It was great to have so many friends and TNT colleagues join me at the white and red checkered tablecloths for German food and beer, bidding on items at the silent auction and just spending time together. The accordion player came around and asked for requests. My friend Sandy for whatever reason told him that it would be my wedding anniversary in two days, when he asked if we were there for an occasion. He played until I awkwardly told him to leave, as it was making me sad and in fact my husband had recently died. Owen and I exchanged awkward looks and laughed silently, thank God or I would have cried at how ridiculous and badly timed this was!

Facebook: Aug. 19, 2013: Big blessed week ahead of me! Tomorrow am staining my wooden dining room table and doing weeks of laundry. Tuesday would have been my 9th wedding anniversary- so girlfriend's dinner out. Wednesday Charlie Mars in concert, Thursday and Friday-catch-up dinners with friends and a weekend trip to the MN Zoo.

CaringBridge/Facebook: Aug. 20, 2013: Today would have been our 9th Wedding Anniversary. We got married on Friday, August 20th, 2004 on a sticky day in the Wabasha Street Caves. It was wonderful and fun. I was really looking forward to the fact that we were getting closer to 10 years, a full decade. Keep Grayson and me in your thoughts and prayers today...certainly a shorter marriage and lifetime together than we had planned.

Facebook: Aug. 20, 2013: Thanks to Cassie, Jenna, Sarah and Kaylee for meeting me in Edina for dinner at Big Bowl. Great food, drinks, friends and laughs. Got a cupcake on the way home. I was dreading today ....it was an excellent day. Never thought I'd feel this single and independent and mentally okay this soon. Am blessed!

I used to count the years until our 25th, when I'd be 47 and he'd be 53, and our 50th, when I'd be 72 and he'd be 78. After this year there was no need to count anymore. Grayson had wanted to renew our vows on one of the old riverboats along downtown St. Paul, with just family and friends for our 10th anniversary in 2014. That was out of the question now.

Facebook: Aug. 21, 2013: Fun evening planned in Minneapolis at Saint Anthony Main: Pracna, Astor Cafe and a Charlie Mars concert. Hanging out with Owen in the waterfront neighborhood in the heat.

Healing Blog: Aug. 22, 2013: As I lay here in the dark in pain, am thinking about how ridiculous social media is, but am very happy it connects me with support, laughter, and all of you.

Healing Blog: Aug. 22, 2013: Am awake way too early, exhausted, tired and in a lot of endo pain. 2 weeks from today I have my surgery. It's going to be 90+ degrees for the next week. God Save the Queen.

Healing Blog: Aug. 22, 2013: Just did major sorting of Grayson stuff in the finished part of my basement, albeit my pain and allergy migraine. Found some funny things, annoyances at the mail from many years that he never opened but filed, and old photos including funny ones of old girlfriends. Found comical stuff, like the pink clear, naked lady razor I bought him as a gag gift when we got married, his old photography magazines and mixed CDs we'd made. Tons to donate and throw out. Thank God I am organized, and have a great friend like Owen who helps me lug it all upstairs and out to the bins.

Healing Blog: Aug. 23, 2013: Greatly appreciate it when people keep up with me on here. Most days am a hermit in pain at home. So it means a lot to be able to just blog, or nearly "tweet" about my day. I feel less alone, and am very, very alone right now.

Healing Blog: Aug. 24, 2013: In so much pain, scary amount, is disabling me to the point where I cannot drive, canceling plans, cannot do desired projects I want. Here's the kicker: Precious Greta just pawed my back to get my attention while I was on the couch on the phone, my back to her. Now I have 3, 6 inch long painful scrapes down my shoulder/back. Also Rufus is being naughty. Hope you don't see me on the 6pm local news.

Facebook: Aug. 24, 2013: Today I spent time with Owen, and My Little Pony playing with little girls which is quite healing! Got out of the house for the first time in days, despite pain and spent a couple refreshing hours with these beauties, oh and their dad.

Healing Blog: Aug. 25, 2013: Here I go. Hardest year of my life, hurdles still to jump, but I have ~Strength~Faith~Courage~ to carry me through. Once you have held your life and heart in your arms as they breathe their last breath, there isn't much you cannot do.

Healing Blog: Aug. 25, 2013: I cannot wait till I am healthy again. It's been a long time. We take so much for granted. Lately, most days I am in so much endo pain I cannot go to the store, have to cancel plans with friends, cannot even lift my cat, somedays cannot get out of bed hardly, walking can be painful. In less than 2 weeks I will have major surgery, and see it as a light at the end of the tunnel. I thank those of you who read this and listen, those who have reached out to me, who have been unwavering in your support. I have a tough road ahead of me, am glad I am doing this, but feel scared, alone and need lots of support, as I will be in a lot of pain and stuck in the house, into this fall. Love, R.

Healing Blog: Aug. 26, 2013: My 13 year old cat Rufus always seems to make things better. I've waited his whole life for him to be affectionate. Finally he is. Grayson are you seeing this?!

Healing Blog: Aug. 27, 2013: Am in mondo pain today- not looking forward to 100 degrees at the MN State Fair, but bought tickets back in March for Grayson, Owen and I to go see our beloved Depeche Mode. Sandy, Owen and I are braving the heat, and will triumph.

I had a great time with my friends at the Depeche Mode concert. As I sat there in the crowd of thousands I had this odd feeling that in that same crowd was the man that someday I would date and maybe even marry. I cannot explain it, but I felt it. I just felt a presence there; that somehow, someway, he- the next Mr. Rachel, was there. I let it go after a couple minutes of feeling it quite strongly.

Facebook: Aug. 28, 2013: Good evening at State Fair last night. Woke up to allergy migraine. Minnesota, how I Love/Hate you! Bah humbug.

Healing Blog: Aug. 29, 2013: Fatigue has been kicking my butt lately, have napped a lot. Just bathed a Greta, Puddin' and Rufus. I have to keep trucking. Thank you Lord for strength.

Healing Blog: Aug. 29, 2013: Life has thrown me curves, twists, mazes, fireballs and much heartache this year. Soon I face another huge bridge to cross, this time without Grayson by my side. It's still odd he is gone forever. Despite it all, and my fragility at times, I am amazed by my strength and resilience, ability to laugh, and desire to be there for others. I owe a lot of this strength of course to God, but also to several great eggs in my life- you know who you are, Thank You

- o You are so amazing and I am glad we re-connected.
- o I hope you like em' hard boiled.

Healing Blog: Aug. 31, 2013: Strength is not something that comes easy. It's acquired mostly unfortunately when you've gone through things like I have. So many things have happened that I've gotten through with God's grace and my resiliency, but I may need reminders with everything coming up. I wish Grayson was here to hold my hand. My upcoming surgery has a lengthy 3-6 week recovery time, and I am scared as hell, alone, sad and depressed right now. The strength I've gained over the past couple years is still here somewhere, but I need it now more than ever, I feel needy asking for help, but I need all of you now more than ever.

- • I agree 100% about how one acquires strength. And my goodness, yes, you were with a loving partner for so many years it is natural to feel vulnerable at times I think. Being alone and ill sometimes makes me feel empowered and sometimes scares the Hell out of me
- o Rachel: Thanks. Asking for help doesn't always come easy for me.
- • It is hard for pretty much everyone (as you know from SW jobs), but you did it! Proud of you
- • NEVER, EVER feel needy, Rachel. Needy is freaking out and wanting sympathy over a broken nail. You have a broken heart and some breaking parts of your body... asking for help is survival, girl!!!!
- • I know I hadn't seen you for a few, but I bet NO ONE in your close friends or family think you're needy. So keep reaching out.
- o Rachel: Everyone, all of your words of encouragement are a pain relief in themselves thanks!
- • Thinking of you, Rachel, with prayers and hugs.
- • I have so much empathy it hurts! Please know your fear of the pain is probably harder than the pain will be! I have found this to be true of my sister & I and several of our cousins as well. When you have it, you just get through it and there will be better days.
- • I don't know much about that level of pain, Rachel. All I know is that you clearly have lots and lots of people who love and care! And there's always more Holy Land take-out where the last came from.
- • I'm so glad you share and tell us how you feel. I don't have the words to express how much I care & am concerned... I love you girl

Chapter 27:
Fall Brings Challenges and New Triumphs

Facebook: Sept. 3, 2013: Listening on repeat to Eric Church's, "Like Jesus Does."

Facebook: Sept. 3, 2013: Ray LaMontagne, "Empty."

I had my hysterectomy on September 5th. I'd been prepped by being part of a Facebook hysterectomy group where I asked questions, and I'd purchased some self-care items online. When I tried to find things out myself online, I found disgusting and scary photos of uteruses on surgical tables, all bloody and gory which made me almost puke, so I opted to seek support from those who had had the actual procedure themselves. From "HysterSisters" I purchased bathing wipes, no-rinse liquid shampoo (dry shampoo hadn't come on the market yet), and a reacher-grabber stick that proved to be handy when I needed it.

I had needed my parents to come take care of me, and had opted to have my dad come first because he would be more objective, when my mom would have been a little too gooey. My dad took me to the hospital bright and early. I sat so nervously in the car, feeling as if I'd throw up. I absolutely could not believe Grayson was not there with me. I woke up in the recovery bay and kept telling the nurses in my doped-out delirious state that my husband was dead and this was such a big deal that he wasn't there to support me. I'm sure they thought I was insane and/or felt really bad for me.

I napped most of the day in my hospital room, waking up less in surgery site pain, but more in the shoulders as the anesthesia wore off. My dad left by lunchtime when he knew I would be okay. By mid-afternoon I was trying to figure out how to navigate my phone when I could barely move, so I could call Owen and ask him to come visit.

We'd had a really big fight the week before and I stormed out of his house, then called him later and reamed him out for the things he'd said that I didn't want to hear. I had convinced myself in my state of loss, despair and impending life-changing surgery that I liked him a lot and that he should date me. I was lonely and somehow my mind had convinced me that he was it, that I loved him, even when I in-fact actually did not. I called him, asking him to come visit, and he was there within less than an hour. We apologized as we both cried, held hands and said I love you to each other. This was not romantic love, but friendship and I've-got-your-back-through-it-all love. Later Sandy came to visit and sat with me until I fell asleep.

Over the next two weeks I rotated between my bed and couch, with the help of my dad. I could not get down off the bed or up from the couch without help. I could not bend my body or I would be in diabolical pain. I had my Fallopian tubes, uterus and one ovary taken out, with the other ovary left in, so I would not hit menopause at age 31. If I had taken it all out I wouldn't have been able to take any sort of hormone for six months, and didn't want to do that as many hormones have bad, sometimes fatal side effects.

Dad and I binge watched a lot of Chuck, and Big Bang Theory, as I ate a lot of Jell-O and fish sticks. Sandy came over and brought the most amazing macaroni and cheese with pretzels on top that made me so happy despite my pain. I found and enjoyed Michelle L. Whitlock's book, "How I Lost My Uterus and Found My Voice," that gave me peace and calm during yet another major life change in which I did not know many other young women who had had a hysterectomy. I later connected with her on Facebook and am friends with her to this day.

One night, a young man in a depression group that I was a part of on Facebook posted, "I cannot do this anymore, I am done. Goodbye Forever." I knew as a mental health professional that meant he was planning on taking his own life. It was 12 a.m. my time, and 6 a.m. to him in England. I spent twenty minutes frantically trying to reach this nineteen-year-old kid via Facebook Messenger to no avail, then bought an international calling card, as I didn't have international coverage on my cell plan. I called the number on his public profile page, but that didn't work either. Finally, by 2 a.m. here and 8 a.m. there, we were chatting online, while I had the Fray's song "How to Save a Life," circling my head nonstop.

At the same time I tracked down a couple of his close friends I had found from tagged photos and posts, looping them in on the situation. By 4 a.m. here and 10 a.m. in the UK an intervention had been set up, unbeknownst to the young man. He told me, "Guess what, my mates are having a gathering today and invited me!" I told him that was great, that I knew he had support and went to sleep. The following night he messaged me, angry and swearing that his friends had had an intervention, along with his family and I'd ruined his suicide plans, then he blocked me. I smiled and knew I had done what was right.

During my recovery my dad told me that he'd received a letter from Victoria with a copy of the police report from the "incident" that never happened. He said "She said in this letter that you were behaving unlike yourself. Per the report it is clear you didn't even do anything, I think her sending this to me was her trying to get to you through me, that your mother and I would get upset and love you less or something. I think it was her way of trying to dig the knife in one last time." That, my friends, is the last time I ever heard from Victoria!

Two weeks after my surgery my mom came to switch shifts with my dad. By that point, I wanted her mom-esque baking, care and babying me, when I still felt like crap but was a little stronger. I took walks around the yard at the initial instruction by my dad, even though it hurt and was uncomfortable. Gus, Sandy, Pam, Hazel, Vera and my former coworker Charlie all came to visit me, which was wonderful. It was a hell of a journey, but my quality of life depended on it, and I had no idea how happy I'd be for years to come when I'd pass the tampon aisle at Target and keep on walking.

Healing Blog: Sept. 30, 2013:

~Paths~

Life offers us many paths

Some are simple choices

Some are challenging

Some surprise us

Some hurt us

Some inspire us

Some enliven us

Some beat us down

Some are stormy

Some are sunny

..It's the attitude and willingness to know that God knows what the next path will be, and to trust that tomorrow can only get easier than today~

Healing Blog: Sept. 20, 2013: Tomorrow would have been 12 years with Grayson. As I struggle in limbo of sadness and moving on, recently prickled more by thorns than roses, I count my blessings, and know I am an amazing person and shall wait for the days of more sun and less clouds in my mind and heart.

Healing Blog: Oct. 1, 2013: I find myself in the juxtaposition of being in limbo of uncertainty, and feeling lost, but also comfortable in the insanity of not knowing. You go to college, meet someone, graduate, get married, have jobs, life goes on…then that someone suddenly is gone, (albeit years of illness). The layers of strength I have acquired over the last couple years and recent months are like a backpack, always with me…sometimes loaded with books, heavy and tough to carry, other times, light and airy…comfort in knowing the strength is packed inside, has been utilized and can grow when necessary. Ultimately am proud of myself a thousand times over for what I have done for love, others and for myself. I believe my unfortunate happenstances have prepared me to live more serendipitously in the present, and given me a gift that only someone who has been through hell and back can fathom. I wear my thoughts, heart and mind on my sleeves...which no doubt can cause me to get hurt at times, but am oh so happy to have evolved so much, especially in the past few months, to be unapologetically me, Rachel.

- You should be a writer. Love your words.
    - o   Thanks, if I could get paid for it I would. I have actually written a lot in my short life.

Healing Blog: Oct. 13, 2013: Today I got the invite from the University of Minnesota's Bequest Program, inviting me to the program where they honor those who have donated their bodies. It's November 19th and the TNT honoree dinner for the 25th Anniversary is the next day. I had no idea the U would contact me so quickly. I don't think I can do both days of this as it will be so hard mentally to wrap my mind around. I want to keep moving forward, I gave him an amazing service in May and am getting worn out by making hard decisions.

- • You know what you can do. For what it is worth, I think you are right.
- • Sounds like you've made a good decision.
- • Sounds like a good decision. Only you understand your situation.
- • Any decision you make is the right one.
- o Rachel: Thanks! Life/this year keeps getting harder!!!!! I will need an armor suit soon.

Healing Blog: Oct. 27, 2013: You all know my story and what I've been through. I'm officially posting that I've begun dating someone. I'm choosing to have some happiness within this storm and am choosing to laugh, smile, giggle and know no one can/should judge me…although I wish I could take away the suffering, pain, death.....God has a plan for us all...mine is to share my story, life, love and keep trucking.........and I keep on smiling.

- • There is no shame in finding love and lightness after such a dark period. Your experience enriches your spirit and I am truly in awe of your strength and perseverance. No one will truly understand your struggles, and, therefore, no one has the right to judge your steps forward. Be proud of yourself and continue doing what makes you happy. Thank you for sharing your story. You are such an inspiration.
- • Love you!
- • You're an incredibly strong woman, Rachel.
- • Girl, i am so happy for you! This made me tear up!
- o Rachel: Thanks, that was really difficult, but releasing to write.
- • I bet. You are amazing. I hate what you've been through, but I admire you so much for the way you process everything, your outlook, honesty, and feisty-ness!!! You deserve every happiness in the world! Xo
- • Beautiful.
- • Love you Rach, so glad you're giggling again finally. It's ok to move on and live life again. In fact it's wonderful. I'm excited to meet the man who made you giggle and smile again!
- • You have such a wonderful, strong, loving soul.

I had no idea how to share the news that I'd begun to date Gus, the big, kind guy I met through Team in Training. We'd had a nice time at the beer festival during the summer and he came to visit me post-surgery, and we'd texted from time to time, just as friends. He was funny and that is what I needed at the time. I later came to know that he was just the lidocaine to my situation, numbing my pain and distracting me from the awfulness of grief and loss. That fall we did fun things together like attend a U Gopher football game, then a birthday dinner with friends that I'd organized for him. We saw Chris Cornell in concert in St. Paul, which was wonderful, and we participated in 5K races around the Cities. He endured a lot of my tears and not knowing what to do with this ever-changing emotional widow. I give him a lot of credit for the months we dated.

Healing Blog: Oct. 30, 2013: Very tough time this week, lots of grief and tears...prayers please...this ebbs and flows and is the latter right now. I thank God for my strength and many blessings.

- Poor Rachel!
  - Rachel: Am ok, got a lot of good people in my corner! The first of each, bday, holidays is supposed to be the toughest....
- Prayers. And I can't wait to give you a hug on Saturday!!

Healing Blog: Oct. 31, 2013: Today is Halloween, it would have been Grayson's 38th Birthday, let's have a moment of silence and celebrate the amazing, funny, witty, caring man and human being that he was....thank you Grayson for a wonderful, yet short life with you, your love, courage and strength has left me a thoughtful and happy girl, despite the pain we endured the last few years together. Blessings of happiness flow from me in new relationships due to the power of the challenges we faced and the strength and positive outlook I have, that is allowing me to move forward and on.

Healing Blog: November 2, 2013: Please pray for me. Tomorrow is All Saints Day at church...they ring a bell for everyone who died this year...I cannot stop crying right now.

- Love to you babygirl!
- Praying for you
- Love to you, baby girl.

Healing Blog: Nov. 3, 2013: I want to fly away like a bird....dreaming of getting on a plane and exploring the world.

Healing Blog: Nov. 3, 2013. I belong to a young widows group online here on Facebook....I rarely check it, as the women are stuck in the loss process, (albeit everyone has their own journey) and/or so sad, crying every day etc. As a mental health professional I know I've been grieving quicker than the average gal- it will be hard for a long time, but I chose to be happy for what I had.....so many women in this group have had such tragedies...a child setting their house on fire with spouse and pets dying inside, many, many stories of suicide, some done in front of spouse, etc. I feel blessed to be able to comment on their posts saying "it does get better, or easier" because it does...the sadness of the tragic illness and loss lingers, but the sunshine of the past that made you who you are, allows the rays of light to reach far from your soul, outward into new life, new relationships and to have renewed strength.

Healing Blog: Nov. 4, 2013: I was just listening to my beloved Bruce Springsteen, and a fave of mine, "Secret Garden," which made me start crying. It discusses being able to forget and remember at the same time. I think that rings true to me as I have come a million miles, I've been fragile like glass, and also under several suits of armor... I have come so far, but am so pessimistic of this world. I have my strength, faith and at times courage, but feel quite tiny and beaten down by my own personal warfare....each day is easier, each month is tenfold better, but it's the journey that hurts. I have a great support system, and blessed family and friends, but it's so hard to be on this journey; so alone, because I am the only one that has lived it every day. Thanks for listening, R.

Healing Blog: Nov. 4, 2013: Decided not to go to church today (haven't been in a few months due to health, so felt bad anyway) but had so much anxiety about hearing yet again, in another way that Grayson is dead. Am working really hard at moving on, being comfortably okay, a little numb, and happy....I feel these things make it tougher...still have a few financial business matters to take his name off of, it is evident he is gone, and I am moving on, but these blatant recognitions of his passing (albeit in an honorary way) throw me back down the rabbit hole. - R.

My good friends Vera and Kent got married that week. I took a girlfriend with me as my date, and had Sandy with me as well, as she was friends with the couple, and had been invited, too. They literally had to hold me up, sitting on either side of me during the ceremony. Bless those angels for holding my hands and keeping me upright, when I was falling apart. I was so happy for my friends, but so sad that my person, my silly weirdo that I had so many inside jokes with and such a connection, as Vera and Kent did, was gone. It was such a difficult experience to be a part of, and words cannot articulate the amount of strength it took to get through it. I was salt without my pepper, ketchup without my mustard, and peanut butter without my jelly.

Healing Blog: Nov. 13, 2013: It's been nearly 7 months since Grayson died. I just emailed Grayson's primary doctor and P.A. of his entire illness, attaching a couple pics from Alaska. I updated them and thanking them for giving me the 2.5 years with Grayson I might have not had, if not for their amazing expertise and care. I think it's important to let them know positivity can come out of something terrible, especially when they were the providers.

In mid-November my best friend Sandy got engaged. It was a very exciting time, and I offered to host an engagement party at my house for her and her wonderful fiancé Jesse. I decorated the house and had thirty people over that I'd never met. They laughed, ate and celebrated my friend's exciting news and major life event. As excited as I was for her, I felt so numbed to it all as well.

Healing Blog: Nov. 19, 2013: Tomorrow is the honoree dinner for the Leukemia and Lymphoma Society's Team in Training, 25th Anniversary. I am quite dreading the emotional flow that I know will erupt. Of the 25 honorees, 24 are alive, mine is not. Sandy is coming with me, thank God. Please pray for me as this is another event in which although I am greatly honored to represent Grayson, (as was he to even be considered an honored teammate), it is another evident, face slapping, Grayson is dead event/occurrence. Thank you to my TNT peeps for every step, swim stroke, bike pedal you take.....I will be doing the Seattle half marathon for TNT next year. And Gus, thanks for sticking with me, especially for your TNT dedication and listening to me when I am in low places about this life and circumstances of mine.

Healing Blog: Nov. 19, 2013.
Each day even if my body hasn't gained full strength,
I am grateful for my inner strength.
The things I've done
Things I've seen
Things I've been through, can cause tears when I think about them, at the drop of a hat.
But they are over and in the past...
I have had huge, gigantic, life altering mental, emotional and physical changes in the past seven months.
I Thank God for listening, and never leaving my side.
This strength is earned through faith and trust, and am a living testament that without it, I would have withered long ago.
Instead I am here, living on, each day new, adventures, even if tiny in the big picture, to be had.

- Love you, girl!!!
- Your articulation of your heart, mind, and situation amaze me.

I'd begun to count the months from Grayson's passing, getting excited as more time passed. It made it less fresh, more doable and added more tools to my survival tool belt. Each month on the 21st I was glad to count the months out from GDD-Grayson's Death Date, which I did for the first few years. It meant I was surviving and getting through it all.

Healing Blog: Nov. 28, 2013: Am very sad and upset. Please pray for me, am heartbroken.

Healing Blog: Nov. 28, 2013:
Kindness is earned.
Thankfulness is a given.
Politeness should be necessary.
Love is earned,
Trust is earned.
Faith is inherent,
But kindness is the building block of a nice, great human experience.

For Thanksgiving that year I organized a "Misfits Thanksgiving," which was wonderful. I had a Facebook event invite to anyone that wanted to come to lunch at Buca de Beppo in downtown Minneapolis. With several friends, some bringing their baby, we shared giant bowls of pasta, veggies, salad, and bread, while creating our own family and own tradition that year. It felt amazing to be with those who would have been alone otherwise. God always has a master plan!

Healing Blog: Nov. 28, 2013: I just woke up after a 2.5 hour nap that followed an hour of crying after I attempted to watch the Wizard of Oz. Ideally I'd like to be a hermit or squirrel away from the world, to unplug and hide, but I need support. I had no idea what this holiday season would bring…but I'm finding it's like losing a limb, in this instance a leg. I have phantom pains that come in the form of memories, or flashes of illness. At times I have pinches of pain like that from an artificial leg at times, and other times I am right as rain, walking around with no issues. I fought the war and am proud of what I did, but those memories sure pinch and cause pain at times. Despite the good things in my life, specifically great friendships and relationships of late, the awful war weighs me down this holiday season, and only time can help heal these battle scars.

Healing Blog: Nov. 29, 2013: I stayed up late, not able to sleep, finally went to bed around 4 a.m.- Rufus and Greta both interrupted my sleep at points. I had to put one downstairs and the other in a crate to get some rest. I woke up to find Puddin' had peed all over the couch to my dismay. I cleaned it up, then watched a cheesy Christmas movie as I ate my Buca leftovers and decorated only a tiny tree and put up baby stockings for the animals and I. I spent last Christmas season running back and forth to the cancer unit at the hospital, decorating and trying to normalize Grayson's room for the holiday, as best as I could. This year is anew, great losses and lots of mental pain, but new relationships, strengthened ones and a new future full of different adventures ahead of me. Now just to get through this holiday season without too many breakdowns like last night, please.

The Holidays: Whether your spouse/significant other is ill or has passed, it's important to seek out support over the holiday season. You will need this more than you know.
- Plan to have a meal or coffee with friends or family.
- Don't be shy at this point. It's important to seek out support, let people know you will be stuck in the hospital with your loved one, or alone. They will want to help you and take care of you! You most likely will reciprocate with those close to you at some future point as well.
- Plan a movie marathon or Christmas themed get-together, whatever makes you happy.
  o It is okay to find joy in the small things, even when you're feeling down.
  o Figure out how to take care of yourself, treat yourself, and do it.

- Look at your circumstance as a time to start something new, adapt and use what strengths you have, try not to focus on what it should be. It's not easy to do that, but if you can find positives within the voids, the sunlight can peek through the clouds at times.

Chapter 28:
Frosty Days and Frozen Nights

Healing Blog: Dec. 1, 2013

Silence is the bitterness that calls the beast,
Silence can also be the solace that protects the bird with broken wings, giving it time to heal.
Either way, silence can be stretched long and wide,
Leaving one feeling so isolated, alone and numb inside.
I cannot wait for the solace and silence of my beloved snow to fall, it provides beauty, wonder and calmness for me, and it helps make sense of the world, time, the greater purpose of it all.
This pending and already begun holiday season has begun to rip the wings of this bird,
The newness, the silence and the numbness, doesn't provide solace at all, it beats the drum of the weight of this year, the loss, the pain, the aching tiredness of my exhaustion inside and out….without ever even speaking a word aloud.

Healing Blog: Dec. 2, 2013: These past few days have been rough. However now it is snowing big, fat, fluffy flakes. Snow always makes me happy/content/renewed in spirit. It snowed on April 22nd of this year, the day after Grayson died. I believed it was just for me. This snow falling now gives me hope and adds a touch of positivity to my weary soul.

Healing Blog: Dec. 9 2013: I have had difficulty becoming motivated to exercise, be healthy and fit. I have 20 endometriosis lbs. that came quickly last year, 10 lbs. at a time in a matter if days, 2 times, add to that caregiver stress then loss and horrible reproductive health issues=lethargic me. I've begun to juice and eat better but needed a kick in the butt. I'm going to start working on my health, so here I go!

Healing Blog: Dec. 9, 2013: So I sleep ALL the time...I told someone the other day I have a PhD in sleeping. I know it's due to inner sadness even if I don't always acknowledge it, as sometimes I do feel super sad and awful lately, sans normal   holidayness/familyness. I am looking forward to and have been connecting with friends. I need a ton of support right now, am feeling a bit lost. If you are in town this week, and can come to my Holiday Sangria Party on the 15th.... I need you and would love to see you!

Healing Blog: Dec. 10, 2013: I looked at some pictures of Grayson today on the Team Grayson page on here. I am so tired from months of crying, I don't even have the tears to shed for the numbness and sadness I feel within. Ironically writing this makes me cry.

Healing Blog Post: Dec. 10, 2013:

The Hounds of Winter

Whistle and howl as this Minnesota winter whips winds and snow around my house.

I sleep most of the time, snuggled in pjs, warm blankets.

Take care of animals

Watch TV and movies

A few days a week I hangout with friends and my guy

Most of the time, I am exhausted, bottomed out from the collective fires, hurricanes and storms of this year.

I ran back to back marathons and endurance events…now this "cheery" time of year I am quite numb, depleted and tucked in from the

Hounds of Winter and everything that swirls around my head.

Healing Blog: Dec. 11, 2013: Cleaning office and in a drawer I found a baby tape recorder....on the 10 minute clip, Grayson states it's 2 weeks before Christmas 2001 (we'd been dating 2.5 months). Amazing timing and a blessing to hear our young 19 & 26 year old voices.

Healing Blog: Dec. 12, 2013: I am having a really tough time, breaking down and crying a minimum of 3-4 times a day now. Please pray for me, and keep checking on me via Facebook or text, I don't answer phone much, but text. And Gus, thank you for being an amazing boyfriend and friend understanding I am happy with you, but am also processing and crying a lot too, your ability to always make me laugh is wonderful.

Healing Blog: Dec. 14, 2013: I am looking forward to a New Year, new beginnings, new adventures. None of it compares to the hollowness I feel, despite the kind words my supporters give me. I am so tired and the collective amount of losses and trials I've been through has made me more tired than I ever thought possible. I am tired of hearing platitudes, albeit I know people are trying to help. This lady at church kept telling me she was a widow, she knew what I was going through. Turns out her husband volunteers and plays golf so much, she feels "like a widow." That is not the sme. Face palm. Please keep up with me, I feel like a wounded bird. Sad, sad girl, Rachel.

- You might be burnt toast and a wounded bird right now, (and all those other things you list) but don't ever forget you're my unicorn too. Love you Rachel!!!!

- Hang on, honey. As I told you Friday, personal experience has shown me that it does get less hard. Hang on to those of us who love you. Surround yourself with those of us who know what it is like to have been in your place right now. I know it is hard to be strong, but you are strong, even though you may not feel it right now.

December 15th ended up being a terrible, let me repeat that, terrible day. Grayson's cat Puddin' had been peeing on everything for the past week because as it turned out, he had diabetes. I looked at my little black fluff ball that I loved so much as he was squeaking in the downstairs basement bathroom where I'd confined him to- when he lost control of his bowels, and knew I couldn't let him live that way any longer. He was thirteen, had lived a good life, and there was no way I could afford the $400/3 months of insulin.

I took my little buddy into the vet two hours before I was to meet my new boyfriend's parents for the first time at lunch. It was awful. I paid the $280, kissed and hugged my beloved cat, then cried in my car as tears and snot ran down my face. I called Felicity and told her I'd had to put my cat down, just like I did to my husband months earlier, as crude as that sounds. My sister replied, "But, Rachel, you gave Grayson his cat back!" I laughed through tears, then called my friend Vera while I waited in the restaurant.

We had a nice meal at a Mexican restaurant, where I was able to keep it together. After lunch I raced home to get ready for the Christmas party I was hosting that night, only to find out that Gus and I both had food poisoning. I cancelled the party and was sick for the next several hours. Worst day ever for sure.

Healing Blog: Dec. 21, 2013: Rachel update: I have horrific head and eye pain, yes have had many losses, but want to reflect on my Blessings! I have amazing friends, family afar (that I of course wish was closer), and a kind boyfriend who doesn't run away from my widow grief. I hold steadfast to my faith and the strength I have hidden in pockets of my soul, that continues to allow me to make it through each day, when the going is rough and tough, like right this second.

Healing Blog Post: Dec. 23, 2013:
Weakness
Numbness
Sadness
Loneliness
Strength
Courage
Faith
Patience
Trust
Fatigue
Depression
Emptiness
I feel like a ravaged, wounded little baby bird, no words can comfort, only time can do the trick.

For Christmas that year, I invited myself to Gus's family's cabin ninety minutes away for their family Christmas. He didn't mind and was surprised that I didn't want to be with my own family. I couldn't afford airfare to see anyone, and they all had their own plans, which was okay with me.

It was a fine time, as his parents were kind, especially his dad. His mom didn't seem to "get," me but that didn't bother me. His sister was mean as a snake, but I already knew that because she and Gus lived together, as he rented the bottom floor of her condo.

We went out to cut down a Christmas tree on Christmas Eve which seemed odd to me as it was a lot of work to decorate a tree for just one day, but I did enjoy cutting down the tree and playing in the snow. That night we had appetizers for dinner, and no one liked the broccoli salad I'd made except Gus and I. We played a trivia game then ended the night, not watching a Christmas movie like I'd hoped, but the new Smurfs movie. After twenty minutes of the loud cartoon voices I retired to the small twin bed in the guest room I was staying in, where I cried so hard for nearly an hour, that I blew big snot bubbles into the shirt I was wearing, as I had no tissues and I didn't want his family to know I'd been crying. The next morning they opened presents, his mom exclaiming, "Ooh, I hate fish!" to the fancy canned garlic salmon from Alaska in the gift basket I'd made his parents, then had lunch with more extended family that came for the day. Gus was very kind and understanding of my grief and crying, but I just felt out of place and wished I'd been with family and of course, Grayson, instead.

Later that evening I drove over to see Wyatt after I got home. We sat in his living room and cried for an hour, me over the loss of my husband, and him over the loss of his dad the year before. It was a holly and jolly old time for sure.

Healing Blog: Dec. 29, 2013:
Super sad
Nothing can rectify this pain in my heart
Haunting memories in my head
Moving through
Moving on
Still applying for jobs:
7 months with lack of routine
8 months as a widow now
But 12 months since I knew life would be different
Strength in my Faith
Trust in my Lord
Supported by my loved ones
But alone in this journey
The things I have done, things I have seen, things I think about as I cry myself to sleep....
I usually am 85-90% okay...
But it can change so much day to day

Pride I have in everything I've done...giving Grayson an amazing life, taking control of my health-making another huge life changing decision and having surgery (now pain free!), working on moving on and finding joy and new adventures with friends and a new man (creating new fun memories for us both)

Still these cold wintery days can bring a chill to my heart...

But overall am so proud of how far I have come...

This New Year as a different person with different roles scares me right now...

But my Faith and inner strength has not led me astray yet.

I wouldn't have been able to get this far without the fight of a tiger inside me....

I was terrified to move into a new year without Grayson. I physically felt sick and panicked from December 28th on. I felt if I moved into the new year, I was leaving him behind. I just couldn't leave him in the dust and move forward. For the first time since 2001 when I was nineteen, the calendar would turn and Grayson would not be there. It was terrifying.

I did make it through okay. Early on the morning of January 1, 2014, Gus and I walked the Polar Dash 5K in negative one degrees then came home and vegged out on the couch, eating and watching movies all day.

Healing Blog: Jan. 7, 2014: I am so Angry!!!! In efforts to keep my computer up to speed, I am going through files to make sure I am saving all my treasured pictures. There are so many beautiful happy and healthy photos, but also so many of him sick and so ill. I am so angry I've been robbed of my certainty, my life, my best friend, everything I knew for the last 11.5 years...my entire adult life so far. I sit here so mad and devastated with tears running all over me and this desk. Only those who have walked in similar shoes understand, and I pray cancer can end one day. Time heals, but cannot take away the PTSD of the war that was fought and the demons of suffering that linger.

Healing Blog: Jan. 14, 2014: A new year has left many negative feelings of heartache and despair that I hope to replace with positivity and moving forward with good health. I've been a grieving couch potato, but now plan to continue to track my food intake and have signed up for several 5Ks and another half marathon through the LLS TNT program. I'm going to Portland for a week to visit friends and I hope that helps even more. My aunt told me that I get a dog year for every year Grayson was sick, so I am really 46, not 31. I do feel like I know things only older adults know with all I've been through. Each day is a gift, we are in charge of our own choices, behaviors, words and destiny...with a major gentle hand of the Lord.

- You are one of the most amazing women I've ever met. You are creative, talented, compassionate, beautiful and full of love and life. You are doing great! You will keep doing great! It's a pleasure and a privilege to be counted as your friend.

The first week in January I had a job interview at the U's public health clinic to be a mental health worker consultant with clients who came in for medical wellness checks. I had great rapport with the gentleman that interviewed me, and thought I had a good chance of getting the job. He said he needed to call my references, then he'd get back to me. The day before I was to leave for Portland I got a call from the interviewer. My last employer said they had a lot of problems with me, and I was told would not be getting the job. I called my former boss and left a voicemail asking what I'd done to receive this kind of negative review. I had done many extra things in that role, such as pointing out when the client forms were low and needed to be ordered, and updated my managers when my clients had extreme paranoia and said things that were not true.

As I gathered my belongings to get off the flight when I landed in Portland, Oregon, I turned on my phone and received a nasty little voicemail from my former boss. She went on and on about how I'd used the wrong forms, and had upset clients. It was amazing how this same woman who came to my husband's memorial service and said how valuable and missed I was, and when I quit, told me that I could always come back to my job, now was rattling on about how horrible I was. I sucked it up, moved on and went to find my friend Hudson.

I spent a week in Portland, one of my favorite cities. I'd been there many times, as Felicity had lived there years ago, and my sister-esque friend Poppy currently lived there. I stayed with Hudson in his small apartment. I spent my days wandering the city as he worked. He is a very talented, earthy and kind furniture maker and designer whom I met when he lived in Minneapolis the decade before. He, Sandy, Sage, Grayson and I used to hang out, Grayson was the guest star as he worked nights. Hudson and I had gotten to be great friends over the years.

I spent hours walking around the town, enjoying Powell's Books, the farmer's market and small shops, all in the balmy thirty-degree weather, compared to the negative twenty-four degrees I'd left at home. We met up with my buddy Zeke, who had been great friends with Grayson for years as well, and went on a mead tour. I enjoyed the crisp honey fermented alcoholic beverage made by a local business, and had great Chinese food. I spent a few days with Poppy, her kids and husband at their home, playing games and eating the chocolate cake she always made from scratch each time I visited. It was a great and refreshing trip that was well needed to feel more connected to those lovies I hadn't seen in such a long time, who had also been so close to Grayson as well.

Healing Blog: Jan. 19, 2014: I am disheartened at the last two jobs that I had, both in mental health over the last five years. I loved working in mental health, but think the politics of those I worked with combined with the burnout of the role, has led me to do something else. I've recently interviewed with a nanny agency, just like I did in my early twenties, and am waiting to be connected to a family. I want to do cancer volunteer work, and in time get back into social services, but Rachel 2.0 needs to nurture her soul and being. I am working on creating the life I want!!!

Healing Blog: Jan. 21, 2014: Today is a tough day.....1 year ago Grayson was admitted to the hospital.....last night a year ago was the last night we were in our home together. He never came home...we left with hopes he'd be cured and our cancer nightmares were over...but also today is the 9 month anniversary of his death.

That weekend I went to the annual wedding fair with Sandy, which was a double edged sword. It was fun to be there with her because she was getting married and starting a new life with the man she loved, but it also hurt because my husband was dead. We had a great time snagging freebies, downing chocolates and treats, and taking photos of ourselves in boas and tiaras, but most of the time I was hiding the fact that it was so painful for me. All around me were shiny-eyed, bride-to-be women, with their engagement rings and lives ahead of them with their grooms-to-be, and my husband was gone, gone, gone. I didn't ever let Sandy know how sad I felt. I pushed it down and put on a smiling face because I was her maid of honor.

When we got back to my house that day she told me in a well-intended way (I believe to her), that I needed to work on being happier and moving on. She said it was time for me to get a full time job and to work on being more cheery, as she knew I could be. I bit my tongue and thanked her for a great day, then went inside.

Healing Blog: Jan. 26, 2014: I am awake, after crying in bed intermittently for the last hour and a half, haunted by images of Grayson at his best, but worst most of the time. Our song, "The Luckiest," plays in my head as I see the crinkle in the corner of his eyes, the way he'd laugh and look at me, us getting each other 100% in person or across the room. Then I see him with sunken puppy dog eyes, on oxygen and infant like. I have feelings of terror and guilt. How frightened he must have felt, how alone, how helpless. I sit here bawling... I know I did the best I could and gave him a good life, yet I am haunted by it all. How am I only 31 and starting my life over again? My ability to trust God has never wavered, not once, but my ability to plan anything is gone. Things I've seen and done during the illness hit my mind when I least expect it. I've lost so much control over things, like I am in the ocean without a boat. Writing it out is helpful...so thanks for listening...

- I'm sorry Rachel
- We'll always be here to listen.

Healing Blog: Jan. 28, 2014: I just got home from my first yoga class that I started from a Groupon deal. Some poses were really painful with my endo pain but I worked through it the best I could. I am tired of crying, lately am on a rollercoaster ride of tears. Some days like

257

today I cannot believe that my best friend is actually dead and never coming back...I am up-then down -then up.

Healing Blog: Feb. 1, 2014: This endless up and down of grief is quite the learning experience. I decided to get my certification in Grief Counseling just for kicks, as I was going through it all anyway. Today I got my first textbook in the mail, "Death, Dying and Mourning," and also bought "Transform Your Loss," for casual reading. I'm hoping to heal myself while I help others!

Facebook: Feb. 2, 2014: I feel extremely proud to be training among the other TNT warriors that are raising money to fight blood cancer. I didn't plan to write this and am now crying. I'm cleaning out the office and making myself toss out unneeded things. I have hung on to Grayson's Van's skater kicks, and have decided to throw them out. He will never be back to wear them. Last week I tossed a pair of his jeans I kept in our dresser. Switching gears-to have my best friend of 12 years Sandy, join me for trainings, as well as Gus who is in TNT again this year feels amazing. We are all working to make sure there are less losses and more life. From the bottom of my heart, Thank You.

Facebook: Feb. 4, 2014: Depression is the beast that bites my back. It zaps my energy, will or motivation to do anything. I nap a lot. I watch a lot of "Cheers," while I pack items to ship as I've started selling so many things on eBay and Amazon to make extra money. It is a lot of work, and turns out people do want your random stuff. I've turned my basement into an organized system of books, clothing, shoes, purses, trinkets and other items that I don't need or won't use. It's been a painful process at times, but I'm forcing myself to do it. I'm planning on having a "Hipster Estate" sale when the snow melts. Each day is a gift, a blessing, one day farther away from my sad past....but depression is still the beast that sometimes bares its teeth and bites this widow's back.

- Ten months isn't very long. Give it time. I think you are on the right track. Grief is hard work.

Facebook: Feb. 6, 2014: I just had a panic attack and am writing to detox. I was just sobbing and sucking in air. I got a cheap Groupon deal to make photo books, and as I was making them of Grayson, my family and I, I looked around the office and had an existential moment of "Holy crap, Grayson will never use this office that he loved, and the computer that he built ever again." I made myself look at photos of him his last months and weeks to show me that yes, he is forever gone. It is hard for me to believe how emotional I get, with so many ups and downs. I never know when I will get bit in the butt with the grief bug. Someone close to me actually said recently, "Set a timeline of when you want to be done with grief, then figure out how to be done feeling this way, get past it and move forward." That is one of the dumbest things I have ever heard. I know their intentions were for me to feel better- but that was not my reality. Grief is something no one asks for, can plan for, or can stop. I have a nanny gig set up, am feeling healthier and moving forward but this really smarts right now.

I nannied for a sweet little baby girl named Emerson for two weeks. She was only six months old and was either napping, crying or eating, or for a small amount of the time, playing. Her caregiver grandparents were on vacation, her dad worked at home and her mom worked in an office. I took her for walks in her stroller, bundling us both up to brave the temps outside. I sang to her and tried not to be too sick from the Fresca and Lean Cuisines that I ate too many of at that time that sent me to the bathroom way too often, I think from their "diet food" ingredients. During the day I'd take care of her, and a couple nights a week I'd meet up with friends or Gus for dinner, tea, or to try out a local brewery. Things were good for the most part and I felt really blessed. I was able to get out and do a "SoleMate" race with Gus for Valentine's Day the weekend before. I started the day crying hysterically at how I thought Grayson would have liked Gus, then ended up much calmer after the race, having reached my personal record race-wise. The ride never stopped.

Facebook: Feb. 11, 2014: Grief is a spontaneous beast. I am in the process of my body adjusting to a medication change, so I have stomach cramps and nausea. The mailman just came, leaving photo books that I ordered online for my family. They are of Grayson's cancer journey, beginning to end, with a small retrospective of good health at the end. The pain I feel in my mind, heart and body at every memory of holding his hand during countless painful bone marrow biopsies, leaving him there alone, sad and lonely each night to go home, and hours by his bedside in stages of wellness, illness and scary ICU times, and waiting for miracles, is terrible. It doesn't matter how successful I am at being positive and moving on…these memories burn in my mind like fresh flames, just when I think they are embers.

- Embers rekindle. Try not to allow them to become forest fires! Hang tough - tomorrow is a new day…your innate optimism will serve you well. You remain in my thoughts and prayers.
- Such a looooong journey! But, that's life. Take your time, develop new routines, just continue to be YOU, and it will get easier with time. My mom passed 12 yrs ago and it gets better.

Facebook: Feb. 15, 2014: I have had a hellacious week. My health hasn't been great. My furnace broke on a Thursday, and I could not get it replaced until Monday, which meant I was freezing in twenty degree weather outside, aside from the two small space heaters the power company brought me. I wore three pairs of clothing as I snuggled in tight with Greta and Rufus, watching movies and drinking hot tea. The new furnace costs $4000. Thank God after Grayson died I sprung for the appliance replacement plan, which will help with $1300 of the cost. What more can happen I ask?!?! I keep walking and training nonetheless for my friends going through cancer treatment, and Connor, you are a beacon of hope, young man in that you finished the ALL clinical trial that Grayson could not! My song of the moment is Pearl Jam's

"Elderly Woman Behind the Counter in A Small Town," as I walk, train and freeze my butt off. Widow Rachel-over and out.

Facebook: Feb. 21, 2014

When the book falls off the table in a quiet room, and leaves a loud "thud"…

When the glass of water tips and liquid spills everywhere and a mess is made…

When the power goes out, and despite knowing this, you still flick the light switch, you instinctively must try...

These occurrences of unstoppable force yet simple occurrences are like the tears that just spontaneously came to my eyes as I wept and shrieked in the pain of actualization, once again, that my best friend Grayson is gone....forever.

- Hang on to everyone that loves you, you have so many of us.

Facebook: Feb. 24, 2014: Early Morning Confessions of A Widow with No Uterus, Awake Too Early In Pain:

o The worst thing that can happen in life (aside from losing a child) has already happened, I can only go up from here.

o My level of inner strength can rival that of a caveman, UFC boxer or the meanest person in the world.

o Despite not being able to have a baby, it is pretty exciting to not have to buy feminine products ever again.

o I will need quite a savings to adopt- I've looked into it, it's quite costly, (minimum $20K)

o It is no longer awkward to tell someone I am a widow, but it shocks them all the time.

o By the time it is the one year anniversary of Grayson's death, I will have dated Gus for 6 months, not kosher to many people, but I'm happy and Grayson would be for me too.

o I consistently surprise myself with my ability to laugh at the little things, even on the days I want to hide in a ball. My ability to write, express myself and get it out to breathe and move on- is wonderful.

o I still cannot believe I stood in the mud at Lollapalooza and saw New Order sing live.

o I haven't had red meat in 15 years, 10 years veggie and am dating a meaty, bearded hunter.

o Yes, I am still waiting on a permanent nanny gig.

o My best friend Wyatt is in a wheelchair and it ticks me off that I cannot get him into my car and just zoom off somewhere whenever we feel like it. Society is so obtuse about the normalcy of disability in everyday life for so many people.

o I love naps! I always have and it used to drive Grayson nuts, but he'd laugh.

- I hate it when I burn through a TV series on Netflix, Hulu or DVDs and you're left feeling like your friends have gone away.
- I really want to live in the middle of nowhere in a Podunk town with goats, llamas and chickens (not to eat!), to hear the crickets, watch the sunrise, the dew evaporate and sit on the porch with a cup of tea.
- I loathe how social service workers get paid crap, and have thousands upon thousands to pay in student loans until we're in retirement.
- I am nearly 32 and sleep with a purple stuffed unicorn my boyfriend gave me for Valentine's Day.
- Despite making a photo book yesterday that took hours, I rarely look at photos of Grayson as they make me feel like crap.
- God is the #1 thing that is keeping me going, has kept me going, and my ultimate anchor in life. My Faith has not wavered once in these hellacious years. I have several atheist friends and would never try to change them.
- I have no idea what my future holds, I have lost my ability to plan beyond family gatherings, running races, TNT practices, and recognizing the vital people and things in my life.
- I hate cancer more than anything in the world (next to intolerance) and want to dedicate my life to helping people through it, past it, etc.
- Each day is a gift. Not enough people know it until it is too late...tell people you love them, what they mean to you, etc., cliché as it is, before it is too late. We don't always get a do-over, we could be hit by a bus any day, anytime.
- I get goosebumps from Billy Currington's "God is Great, Beer is Good, and People are Crazy" song...sounds silly, but it is a profound song, Google the video.
- I love Eric Church, Bruce Springsteen (Gus doesn't...The Boss is my boyfriend!!) most sitcoms and John Hughes movies so much.
- I could drink Coke and eat mac and cheese and green beans every day.
- TNT has been a life raft for me. I can be really hard on myself about being unfit and unhealthy, but I adore that TNT has people of all different experiences, shapes and sizes.
- I think we don't take enough time to be truly kind to ourselves....I have worked well on that, in acceptance of myself, where I am in life, and going at the right pace for me, Not anyone else. Grief is a butt-kicker that takes time.
- It's hard to believe I went to Alaska solo for 2.5 weeks last summer.....beautiful, healing, amazing...I want to go back...have never been to Florida, Mexico, Hawaii, any islands, and would choose Alaska or the mountains anytime.
- Despite my tears and sad desperate words on here at times, I Am Okay! (And told people shortly after Grayson died that I would be). A great love that I had, to be loved

like that, to love and fight for/with someone only makes you stronger for another love and new adventures.

o   I have very painful pelvic pain from heavy shoveling and TNT walking, but I am Rachel 2.0, hear me roar, here I stand, every day a gift, another day I   survive.

Chapter 29:
Ashes to Spread

F acebook: Feb. 26, 2014

I am not always sad

I am not always cheery

I am not unapproachable

I am not scary

I am not defined by widow

I am funny

I do cry randomly

I do laugh ALL the time

I am bitter at times of my hard life vs. the norm of marriage and kids all around me

I am super strong

I can be super weak

I don't ask for help well

I do think I expect too much of others, and other times not enough

I know that life is changing, revolving, and cyclical

I know things will get better

I know things ARE better, so much has happened

I am proud of my experiences

I am proud of always being authentic and blunt-even though it can get me into   trouble

sometimes

I am busy every day in my own ways

I am moving on

I am doing ok

I am RACHEL

- Word. I love you!
- You rock!

Facebook: Feb. 26, 2014: I feel blessed, I feel grateful. Despite where I am at and where I thought I would be, I am here, doing okay, laughing at the little things, and working on being a healthier me.

My husband was returned to me in a box on my porch one sunny winter day. I signed for the heavy brown wrapped package that contained a black plastic box with "Cremated Remains for Everett Grayson Thomas," on a white sticker. Inside was a large plastic bag full of ashes and teeny bone fragments that was simply tied with a white twisty tie. I stared at it for at least fifteen minutes, then opened the bag and felt the sandy ashes with my fingers, touching the remnants of what used to be my husband. I had the U send half of the ashes to Victoria, so he could be buried next to his dad as he had requested. I really did think that Victoria would send me some sort of thank you note, but that alas did not happen.

I called Owen, telling him that I'd received the ashes and wanted to go on an adventure around the Twin Cities to spread Grayson's remains in places he had loved, and we'd loved together. I bagged up Grayson's ashes by spooning a few table spoons into little snack baggies that would be scattered at each location. When I did this I looked at the ashes, saw the teeny little white chunks of bone and ran my fingers through it. I was not grossed out or horrified like I thought I would be. I grabbed a glass of water, then took a pencil eraser-size amount of ashes and ate them, then washed it down with water. I guess I thought I was reconnecting with Grayson one last time. I still had a gritty taste in my mouth so I chugged a little Coke, then kept on bagging.

Owen and I met at a pub, which was awkward at first, as it was the first time we'd seen each other in months. We had another blow up in the fall, after I again tried to convince him to like me, when I was so deep in my grief and not seeing clearly. I knew in a way he did. We both had admitted we liked each other in the past, but had moved on, although we both knew and had each said more than once, that it would have been easier to be together than to date other people, but it just wasn't right. As much as I adored him, he wasn't "it" for me and he "couldn't mack on Grayson's wife," as he'd said.

We hadn't talked much from October until that February, when I threw in the towel. I missed him too much, missed my best friend and didn't feel that way about him anymore. We'd been chatting a lot on the phone, but this was the first time in person. Over fish and chips and beer at Kieran's Irish Pub in Minneapolis, we talked about Grayson and how odd it was that it'd almost been a year since we lost him.

After lunch we scattered ashes first in front of the First Avenue music venue, Grayson's favorite place to see live music. We took photos everywhere we went, and at this stop I cracked up so hard, because I ran past a policeman, initially not noticing him, as I took the bag of ashes out of my pocket in front of the famous Minneapolis stomping grounds. It was illegal to scatter ashes, and it was kind of a funny thing we were doing. Next we went to our old apartment in St. Paul, where I scattered around the house, then sat on the front porch for a photo. I had to run to scatter them in front of the Wabasha Street Caves, as staff was sitting in their offices and looking out the windows as I dropped them, then ran back to Owen, who was driving the getaway vehicle. I scattered them on top of the brick in front of the garden with our names on it, and lastly around the front and back gardens of my house. We took photos of

Owen and me together, smiling and laughing as newer best friends, who were honoring and missing our dearly departed best friend.

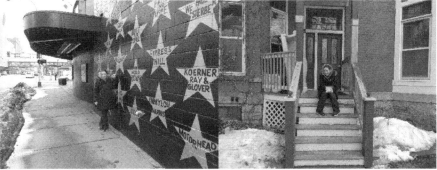

Spreading Grayson's Ashes

In my mission to raise funds for the Leukemia and Lymphoma Society's Team in Training while I was prepping for another half marathon, I somehow became a broken record of negativity, despite my heart's intent to help others. I had written the "ask" letter and sent it out to supporters, but hadn't received many donations, which was understandable because so many people had donated to my first marathon, during Grayson's illness and to me after he died. I was asking for a lot, and in my grief I couldn't see clearly, I was more focused on wanting people to donate to LLS so they wouldn't have to be like me, and less on the positive things like LLS's advancements in treatment drugs and research or increases in survival rates. I actually had this pointed out to me, when I expressed my frustration at not getting many donations. I was so zeroed in on losing Grayson, I was like a carriage horse with side blinders, not able to see the good that was still coming from cancer research and beyond.

I learned that I was living my own internal battle of what was and what is and what will never be. It was like starting college over again at eighteen. I was as in the dark about where to go from there, as I'd been as a ten-year-old who used "Teen Spirit" deodorant on the outside of my t-shirt, to the shock and chagrin of my mother, when I didn't know how to properly apply it. I knew that somehow I had to suck it up. It was up to me to channel my own positivity, to turn this boat out of the harbor and to move it forward into the ocean of my life. I didn't have an example of what to do; I was alone in that. I had to create and stake my own path, and that is what I decided to do.

Facebook: Mar. 27, 2014: I am tired of crying, I am tired of living two lives…the one where I am ok, have a cool house, pets, friends, family, amazing boyfriend…and the one where I fall apart at the drop of a hat…where I feel lost and so alone...like I am friggin' Tom Hanks in "Castaway." I know grief takes a loooong time, but I am tired of being tired and feeling shredded, despite how good the other me can be/feel sometimes.

- You don't have two lives; it is all authentic. And not many people can be that way; it takes a lot of grace and maturity. Keep it up, you're bound to have a lot of ups and downs. Keep reaching out, we all Love you and admire you. Wish I could take the pain away, tho!

Healing Blog: Mar. 30, 2014: I just watched the 1.5 minute video of Grayson I have, I found the night before he died that he made on the iPad in the fall of 2011. He has hair coming back and a teeny beard of red hair. At the end of it, he says, "I love you." What a gift.

- Oh honey, this is so hard. It is the time of year

- I'm glad you made this group thing, I'm glad you have a place to let all this out without worrying about what people will think.
- You're so right, none of this is fair. You're so amazing to be as far as you've come but I still can't imagine how hard it is.
- We're all here for you.
- *Hugs*

During this time I had three short-term nanny jobs. I got gigs on Care.com- the website that I'd successfully used in the past. I was hired by a fiancée of a father, to take care of two little girls full time. They needed a caregiver when she and the father worked; the girls had been taken away from their mother by Child Protective Services. I was hired to work forty hours a week, and after only two days, was called to say that the mom got the kids back and that I was out of a job, to my shock. Thank God I brought my My Little Ponies back with me and didn't leave them there at the little girls' request!

I babysat twins for a day while their mom ran errands, missing my friend Mike's funeral, as he, too, succumbed to cancer after his eleven-year fight. I found out after the fact, and was just a mess that I missed it, and could not support my friend Jenna.

For three weeks I worked for two wonderful women to watch their nephew who was visiting. Lisa and Lisa were a wonderful couple to work for, and are still my friends, to this day.

I answered a guy's ad on Craigslist and helped sort hundreds of stuffed animals and vintage toys in his office in the basement of a law office, and listed some vintage baseball gloves on eBay. I did that for a week and never got paid, despite my attempts to collect for my troubles. It was terrible.

Facebook: Apr. 4, 2014: I am in bed, sobbing and wailing at the loss of Grayson. The loss of security. I look at the photos of us in the office, the only ones I have up, as it makes me so sad. We were so in love, alive and happy. Lately I feel like I'm a piece of paper that has gone through the shredder. I have terrible emotional pain, and physical as I have gut rot again and puked, so I had to skip TNT. This upheaval of loss is killing me. I have been through too much to filter my mouth, I am honest and raw. I have lost 75% of my support in the past 6 months. My family is amazing, but far away. I need people to send me kind texts, messages, cards frequently please. I am not doing so good. I never imagined I would feel so much grief and sadness now more than I did a year ago. I was like a mechanical robot during the last month pre and post death. I'm so lonely and never thought I'd be here.

Ok, it was flat-out embarrassing at first to seek out support. I didn't want anyone to feel sorry for me, but knew I had to ask if it wasn't coming to me. All of the support I'd had when my husband was alive and right after he died had gone away. I know this happened for several reasons. People went back to their normal lives and families when the formal crisis was over.

No one knows how to navigate times like these. I was learning more and more every day in my grief courses, how loss could be so hard for someone to grasp, if they themselves, had never been through it.

I had a very kind friend from TNT come over and take me for a walk. Yes, she took me for a walk, with my dog, but like a dog. Not her words, but mine. She had to coax me out of the house; I was so sad and could barely get off the couch. She encouraged me to keep reaching out to those who cared about me. They wanted to help, but many did not know how. Some of my closest friends now are ones that weren't always there for me during all of this, as a few didn't know what to do. They later told me they didn't know what to do, so they gave me space. I wish I'd asked them directly for what I needed, but alas, it all is a learning process.

~

Self-care When You Need It Most: Do things that make you happy, give yourself space and a place to get out of your head. You need this sometimes more than you know.

- Read a book
- Watch a movie or binge a TV series.
- Exercise- get the feel good vibes flowing!
- Seek God or your spiritual higher power, ask for help and guidance.
- Scream and yell, then go for a walk or take a nap or meditate.
- Know that each day is a gift no matter how scary or unfair the outcome is. You keep waking up every day-which means you are a survivor!
- Take up a new hobby. Join an exercise class, paint, make pottery,
- Check out MeetUp.com groups online. They have tons of options to choose from. Single people meet up in groups to share their common interests.
- Do a jigsaw puzzle. I started doing these the last year or so and have no idea why I didn't start earlier. They work my mind and make me so happy.
- Do a word search, crossword, or Sudoku. Work that mind!
- Volunteer. Helping others creates endorphins and gives to those in need at the same time.
- Change up your appearance if you're up for it. Cut or dye your hair, or shop for some new clothes. You don't have to spend a lot if you don't have the means, garage sale or thrift shop (two of my favorite things!)
- Rachel Do's: The first two years as a widow, I re-watched shows that made me laugh again. It was healing to heartily laugh and feel whole from my head to my toes. I watched Cheers, Frasier, Roseanne, The Office, Friends, Everybody Loves Raymond (I could not watch that when Grayson was alive as Marie reminded me a bit of Victoria!)
o I know it is cliché, but laughter is so very healing and smiling feels so good. Laughing alone is such a fun victory. I'd sit on the floor and package up items to ship all over the country and world, and just watch and laugh.

~

Asking for Support: This was very hard for me to do. I had to suck it up, bite the bullet, whatever you want to call it. I was alone and flat-out asked for help. So many widows or widowers have children. They need even more help! It is OKAY to ask for help -- it means you're human!

- When you're down and need help, it is not the time to be humble or hide.
- It's okay to need help, everyone does from time to time.
- Ask to be invited over for dinner- it's ok, not rude!
- Ask for cards to be sent in the mail.
- Ask someone to meet you for walks around the neighborhood.
- Ask for someone to run to the grocery store or pharmacy if you cannot.
- This is all interim, it won't last forever and you'll most likely reciprocate in the future.
- Look for support groups, self-help books, online forums or Facebook groups. So many people are going through so many things similar to what you are, even though you feel like you're alone in this. You are not! Seek support, and you'll more than likely find more than you ever thought possible.

It was around this time that I found my little red and golden Sarah McLachlan "Afterglow" journal that I'd written some wise notes in, back in 2012 during and after the silent retreats I'd been on. I reflected on the need to practice what I'd preached or written down in this case:

- ❖ God help me to understand those family members and friends in my life, and what my part in working on/repairing relationships is.
- ❖ Please help me to continue to reflect and connect through my imperfections, to see what is important.
- ❖ Thank you for the serendipitous learning experience of being a cancer spouse and what is really important in life.
- ❖ Strength comes from God, but forgiveness comes from a power, greater than our willpower.
- ❖ Be honest, own what you need to work on, and work through.
- ❖ You can be bitter or better, always choose better in the end.
- ❖ There will be stumbling stones. We all stumble, get up and learn. It reminds you that you're human.
- ❖ There can be moments of grace in letting things go.
- ❖ We all have to know that we need to do what we have to do, in order to move on.
- ❖ There are some things in life that there is no way out of. It may not be in God's will to fix what you want to be fixed or the problem to be solved. It's how we choose to deal with what happens that makes us strong.
- ❖ We are so hard on ourselves most of the time. If you arrive late, so what. It's how you connect when you get there.

Facebook: Apr. 11, 2014: My neighbor whose name was also Grayson, my friend Mike and a cousin all died, within a few weeks. I feel unbelievably strong, but am having a hard time not scooping up my 35 yr. old friend Jenna that is now a widow. We both recognize the support is great now, but it will simmer down as time goes by. She is in the eye of the hurricane and has to wait for the storm to pass. My heart hurts so much for her. I just went and brought her some tea and her 5 year old son suckers, then hugged them and left. Until you've clung to the ditch during a tornado, you can never truly know this pain. But then again, sometimes the calm presence of just being accepted and heard is all that is needed, when one is on the raging waters in a boat at sea alone.

- You're amazing, kiddo

I held a TNT fundraiser with donated coffee and bagels from a local business, in honor of Grayson. Although I had ten friends come over, I was so upset that more did not. I felt like I'd been so wronged and asked the Lord why more people didn't come, didn't care. My blinders were up again and no one could take them off for me, or help me see that at the time.

Facebook: Apr.14, 2014: Am tired of friends that say they want to be there and aren't. Sunday was a really important event and friends of decades did not show up, many said they'd try to make it. It is just weird, having to be okay…dropping people. New people are great, but such resentment and bitterness spews forth a bit- due to these life lessons, changes.

- Rachel: I got used to the friendship and support of people, now they are turning like wild dogs it feels like…..

~

Anniversaries: It's very important to mark the anniversaries and milestones that you had with your late spouse/significant other.
- Get together with friends or family, get out of the house and go do something fun.
- Make your own annual tradition that can replace whatever you did when your loved one was alive, or adapt what you did with them, and make it new and yours.
- Have a party or celebrate the occasion with friends or family, honoring your dearly departed.
- Even if you just have a movie marathon and cry, ask a friend to be with you. Please, don't go through it alone.
- And if you're like me and someone of faith, ask for prayers during this time.

My sisters Felicity and Diana came to visit, along with Felicity's four-year-old daughter, Ione. We went to El Loro for lunch with Gus, watched movies at night and just spent time together. I had a 32nd birthday party, on my actual birthday, the day before Easter that year. I had done a big Facebook event invite and nearly forty people came over the course of my five-hour gathering. We laughed, hugged, listened to music and talked about life, and Grayson, as the one-year anniversary of his death was coming up in two days.

271

It felt great to have my sisters there, along with many other good friends that had become my family over the years. On Easter Sunday Gus came over to celebrate with us, which was a bit awkward as we planted an urn in my front yard with Grayson's ashes in it that would spring up into a tree in the coming years. (I later accidentally mowed over that dang area and the tree never grew!) After an hour or so he left, and I spent the next few hours crying.

Facebook: Apr. 20, 2014: I would give anything to talk to Grayson again. To hear his voice, have him call me Rachie or Pony. I called his cell phone and someone picked up, they'd given his number to someone else. I feel like I am successfully moving on, yet emotionally bleeding daily. All my plans have gone away and I've left here wondering where it all went wrong. Today I feel bitter and broken.

- I wish I had something helpful to say or do. I can only thank you for reaching out, telling your trusted ones what is on your mind. I Love you so much and I wish I could take the last 4 years away.
- Oh Kiddo....

Facebook: Apr. 20, 2014: Heartbroken to the core in a way I cannot even explain. I feel gutted and shredded.

- So sorry dear
o Rachel: Thanks. My sister and niece are here, but I feel so alone, so terrible, so very very alone.
- Call me.
- I'm so sorry Rachel... I wish I could say or do something to make you feel better. But know that so many people are thinking of you and sending comforting thoughts your way.
- So sorry. I hope the pain lessens. Lmk if I can help.
- This is probably the roughest time you'll have, you are strong, you are my unicorn. You will make it through.
- Hang in there, Sweets.

Facebook: Apr. 21, 2014: One Year Anniversary of Grayson's Death: I am so sad, heartbroken, pissed, bitter.

o Big, ginormous, huge, loving hugs to you today!!!thinking of you and praying

My little niece asked her mom a few times, "Is Aunt Rachel crying because Uncle Grayson is dead?" which made me cry even harder, bless her little heart. My sisters took turns rubbing my back and talking to me as I cried late at night and the next day. On the 21st, we went to the Minnesota Zoo for a fun field trip, enjoying the baby animals at the farm exhibit and the wild animals throughout the park. I don't know what I would have done without my sisters there. Every year I try to do something fun on that day.

272

Chapter 31:

A Brighter Outlook is Upon the Horizon

I spent the spring and summer of 2014 figuring out who I was as a widow and single woman while learning about grief and loss and attempting to move on.

Every Thursday through Sunday from late April to mid-June I held garage sales which were fun, tiring and a lot of work. I asked for donated items from friends online and received several to add to my "garage store." I spent hours pricing items and setting them up on tables around the garage and into the adjacent three-season porch. I arranged things to look nicely, had a huge bookshelf full of books, and racks of clothing. I also had items listed on the "Offer Up' app, which brought people outside of my neighborhood to the sales, signs and via Craigslist advertisements.

I sat in the chilly winds that later turned into blistering heat, from 8 a.m. to 4 p.m. four days in a row each week. When I obtained a job in June, I ran the sales from 8 a.m. to 3p.m. on Saturdays and Sundays. I learned a lot about people as I sat and listened to the radio while I studied hour after hour for my grief counseling certification. People felt free to step on things; bring their dogs; fart, then walk away; and come and go without saying a word or even a thank you.

One older gentleman who lived in the neighborhood came by a few times. Somehow we got to talking about cars and he said he had purchased the car that the Spice Girls had used in the British MTV Awards in the late '90s. He left, then came back in that actual old timey slate gray car with glitter sparkles, with a photo of the band in it during the show. I sat in it and had my photo taken. He printed it, then brought it back later for me to keep. It was funny and delightful and I couldn't believe the things God brought into my life at random. I still worked really hard at my Amazon and eBay sales, shipping items Victoria had given us that we'd never used, or Grayson's synthesizers and music or computer items I'd never utilize. I even shipped some of his techno records from his old DJ days to people as far as Germany, Russia and Prague. I was doing what I had to do to hustle and make a living in this house bought for two, but lived in by only one.

I broke up with Gus in May. I realized how much I really didn't get along with him, how immature he was and how we weren't right for each other. I called him and asked him if he'd ever love me, as I delusionly in my grief thought I loved him. Three days prior we'd gone to cheer for the Minneapolis Marathon for TNT, but it had been cancelled due to thunderstorms, so we went to Perkins for breakfast instead. When I ordered my food I said I didn't want the side of meat, as I did not eat pork, and I'd apparently offended Gus. He said, "My other girlfriends have always offered me their bacon or sausage if they didn't want it." So a week later when I called him frustrated and not sure what was going on with us, he told me he'd never love me for reasons including the fact that I didn't offer him the breakfast meat, and I didn't freeze any eggs before having my hysterectomy. Yes, that is correct. It all came down to bacon and eggs.

When Gus and I broke up, I sent a group Facebook message the next day to my best friend Sandy, along with a few other of my friends asking them to "unfriend" him as we were no longer together. They all did immediately, except Sandy. She sent me an individual message telling me what I did was not okay that "I have to go back to work, but we are not done talking about this, we will finish this later."

In that moment, I made another big life decision. Sandy had been saying things that in a small way, had contributed to the feelings I was having of despair for months, telling me to be happy and move on, belittling my decisions and just being a bad friend, although she was trying to be a good friend in her own way. I'd helped her try on and pick out a wedding dress, was her maid of honor and was planning a bridal shower, but was being treated like a naughty little child and sometimes shamed for my actions. I prayed about it, asking God for grace and guidance. I did what I felt in my gut would be best for my life and mental health. I pulled the plug after twelve years of friendship. It had become toxic. I backed out of being her maid of honor and ended our friendship.

I received a nasty message from her longtime friend, Jenn. She pointed out that when our mutual friends got engaged months before, I didn't look happy and could not be happy for others. I pragmatically replied that this birthday party for our friend that had turned into a surprise engagement had been wonderful for our friends, but that she, Jenn, had sat there with her new husband, Sandy with her fiancé, and our friends newly engaged, and my husband was dead. I was crying as they were all full of love and I was at a loss and alone in my grief. It was very odd to have Gus and Sandy both gone in a matter of two days, but I felt so free, as if twenty pounds had been lifted off my shoulders.

In June I went to Seattle for the Rock and Roll Marathon and hung out with Gus, just as friends as he was one of the only people I knew there, as we explored the city, and met up with Yelena, my friend from the Stupid Cancer conference, who lived there. I had a great time at Pike Place Market and walked around the city, before participating in the race, where I rocked my own socks off, actually running for short stints within the 13.1 mile race. The night before I lost my temporary crown when I bit into baklava, so I had to do the race with an open hole in my mouth, to my chagrin. I had a great playlist and was quite proud of myself. I thanked God for getting me there and doing so well. The night of the race I smoked cigars with Gus and pondered what next. The next day I could barely walk, and on the plane ride home in a moment of grief and forgetting how not great things had been when we dated, had thoughts of getting back together with Gus. I pushed that down. We hugged as we got off the plane, and have neither seen or talked to each other since.

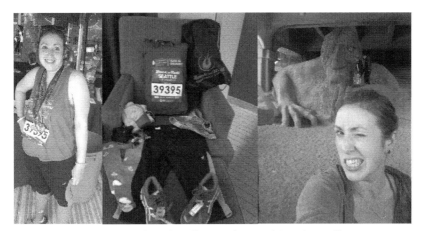
Seattle Rock and Roll Marathon and Seattle Troll

Facebook: June 11, 2014: My hope is that you'll take 10-15 minutes each week to rest, reflect and connect...I have had more time than the average person to do this in the past year, months; and it's wonderful!

Facebook: June 11, 2014: 5 things I learned in the last 2 weeks, or month: Some are no-brainers but life sometimes provides these sudden surprises:
1) At age 32 I realized sleeping in a T-shirt when it's hot out is better than pjs.....lol. who knew?
2) Breaking up with your significant other, after going through something as hard as the death of your spouse sucks and is hard, but it's so much easier to heal, knowing you tried, put yourself out there and are better off being true to your heart!
3) Forgiveness of said break-up occurs at lightning speed when you know you need positivity in your heart and mind.
4) Ending a long friendship with someone isn't easy, but you have to do what is right...we need people to pick us up, not tear us down.
5). Nothing, nothing is better than a warmish summer night listening to '80s tunes with the windows rolled down on the way home from an excellent hangout with good friends!

From mid-June to the end of August I nannied for an Indian couple who were both doctors. The mom worked nearby and the dad was an MD at Mayo in Rochester. I spent 7:30 a.m.-3:30 p.m. every day taking care of a teeny little thirteen-pound six-month-old Darsh. He was the cutest little thing and was fun to play with and was not too heavy to hold, as I'd recently been back to my gyno surgeon to tell him about all of the pelvic pain I was having, only to be told I could not lift more than fifteen to twenty pounds until I hit menopause or I'd have pelvic pain. Sadly, he was right.

Darsh and I would go for walks in the stroller and play and sing. His maternal grandmother was visiting from India the first three weeks I was there, which I thought would be awful, as

I'd be watched like a hawk, but it was wonderful. She taught me a lot about her culture, how to cook traditional Indian cuisine, filled my belly every day for lunch with her amazing cooking, and taught me Indian lullabies to sing to Darsh. I had planned on working for the family long-term, but they moved to Rochester at the end of the summer, causing me to panic to find another job.

I spent three nights a week from 7-10 p.m. as a personal care attendant (PCA) for a wonderful woman named Florence, who went by Flo. She was in her early fifties, had Multiple Sclerosis and was wheelchair-bound. She lived in an apartment that her sister had built onto her house out in the country, ten miles from my house. I loved driving out there among the corn fields and silos, seeing tractors work the land as the sun set, and at times seeing rainbows over the fields after it had rained. It made me feel smaller and more secure in the big picture, made my mind slow down and gave me time to appreciate God's beauty. Over the course of the year and a half that I worked for Flo I would tell her about my other jobs, and my adventures dating while helping her groom, toilet, watch TV, get ready for bed, and get positioned in bed. We became close friends and allies as we analyzed the men that I talked to and met, as well as shared our life stories and prayed for a better future for both of us.

I spent the summer getting out and about and doing more with friends in those months than I had in years. Vera and Kent had a backyard beer festival where I connected with their friends who later became friends of mine, too. I went to a battle of the bands with my friend Sarah at the Fine Line, listening to old school hip hop played live versus the original records, where we were silly and carefree.

Owen and I went to the annual Pride Festival that celebrates the LGBTQ members of our communities. We listened to live music, ate food, drank local beer and hung out. I introduced myself to the tall, shrieking singer, Jonathan, of the band Black Diet, as I thought "Why the heck not, make new friends everywhere!" He later became a friend online, and someone who I saw a couple times live in the future and we're still connected today even though he now lives in another state.

I became a blossoming flower that was open, raw, honest and just didn't care what people thought of her. I had been living in the trenches, working two jobs, three if you counted the garage sales, four if you counted the online selling, all to keep my house, and I'd seen and been through the worst. When I was out and about I was alive, felt young, and lived my best life… most of the time.

When my best friend Sage came to visit her hometown of Minneapolis and her parents, we hung out and had a great time. We would see each other each summer and during Christmastime, and it was wonderful to see and know her, as she'd been a close friend of Grayson's. She and her friend Frank and I went to the Saloon during the Pride weekend and danced until 2 a.m. outside among the thousands of people there celebrating hope, life and love. I danced and danced under the Minneapolis summer nighttime sky, took photos in a photo booth with my friends and felt like I was twenty-six, not thirty-two. I felt young and free and weightless, not the widow who had been dragged through the mud.

Chapter 32:
Dating: The Good and The Ugly of It All

I could write an entire book on dating, but will do my best here to describe the mess I got myself into and out of during the year and a half that I dated after Grayson died, starting the summer of 2014.

I'd met Grayson so young, I hadn't really "gotten out there". My sister Felicity put it best by saying, "You had a really rough dating life from ages eighteen to nineteen and a half!" I had no idea what I was doing, I was too open and honest to a fault at times, and was way too trusting. I wanted to get out there and have fun, go to dinners, go to concerts. Throughout this process of talking to dozens of people online that I'd never meet in person, several that I'd text and fifty-four that I actually met for face to face dates, I learned so much about myself. It was like interviewing for a job, or looking for a house. The photos and job descriptions don't always do justice to the actual job, home or in this instance, person. People tend to hide a lot about themselves, just like those photos of the house hid the black mold or the "second bathroom," that's a toilet in the basement that's out in the open.

I'd been used to my favorite lunchbox, the Wonder Woman one that was metal with the matching plastic thermos, which was Grayson. Now I had to get used to the soft-sided zipper ones with Sponge Bob Squarepants or Paw Patrol on them. Everyone at my church was already married with kids, if they were even close to my age range. Those on Christian dating sites were far and few in between of what I was looking for. In 2014-2015 the pickings were slim, so I thought I'd try OKCupid and Plenty of Fish.

I enjoyed the plethora of random questions about food preferences, hobbies, habits, etc., that OKCupid asked to match you with someone. Plenty of Fish was a little less stellar, but from there I had many dates…which I guess may have been the problem.

I was an equal opportunity dater, going out with guys that were white, African American, Asian, British, Eastern European, African, French, tall, short, and all kinds of different backgrounds. God made us all and you'd never know who you'd meet. I often used the words "zany, funny, whip-smart, compassionate, caring, authentic, genuine," to describe myself, and posted cute photos of myself, modest, not scantily clad like so many other women. I went for nerdy nice guys, skipping over those with beefy muscles and flashy cars to match. Here in Minnesota, so many guys had profile pictures holding up fish they'd caught, or standing behind deer they'd hunted, and/or the car they owned. I was what one would call a "sapiosexual," which means I was attracted to intelligence.

Over time, I crafted a system of how I'd decide who I'd actually meet. We'd talk on the dating website, then move to text in a day or so, then meet up in person, or talk on the phone first. So many people are not into talking on the phone, as we live in such an instant messaging time. There were many men who did not make the cut past the texting or phone, and I am glad I was able to filter them out that way before I wasted more of my time. I found out pretty quickly that being a widow was quite intimidating to men. I didn't have an ex, a horrible person that I'd broken up with or divorced that was gone, good riddance. I'd had someone I had tragically lost and that was hard for men to get past. The looks on their faces, or the "…" in texts of not knowing what to say was quite clear. I still loved Grayson, he was still a big part of who I was and he wasn't someone I would or could just forget.

I either met dates at a Caribou Coffee location, Liquor Lyle's (nice little Minneapolis bar on Hennepin Avenue with affordable drinks, old school red booths and retro wooden tables and chairs), Pub 42, or other agreed-upon public places. I always had my keys in hand, had a pink bedazzled lipstick-looking bauble on my keychain that had mace in it, and my phone was always in my pocket, not in my purse.

I met a guy in his late thirties, father of two girls under fifteen, at a Caribou twenty-five minutes from my house. We talked on the phone for hours the night before and he told me that he'd seen I'd been online earlier on the dating site and said, "After we talked for hours, you must be a messed-up chick to look at other men." Excuse me, I was not his property and didn't appreciate him commenting on my breasts during our date. He texted me on my way home and said "Nope!," which was fine with me.

The guy I talked to for a week via text who I thought was so kind and sweet, that I met up with four times, including once with his friends, turned out did not want me for my mind. Sigh. That was my first insight into men lying, as he stated on his profile that he wanted a relationship, when that hadn't been the case after all.

I talked to a guy one night on the phone that was a dead ringer for Wyclef Jean. As he was driving around in the rain, I heard him ask above the flap of his windshield wipers, "Did you catch your husband's cancer?" Oh my. I hung up and said, "Lord help me!" aloud.

A sweet country-listening, Daniel Dae Kim -looking guy who I connected well with for a couple weeks, got a tattoo covering his whole hand of a glowing skull face to hold up to his face, then made a creepy noises. No thanks. Insert the old AOL logging off message of "Good-bye!"

I met a really nice zookeeper who I hung out with several times, but he lived seventy miles away, which made it hard to really date, to see each other much. We decided to become friends and that worked out well for awhile.

I met a great guy who was on both of the dating websites I was on. He had only photos of himself from the waist up, which I didn't really notice until he pointed it out. He told me via text that he'd lost one leg in a motorcycle accident, two years prior. I hung out with him several times and we really hit it off, but he was just so down on himself and not able to fully enjoy life or believe he deserved a great life. I joined an online Facebook group for amputees, where I asked questions to be more supportive. I met Selena in this group, a feisty Latino cancer survivor who lived in California and had lost a leg to cancer. She gave me great advice and became a friend that I talked to almost daily for two years when we were both going through hard times. It didn't end up working with this guy, but I got a great friend out of it.

That fall I talked to a guy online who disclosed, after we'd been talking for an hour, that he was in fact at the Minnesota VA Hospital in Minneapolis. He'd been blown back into his comrades when a bomb went off during active duty in Afghanistan, and had suffered a broken leg, knee, ribs, and had quite a bad traumatic brain injury. He woke up in Germany and was handed a letter, discharging him from the Army after six tours, and sixteen years of service. He was a kind southern gentleman that I sprung out of the VA hospital for a couple dinners before he was moved to another hospital in another state. He and I got along great, and I was devastated when he left.

I joined a Facebook group for women in relationships with soldiers to ask questions, and had been told explicitly to not date anyone in the services, that it was too hard, and more than anyone would ever think of difficulty wise, in so many ways. It led me to read some really interesting books on war, soldier PTSD, and I again gained a new friend who I talked to quite regularly for years, as she was engaged to a soldier with terrible PTSD and a TBI.

I spent a lot of time sitting on my porch and looking at the trees sway across the street and wondered what I was doing wrong. I learned, in time, although not soon enough, that it was not me...it was never me...I chose people who saw someone that was an easy target to have fun with, then wad up and throw in the trash can. I spent so much time chasing after people who didn't want to get caught. Over the next year I would find myself, a well-educated woman in her early thirties, reading magazine articles online about "How to Get the Guy," "How to Find a Nice Guy," "How to Successfully Date," ad nauseam. Grayson had always been the one constant I always had in my life, outside of God. I was so lost. I kept looking for validation in earthly ways and wasn't finding it.

I also made a new friend, Candace, from TNT and I met up with her at bars like Pub 42, and Psycho Suzi's tiki bar, where we'd have a cocktail and talk about men, as I was boy crazy at the time.

Most of my friends moved on with time and I was stuck in the unknown of what was to come. I had no idea I would be a Sad Sally Sack of low self-esteem that would lick the bottom of the barrel of despair in my sheer loneliness. But I did it, and I am strong enough to tell the tale. I would listen to Dierks Bentley's album "Riser," on repeat every chance I got, and adored Frankie Ballard's, "Sunshine and Whiskey," and "Helluva Life," so much that summer. I would lie in bed and listen to Kenny Chesney's "Come Over," as well as the entire Ben Howard "Every Kingdom," album, just sinking my teeth into the lyrics and letting the music flow over me. Often I would write or read magazines sitting in bed listening to Iron and Wine as well. Music was healing to me in a way that nothing else was. It was my friend, my companion and my soothsayer into being okay. I prayed and trusted God and knew I'd somehow be okay.

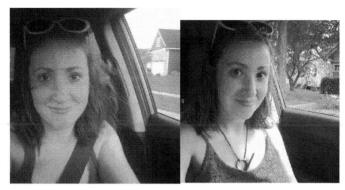
Summer 2014, Smiles as I'm Starting to Feel Healed

~

Instagram~ In the interest of making my actual posts easier to understand, I have taken out the # hashtags, but left in the words I wrote at the time, without photos, as they reveal my raw thoughts and emotions.

Instagram: July 22, 2014: ~Beneath the Stars~ I spin & revolve below ~A sky full of stars~That burst and crackle fragments of light~Beyond what one can see or plan.~We live, laugh and revel in delight~Whether we see them falling at our feet.~We dream, venture & take flight.~Shattered bursts of laughter, smiles & life's pleasures~Twinkle in the skies of my mind.~Beneath the stars I continue to twirl, be brave, Unapologetically me & adventurous~Trusting and unknown and greater plan

Instagram: July 25, 2014: Happy girl, new life, my heart bursts with love for Rachel 2.0, thank you my angel Grayson for watching over me, new adventures.

Instagram: July 27, 2014: I continue to listen to Coldplay's new album and adore, "Magic," and "Sky Full of Stars," they make me quite happy and hopeful.

Instagram: July 28, 2014: I find such inner peace when I listen to Luke Bryan's "Play it Again," and Lee Brice's "I Don't Dance."

Facebook: Aug. 16, 2014: Daylight breaks and I'm too tired to get out of bed, But the cat meows, the dog barks and it's time to start anew again. I am often tired but excited by the fact that I have come this far, I've made it. Survived. Sunset sets in, the lights go down- And I snuggle in bed, pass out alone, knowing there is a new day tomorrow ... Hope for work, love and continued inner peace I have worked for and work on daily.

Instagram: Aug. 17, 2014: Today I received my kit in the mail to register to be a marrow donor. All I have to do is swab my cheek, put it in an envelope and return it. Leukemia sucks, delete blood cancer, save lives, honoring my late husband and friends. Donate, save lives.

Instagram: Aug. 19, 2014: Wyatt and I saw the band Strand of Oaks at the 7th Street Entry. Best friends, summer, Minneapolis.

Instagram: Aug. 20, 2014: Today would have been my 10th Wedding Anniversary. I was a young shiny 22 year old that stood in front of family and friends, as Sarah McLachlan's song "Answer," played. My life story with this man is incredible, and I know God put us in each other's lives for a reason. He had a plan for me to help this man, to hold his hand and love him through illness to death. I am Happy, Healthy, Strong, have successfully moved on, am meeting people and dating, enjoying and loving life. Because of the real love I had from 09/21/01-04/21/13 I am able to be where I am.....complete, whole, healed and Rachel 2.0. I am a bit sad but happy, blessed, love.

Instagram: Aug. 23, 2014: Quote on the sketched art of a city line at sunset, "Tough times never last. Tough People Do." (Source of Quote unknown). #takenocrap #healing #timeheals #believemehavebeenthere

Chapter 33:
Ready, Set, Can I Really Do All of This? Go!

T hat fall I began a work schedule that would work me to the bone and barely keep me up to date on my bills, but somehow I made it work.

Three days a week I drove sixteen miles to a Catholic elementary school to help a little girl who had ADHD, ADD, was on the Autism spectrum, and had poor impulse control. Lexie was a teeny little thing for her kindergarten age and a little firecracker. I would meet her in the office, help get her to the staff bathroom, as the toilets were too loud in the kid's bathrooms, then watch her at recess so she wouldn't run off or jump off high up playground equipment. I took her back to her room for thirty minutes, then sat with her at lunch, and made sure she got on the bus that took her to the special education program at another school, or I took her home, made her lunch and hung out for two hours.

I helped her mother in the library some weeks, going earlier than usual to move and re-shelve books, set up for book fairs, create and draw kingdoms, castles and aquatic scenes depending on the theme, on huge sheets of paper around the doorway for the events. I liked using my brain to be crafty when my body was so tired from all of the driving. At home with Lexie, I burned out on episodes of Caillou and playing dolls or dress up. I was so tired working three jobs; however, I enjoyed her sweet little smile and creativity. Over the nine months that I did this, I became great friends with the school nurse, one of the administrative assistants, and Jackie, the school's chef. While I waited for little Lexie, I would talk to these ladies about life, love, work, and get advice on who I was dating. Jackie was a whip-smart mix of Wanda Sykes and Oprah, authentic, funny and wise.

After the first job I would usually go home and take a nap before I drove twenty-four miles in traffic every weekday to the Minnesota Autism Center to pick up young Steve from school. He was fourteen, Autistic, smart, kind and funny. His divorced parents hired me to take him either the thirty four miles in rush hour to his mom's house or twenty four miles in rush hour to his dad's house. It was a lot of driving, quality care time and definitely increased my skills in patience. Steve became obsessed with the song "Bad," by Michael Jackson, so much at times that we listened to that six to twelve times depending on the day, if he needed it. He'd sit in my front seat and eat the snacks I brought him, until we got home where he'd free play until we did homework, then play a game or play outside. Then I'd serve him dinner and wait until his mom or dad got home. Many times, if his dad was out of town, I'd also pick him up before school and drop him off there as well, sleeping in my car in the Catholic school parking lot until it was time to care for Lexie. Then, of course, I would also go to Flo's three days a week and get her ready for bed. It was so exhausting, but I managed to make it all work.

Instagram: Sept. 9, 2014: "Someday everything will all make perfect sense. So for now, laugh at the confusion, smile through the tears, and keep reminding yourself that everything happens for a reason," (Source of quote unknown). Bah. Waiting, really is the hardest part.

Instagram: Sept. 9, 2014: Tom Petty "The Waiting," rings so true to me right now.

Instagram: Sept. 15, 2014: Fighter, survivor, tears tonight, life not planned 2.0

Instagram: Sept. 15, 2014: The amount of craptastic things that have happened in the last 24 hours is astounding. Job issues, sick- bad cold again, too sick for work tonight at 2nd job, boys, financial, scary issues. Life keeps throwing me grenades…I don't know where I get my gusto. So much has happened by age 32.5 that most people don't ever have happen. The new Ryan Adams album is healing me.

Instagram: Sept. 16, 2014: Tonight I saw Eric Church in concert with Wyatt. A welcomed reprieve. "Springsteen," "Creepin," "Like Jesus Does."

Instagram: Sept. 26, 2014: Please pray I am finally rewarded by karma and God for my trials and losses. I need something good please.

In mid-September I began cleaning my friend Ivy's house once a month between my first and second jobs. I made $100 in three hours and it was worth it despite my fatigue. I came to know Ivy better and as I scrubbed the blue toothpaste off her children's bathroom fixtures, I reflected on how lucky I was to have supportive friends and people who knew I needed opportunities like this to make ends meet. I needed the release to splurge on concerts or a dinner with friends, and doing extra gigs allowed that to happen.

Instagram: Oct. 3, 2014: "You cannot always wait for the perfect time, sometimes you must dare to jump" (Author Unknown). I continue to be inspired by the plethora of topics in the photography here on #instagram. Some simple, some complex, some with raw emotions, captioned or not. I have been fortunate to meet some truly amazing people…truly.

Instagram: Oct. 11, 2014: First concert of 4 shows in 6 days that I am going to alone. Life is a gift. Be brave. Pave your own path. Life is a gift. Joseph Arthur and the Afghan Wigs at First Ave., then Ryan Adams and David Gray both at Northrup Hall at the U, and Sondre Lerche at the Turf Club in St. Paul.

Instagram: Oct. 14, 2014. Happiness through the storm.

Instagram: Oct. 21, 2014: Today is a big milestone, as 18 months ago to the day I held my best friend and husband as he peacefully died. That will always be my proudest accomplishment-loving him through illness and holding his hand as he walked through fire and hell. I am grateful for the passing of time and my strength, but my will to be blunt and authentic does cost me mistreatment and heartache at times. I am the antithesis of the Grinch... my heart is too big, but I wouldn't change a single thing. I somehow chose/am on paths to support others and that isn't easy, but life is hard and I was gifted a love years ago that has made me 4x4 solid steel. I am a survivor and fighter.

The three jobs made me so tired all the time. I'd come home at night, pet my animals and crash on the couch, getting in an episode or two of a show before I'd go to bed. Most nights it took me several attempts to drag myself off the couch to go brush my teeth then make it into bed. I'd count out loud, not get up, and start all over again.

Instagram: Oct. 22, 2014: My work is joyful and purposeful.

In October my parents came to visit for several days, which was a wonderful time to connect and recharge. My dad came to cheer for me as I did the Monster Dash 5K in St. Paul, watching me run and walk among all of the funny and neat costumes. I had fun picking up candy and putting it in my jacket pockets and hearing it move up and down next to me. We also went to an apple orchard and pumpkin patch and had a great time together.

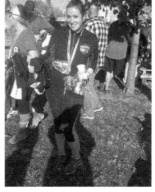
Monster Dash

Instagram: Oct. 27, 2014: The 2nd greatest love of my life is my 14 year old cat Rufus, we've been together 12 years.

Instagram: Nov. 9, 2014: Dance party with my dog tonight.

In November I went to see Interpol in concert at First Ave. with a date who got us in free and into the VIP box, as he was the tech guy for the club. I saw Stars there as well with Owen. I made dinner for Wyatt and many times that fall and winter spent time hanging out with Owen and his daughters playing, watching movies and having dinners out. Owen graciously paid many times. People often assumed that we were a family to our amusement when wait staff would say, "Mom, what will the kids want to drink?" We were not a family, but family indeed.

From time to time between my crazy work hours, I had tea dates with girlfriends in our homes or at funky little coffee shops which provided moments to detox, reflect and collect myself. I had a few dates that ended up in fiery crashes and burns, one in which a guy had a friend call with an "emergency" that clearly was not, and another who had to leave right after we ordered food. Both resulted in me taking fish and chips home that I hadn't had to pay for, that I shared with my dog Greta.

I kept trudging on, working, running to the grocery store late at night after my PCA gig with Flo, when the rest of the world was tucked in for the night with their families. I had a rhythm of going, going, going and that routine was something I was so used to despite the craziness of it all. I knew I could keep going because Grayson had brought me such amazing and unexpected gifts from his afterlife. Who I was, was a direct product of how much I'd been loved and the security he'd helped me build in myself as an individual in the world.

There had been times in the past months when I'd made myself cry in front of the mirror when I'd been crying… to see myself experience the grief process. I had to see and know what I was doing and how I was moving through it all. Sometimes when I was so sad and wished he was there, I'd go into the kitchen, exactly where he and I used to stand, and I'd get up on my tippy toes like I would when I hugged him, and I'd reach my arms up around his imaginary neck and hug the man who wasn't there. I would see him standing there in his Mr. Rogers red or navy blue cardigans he liked to wear, and in jeans or khakis with a smile on his face. Even nineteen months after he died, I still looked at the front door sometimes, expecting him to walk through it at any moment.

Life certainly had changed as I moved forward. One time when I'd just laid down to nap between my first and second jobs, I lifted my head and did a sharp intake of breath in excitement, when I realized I never again had to have holidays with Victoria and Bernard. I had moved past all of that and was on to greener pastures. I still talked to Dean online and via text from time to time, but the rest of his family had dropped me for the most part.

Instagram: Nov. 27, 2014: "The darkest nights produce the brightest stars," (Source of quote unknown). Very tough last few days…was solo today, friend plan fell through. No fam here. Missing Grayson. Grief sucks. We were a fam of 2…..

I was at the depths of darkness some days, despite my sunny disposition most of the time. People who met me said they had no idea that I was a widow or had had a hard life, based on how healthy I looked and how positive I was. One cold fall day as I arrived at the school parking lot at the same time as Lexie's mom, I asked her for a hug when she got out of her car. She seemed to think it was weird, as she raised her eyebrow and asked why. I told her I had no one else to hug and was having a hard time. She awkwardly hugged me, not satiating the void inside me. Many times I'd hug my beloved dog Greta, wrapping my arms around her neck and just crying. I needed affection and contact so badly. I would feel her breath on my arm or neck and miss my family and Grayson. I occasionally would lie on her chest and listen to her heart beat. Even just to write this makes me cry. It was such a painful time. I was trying to keep it all together, doing the best I could, and still felt like a sinking ship.

Every night before bed I'd read my "Jesus Calling," or "Jesus Today" books and would have tears streaming down my cheeks as the passage for the day usually was spot on with what I was going through. I'd laugh through my tears at the kismet match to my current situation, and ask God to keep me afloat.

I'd reflect back on Grayson, of all of the silly things he used to do, like making me buy fancier shoes one time when we went to dinner at the Olive Garden, as "flip flops are trashy, not for nicer places." We stopped at Target on the way there, where I bought a pair of dress sandals that would later only be worn a couple times as they were uncomfortable. When we were seated forty minutes later; I pointed to three tables in the restaurant where women were wearing flip flops. He hated that as soon as I got home from work I would put on sweat or yoga pants, to the extent that he said, "Can you at least wear jeans until like six or seven at night, then put on pj pants?!"I thought he was ridiculous and he later had to eat crow when the majority of what he wore during his illness when he was home was pj pants. He told me how I'd been right and they were so comfy.

During Grayson's illness, the meds often made him mean and not like himself. One time I'd gone and purchased a Rubbermaid drawer storage unit to put in our back closet to keep pet items in, that sent him into a swearing angry rampage. He couldn't believe "You didn't consult me first!!!," which I thought was odd as the $20 item would help organize the closet and wasn't a big home purchase in my eyes. Another time there was a major blowout over picking out new bath mats. It was ugly, lol.

The steroids made him crazy mean, just like the time in the hospital months before he died when he was unable to articulate what he wanted to say, and I answered the nurses' questions when I knew the answer. He pointed to me and said, "Don't listen to the talking head over there, I can answer that myself." He really hurt my feelings sometimes, but thank God, I had the ability to recognize that it wasn't him talking, it was the cancer and the meds. Even back then, parts of Grayson were slowly slipping away right before my eyes, when I'd not even known it.

Cancer is so manipulative and deceptive in that it tricks you, keeps coming back and portrays things sometimes not as they really are. When those moments would creep up in my head after his passing, I'd tried to replace them with happy ones. Every time I filled up my days of the week vitamin pill box, I'd think of our dance party. During Grayson's last Christmas, at home I was filling up my vitamin pill box, when I heard him turn on Wham's "Last Christmas," coincidentally, and said, "Pony, come down here!" We laughed and danced and had a great time. That memory has lasted forever in my mind, creating joy in ways I try to grasp when the bad memories and images creep in.

It took about a year and a half, but there were some days when I'd realize I hadn't thought about Grayson for a day, or even several. I knew it didn't mean I hadn't loved or cared about him; it meant I was surviving and moving on, focusing on my life now and feeling secure enough in who I'd become; to keep going on without him.

Instagram: Nov. 29, 2014: Today I walked/ran the annual "Mustache Run," at St. Anthony Main in Minneapolis, along the cobblestone streets in the frigid temps. Challenges. Keep going.

~

Self-Care Check-In: As I'd discussed before, around the holidays or anniversaries, it can be really tough whether your spouse/significant other is in treatment, in remission or has died. Make sure you are taking time for yourself to work on that hobby, going for coffee with a friend, going for a walk, or enjoying a book or TV binge.

- Know your limits- you can only do so much, and need to take time to rest, reflect and recharge.
  - o Even if it's only for an hour or two a week if you're balancing work, family, etc- take that time just for you, before you burn out. This journey is incredibly long and difficult at times and it's important you give yourself the space and freedom to rest.
- Reach out to loved ones or friends and ask them to go to dinner or coffee with you, or even for just a check-in text or phone call.
  - o Still to this day, all these years later on Grayson's birthday, our wedding anniversary and his death anniversary- I will do a Facebook and Instagram post commemorating it, and usually often text my parents and siblings as well.
  - No matter how many years have gone by whether your loved one is alive or has passed, those milestone reminders are hard- what was and what is/should be, are two very different things even if your life circumstances have moved on into a more positive and healthy direction. You cannot take away the past memories and for some like myself- scars of the past struggles through cancer life and loss.
    - I have learned it's better to over-prepare then under-prepare for emotions that might come up over holidays and anniversaries.
    - I was knocked on my feet more on Grayson's birthday the year I turned 37, (6 years after his death) as he died at 37, due to realizing that I had surpassed him in age, than I was in those years closer to his death.
    - Preparing for these milestones ahead of time by taking a day off of work (if possible) and letting your support system know you might need back-up, has worked very well for me over the years.

  - Give yourself GRACE! This is an ongoing, uncharted journey and know that only you can listen to what your mind and body need- to help you get through it.

Chapter 34:
Breathe, Sleep, Eat, Work, Repeat, Oh Yeah…and Enjoy Life

In December I happily decorated for Christmas while watching holiday movies with my pets laying around me. I've always felt that Christmas was a magical time of year, and that year despite my isolation and sometimes grief, I felt cheery most of the time.

I had dinners with friends, caught up with Vera and Kent, hung out with Wyatt at a Mike Doughty show at First Ave., and went to a birthday party for my friend Lisa. I went to Half Price Books one day in between jobs and bought Cab Calloway, Bing Crosby and Edith Piaf CDs, enjoying the old school sounds of these artists as I drove from job to job. For a few weeks I loudly sang made up French accented words along to Edith's singing, as Greta lay there staring at me, not seeming to mind my loud outbursts. I was used to doing things on my own a lot. I'd go to dinner or a movie and have a great time alone. Steve's mom took him and me out to dinner at the Rock Bottom Brewery, then to a Christmas show at the State Theater to see those guys who wear all black then light up and dance and make shapes while music plays.

Instagram: Dec. 18, 2014: Busy Week! I am powered by Weezer's music and new Mango LaCroix water.

Instagram: Dec. 21, 2014: Today I got a five inch long by two inch tall "Blessed" tattoo on the inside of my left arm, with Wyatt watching. As I was sitting there enduring the well-worth pain, I told the artist that it had been a really hard year and I was looking forward to the new year. He looked at me quizzically and said, 'Well then why are you getting this tattoo?' I told him that I had been blessed despite everything I'd been through, and that this was an important reminder for me to remember where I'd been, where I was, and where I was going. Blessed. Widow life. Truths.

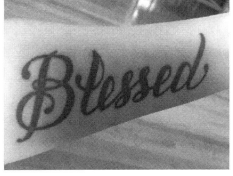

My New Ink to Mark my Thankfulness

A friend house-sat for me and took care of Greta and Rufus, while I drove six and a half hours with a car loaded with presents and Trader Joe's treats to my brother Jack's house for Christmas. Over the course of three days I played games, ate meals and watched movies with Jack, his wife Maddie, their girls Emma, Tabitha and Samantha, as well as my sister Felicity, her husband Aiden and their daughter Ione.

I often felt separated and alone despite the company and togetherness, as I did not have a spouse or children. I was the outsider. Like a numbnut, everyday I drank hot chocolate with amaretto in it, and one day spent hours online trying to find someone to date me. I was so successful in so many ways in my life in how I was moving forward, but just wanted so badly for someone to give a crap and care about me in that intimate, connected way. I missed having someone to share the day's events with, that wasn't my dog or cat. My friends and family had their own lives and it just wasn't the same.

The day before I left to head to Jack's, December 22nd, I took down all of my Christmas decorations. There was no holly or jolly in this chicky, and I didn't want the cheer to be on my walls or around me any longer. I knew it'd be a part of the holiday with family, but felt I had to remove it from my house.

Instagram: Dec. 24, 2014: I am nestled amongst an insane amount of stuffed animals on the bottom bunk of my niece's bed, with three of my nieces 8, 5, 5 (the youngest are a day apart one from my brother's wife, one my sister!) and the 10 year old niece above me. I am so grateful to be in a better place this Christmas. These little giggles and excitement for Santa are so fun. I know I am blessed but also feel so robbed. I know there is a lobster out there somewhere (Friends show reference) hopefully, that will take on this strong unicorn. My 10 year old niece told Santa on the note she left out to "Bring my Aunt Rachel a boyfriend and world peace," as that was my answer when she asked what I'd wanted. Happy, lonely, sad, life is wonderful despite the pain, it gets better every chance you take.

Instagram: Dec. 26, 2014: My amazing parents left these gifts wrapped up when they visited in October. I just opened up Ernest Hemingway's Islands in the Stream, A Reader's Guide to Ernest Hemingway, A Collection of Critical Essays (Hemingway), For Whom the Bell Tolls, and an angel figurine. Yes! Happy girl! I am an Ernie freak.

Instagram: Dec. 27, 2014: "Footprints" has always been foundational for me and my go to for grace.

Instagram: Jan. 1, 2015: BLESSING JAR: Today I opened up the little scraps of paper that I'd written down of people, places, events and things I'd been grateful for in the last year. God is so good!

Instagram: Jan. 14, 2015: Today is going to be a great day despite the fact that I partially threw my back out 2 days ago and I work 12 hours today….keep on trucking!

In mid-January I flew to Boston to spend time with Felicity and Diana; Felicity bought my plane ticket. We spent several days making food, playing with my niece Ione, going to the Children's Museum, a neat indoor farmer's market and finding a really cool, large poodle lamp for Felicity's new house. This sister time was always a gift and a lighthouse in the storm of my life.

Instagram: Jan. 22, 2015: Greta: This chick drives me bananas, terrorizes my geriatric cat, wakes me up around 4 a.m. everyday which gets her butt crated with a treat, but she is my baby girl for better or for worse. #greta #underbite

Instagram: Jan. 24, 2015: From within us all stems a creature that be. We must foster it with knowledge. Foster it with love. Foster it with patience. Foster it with time. But adopt a permanent form of gratitude for the Faith we have in the one above -that provides the soil in which all blessings begin from. Where the water must first flow. It is within this creature we learn to hold the hand of what we are unexpectedly given and rejoice at the Grace of it all.

At the beginning of February I came up with the idea to start a business where I'd help people figure out the cancer process, support them in resources, and do the same if their spouse died. I made a cheap website and got some business cards. In the end, I only had one client. She was the administrative assistant at the Catholic school, and was also a cancer wife. I cleaned, organized and got things ready to donate in her home while charging a pretty penny. I wish it had taken off, but I couldn't afford the startup costs. I needed to pay my bills, so I kept taking the jobs I could find.

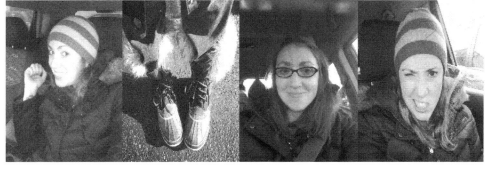

Hustling to Work 3 Jobs and Keep Going!

Instagram: Feb. 3, 2015: Read Siddhartha by Herman Hesse. Amazing. Sometimes I really do feel like Sisyphus, pushing that dang boulder back up the hill again, and again, but I keep going.

Instagram: Feb. 21,, 2015: Wyatt and I went to see Catfish and the Bottlemen tonight at the 7th Street Entry, braving the cold as we stood bundled up outside to get in. Best friends. Minneapolis.

Instagram: Feb. 26, 2015: This morning, I reluctantly got out of bed at 630 a.m. for another crazy long work day of an unusual 4 day stretch of 15 hour work days, 490 miles driven in 60 hours so far. Kendrick Lamar and Childish Gambino are playing on repeat.

Instagram: Mar. 2, 2015: If you know me and my last few years, you know I'm a super trooper. I have a few constants in my life…4 to be exact: 1) my family and close friends 2) my intelligence and perseverance 3) my Faith in God and the greater plan And 4) Greta…this little chicky as annoying as she can be, unconditionally loves me with her under bite and smile, she is always there when the world turns pear shaped. and Rufus my minxy, 15 year old cat.

Instagram: Mar. 4, 2015: KINDNESS IS KEY. Just got my car stuck in a snowy ditch in rural Maple Grove on the way to work. 2 people tried to help and gave up. Another man went home, came back with a shovel and helped along with my client's family that helped me too. Kindness is Key in my world.

Instagram: Mar. 5, 2015: Tonight I went to see The Church with Owen at the Cedar Cultural Center. It was great to hang out with my best friend that I hadn't seen in a while. We drank Surly and caught up. I've been listening to "Under the Milky Way," since I was little, so it was great to hear, but it also brings up events and memories with Grayson, which made me a bit sad. Life is bittersweet.

Instagram: Mar. 7, 2015: I have been asking friends for a word lately and spinning it into a poem in 5-8 mins, this is one I wrote for a friend: Morning beckons, the sun peaks through the cloud, "Thank You Lord for another day," she says aloud. A smile hits her lips, life is good ~ In Minneapolis. ~Systems change. Culture change. Helping others get the most of their education she works on an impacting rearrange. Smiles and enjoys what she does, not what everyone could do, like her, she enjoys social services work. It's the vantage point that has allowed her to see beauty and reward in the craziness and in the niche of it all, the quirk. ~All in Minneapolis. ~City lights, days move on like the speed of light or snail slow. Depending on the day, was gone for a couple years, but she is forever homegrown, back to stay ~ in Minneapolis. ~It's the beauty she sees in life's unwritten, rough and tough edges. She works to help others now, not always on fast forward looking beyond the hedges. Loving life in Minneapolis. Family, friends, festivals, music and drink, so much positivity, her sights on what is real, never lets her spirits sink. ~In Minneapolis. ~She waits patiently to make herself a better woman, waiting for the real deal. Rather than make an incoherent mistake, and easy steal. Real life and love she looks for- she'd rather wait, than settle when she hasn't quite found that important trait ~In Minneapolis. ~Authenticity, faith, honesty is key. Hmmm she thinks…what does he think about me? ~ In Minneapolis.

Instagram: Mar. 10, 2015: 65 degrees on March 10th. Late night Rachelism rhyming: Spring…has it really sprung? In my mind I hear the rat a tat tat of something positive to come…Gotta live & believe that way…each and every day. Blessings.

Instagram: Mar. 13, 2015: Take your negative experiences as GRACEFUL lessons and make POSITIVITY the KEY to future locks… Life Lessons. Positivity.

Instagram: Mar. 15, 2015: Just finished 54 work hours this week. I've got 2Pac on the stereo, and reflect on how I still hung out with friends, swam ½ mile my regular 2x a week, ate well, loved my pets, and yes I do have on the Wonder Woman socks my sister gave me, with a cape on the back!

Instagram: Mar. 16, 2015: Food for Thought: Tired. Physically, mentally, tired of people that aren't authentic. Leaps of Faith are called that for a reason. If I hadn't taken a gamble on someone when I was a baby of 19, and had an amazing 11.5 years til cancer bit and stole him away, I'd never know the realness, joy, grace and serendipity of life. Hard knocks. Truth.

Instagram: Mar. 18, 2015: I had a 6x6 inch rock made for Grayson to put in my front garden with stars on it that says, "GRAYSON the Luckiest." From Death, Life Renews. To See the Process, Feel the Process and Get the Preciousness of Life Renews the Soul. Widow life. Truths. Joy. Hope. Faith. Renewal.

Instagram: Mar. 22, 2015: Hey ladies! Women often downplay intelligence, who the heck knows why. I've been told to play coy, to be less smart with men. No way Jośephina! I'm proud of being a smarty pants!

Instagram: Mar. 25, 2015: Each day is a new opportunity. Wake up grateful, go to bed feeling BLESSED. Truths. Lessons. Faith. Grace. Trust.

Instagram: Mar. 27, 2015: Early morning-have a cold-insomnia. Most days are 97%... Most of the time I don't think about it-the hell I have been through, things I've seen and done for love, through love…things I wouldn't wish on my worst enemy. However it is these experiences that have made me strong, fierce, unicorn me, with strength, faith and courage. Sometimes the weight of it crushes me and that's ok…I believe it's God's reminder that what I had was cosmic rare and never to settle for less. My purpose of helping others and being positive and not following the crowd is clear. Walk by Faith. Unapologetically me- Rachel

Instagram: Mar. 27, 2015: Sick Day Reflections: Rachel's Goals:

- Realistic Goals: Breathe, Pray, Love, Live, Exercise. Finish 2 classes in Grief Counseling Certification, make my business work, travel to family and friends, write two books from outlines, start volunteering for hospice, pay off debt, keep paying for amazing retro house, catch up with local friends and do an oncology research project. Little goals right?
- Dreamin' Goals: Find a good, honest, sweet, smart, communicator man to stand by me and do nice things for me that I haven't had in years! That I can do vice versa for! Only God knows.

~

In my rare downtime I filled my time watching "A Different World," "Broad City," "Will and Grace," and baking. I went to a Stevie Wonder concert with my friend Jackie, and loved that she and I were more like sisters at that point, and met up with friends or had a date when I had the energy. When I had spare money, I'd go to Goodwill and thrift stores and excitedly score deals that delighted me to no end. My spare back bedroom had become the catch-all for all of my clothes. I'd wear something, then, if it was wearable again, I'd chuck it on the bed after I took it off. Once every few weeks I'd hang everything back up. I was exhausted, it was only me and I didn't have anybody to impress. My house was clean and tidy, but that bed was not!

Chapter 35:
Reflections in the Sun

Instagram: Mar. 30, 2015: I continue to work on my grief counseling certification. Life kicked me in the teeth… you can be bitter or better. I chose better, honoring my angel, late husband. Future business woman. Wonder Woman.

Instagram: Apr. 6, 2015: Sometimes things aren't too good to be true…they are actually true in kindness, goodness, courage and what you always wanted, but don't expect to find. *Magic*.

Instagram: Apr. 7, 2015: Love provides simple truths…this is something I had in the past, and it makes me sad others don't know the beauty of it…but I know God has a plan for each person even if we don't know it, wanna believe it, etc. I came from goodness and have much goodness to give and receive. This is all life is about...the rest is just icing on the cake. Unicorn. Leaps of Faith. Widow life.

Instagram: Apr. 13, 2015: Having your spouse die is the equivalent to losing your job, having your home set on fire, a limb cut off and being gutted like a turkey-but it's one's choice to be bitter or better, sink or swim. 2 years ago I was floating in uncertainty, living in hospitals, clinics, waiting for a bone marrow transplant to save, cure, etc.… God gave me an angel to live, love and learn with and from… Everett Grayson was my best friend and my experience has made me the rock star I am today. There have been days I don't think much about him or our life at all, other days I wonder if it was real... friends have told me what I had was cosmic rare and not real life…to me it is fact.. what love life should be. Real stuff. Cancer sucks. Widow life. Either way…I am forever blessed.

Instagram: Apr. 15, 2015: It's the times we had greatness and the memories of what life is, should be and can be…that we know to be the steps of life. We've had security, consistency and blessings that help us acknowledge that as cliché as it is to know: that hard things do pass in time. We smile at the simple things…Growth of spring's flowers, sunny not dreary snowy days and friends from afar that although we don't see them or talk much, we know we're not alone in our 'kazaam' moments in life.

I flew to Los Angeles on the 17th and spent the next four days with Sage for my 33rd birthday and the second anniversary of Grayson's death. We went to the Getty Art Museum, the LA Zoo, and ate sushi. We went to the Pacific Cheesecake Company where we picked out baby desserts that we had later with sangria and a dance party of 2; to thrift stores, the farmers market and watched movies. Sage is one of those friends who, no matter how long it has been since you've talked or seen each other, you can pick up where you left off and things are still just as great. On my birthday I wore a cute little green eyelet dress, sandals and a candy necklace in the warm spring weather, bought myself a little stuffed Rainbow Dash My Little Pony and told everyone I saw that day when I bought or ordered something that it was my birthday. I was a happy girl, felt amazing and had a blast with Sage.

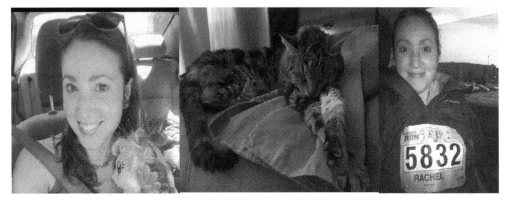

Spring 2015: My 33rd Birthday a Resting Rufus and the Gopher Run

Instagram: Apr. 19, 2015: Today is my 33rd Birthday…Have been told a lot lately I look 24. Woot! I am having wonderful best friend adventures in LA, feeling young and alive and so free. Thank You God, for good friends, healing, laughter, love, life and second chances. Rachel 2.0

April 21, 2015: I walked along the Santa Monica pier, felt the salty air in my hair and reflected on how odd it was that time had flashed by so quickly. The day before, I laid in the sand and felt in awe of how far I'd come in two years. Only two years. As I heard the ocean rolling behind me, a rare treat to behold, I reflected on how precious life is and how I had really done it…I really had survived. Cancer wife at 28, widow two days after turning 31. I had had job losses, huge, life-altering health issues and surgery, terrible dates, broken hearts, lost friends along the way, met incredible people, people who have grown along or with me, and those who have been there with me from the very beginning, in a part of Rachel 1.0. All those things made me who I was, on that day, the girl who ran her fingers through the sand, staring at the tiny grains as she smiled, feeling so close to and so far away from Grayson at the same time. I had made it. No matter what else may come, I had made it through the worst of the worst, and was so thankful to be where I was on that day.

Instagram: Apr. 21, 2015: 2 years ago today I held my husband and best friend in my arms as he died after a warrior's battle against leukemia, after bone marrow transplant complications. I would have never, ever imagined I'd be this healthy and okay, where I am today. I just spent the last four days in Los Angeles with my best friend Sage who drove me around and has showed me love and life and true friendship over the years, and giggles at the goober, kind Grayson she knew and loved. Tonight I'm having fish and chips with another bff Owen. Life is good. I owe it 100% to God, faith, grace, hard work, healing and friends & family. My Angel in heaven Grayson, I know you're up there with two turn tables and probably also a microphone. I love, work and breathe from the love and experiences I had in my 11.5 years with this person. Thank You Lord.

Instagram: Apr. 24, 2015: This week: Checked tire pressure, put air in, tire blew up in my face. 3 days later drove kid to Saturday drop off, crunched curb, other kid peed her pants in the car, had to get new tire, and got bit by her very badly on the arm, then got home to find a $1200 health bill in the mail. Cannot make this stuff up.

Instagram: May 6, 2015: It's taken a lot of grace and strength, faith, and courage to get me thus far. Happygirl.

Instagram: May 8, 2015: Trip B: 583.6 mi, and my gas tank on empty. Add 20 miles and that's my week just for work. Ayayayay. Off to sit in traffic to home for an hour probably. Luckily it's Friday and I have Noodles n Co to eat on the way home and that Surly beer I've been saving in my fridge too.

Instagram: May 8, 2015: The uncertainty of the future is a gift of trust, optimism and faith.

Instagram: May 11, 2015: We can only see so much ahead of us- with our minds, the gift of sight and experiences we have. We have to take the gift of grace and faith in knowing that there is a bigger plan, a greater plan. One we don't necessarily get, understand, that isn't tangible, on our own timeline or at the whim of our desires, but crafted for us...despite tragedies in our own lives and globally that are incomprehensible, we must believe...or at least I do...that someone holds the lantern, faith, grace, purpose and plan.

Instagram: May 15, 2015: Today I cut off six inches of my hair in my bathroom. It's been freeing to be able to cut my hair whenever I feel like it, to give myself a lift then move on. Freedoms. Gifts.

Chapter 36:
Movin' on and Creating Anew

Instagram: May 16, 2015: I'm selling my house I've had for 6 yrs. Bought at age 26, now 33, and 2 years post the death of my late husband. Life is precious, don't be a jerk, tell those you love, you love them and take leaps of faith.

By early May I made the decision that I had had it. I wasn't finding jobs I loved. I was tired of putting together several jobs to make ends meet. Dating had been terribly unsuccessful and the sheer number of difficult things that kept happening was astounding. My sister Diana told me over the last couple of years to stop tallying the number of bad things that had happened, but it was hard not to do when it was my life.

I had thought for quite some time before making this decision, and mapped out how I would move to the little artsy town of Portland, Maine. I'd always wanted to live along the seashore, and now was my chance. I felt so positive that I could start over, sell my house and most of my things, rent a truck and drive out to Maine. When I told Owen, I cried, then he got teary, but he said he understood why.

It was hard to imagine not living near each other as we talked almost daily and hung out nearly once a week, sometimes two, but I had to make a change for myself for the better. I didn't want to leave Wyatt either, my partner in crime, so close to my heart, or Vera or Hazel, and so many friends as well, but I had lost so much and felt like I kept losing and wanted to start over. At one point that winter I'd thought of jumping ship, putting my stuff into storage and moving in with my parents in their little retro house in Georgia. I'd even thought of renting out my house and moving into an apartment in Minneapolis. I was desperate to start over.

My friend Jackie was a part time realtor and had photos taken of my house, listed it online and had several open houses. I cleaned, cleared things out with the help of Owen, and gave my beloved stuffed animals I'd had in storage and childhood books to his little ladies that I'd played with, painted nails with, gone to parks, and chased through slides. Between all of my jobs I sorted what I wanted, what I didn't and was paring down to strike it all anew on the East Coast.

I had garage sales every weekend from 8 a.m.-4 p.m. Saturdays and Sundays, selling furniture, clothes, household items, anything and everything that I wasn't going to take with me. The month before I'd spent weeks organizing, consolidating and cleaning out the house of an older gentleman that Jackie introduced me to through a friend. I spent three weeks going through Tyrone's house between my first and second jobs. I held a pretty unsuccessful estate sale, as not many people came for some reason, so I took his items and sold them online, and added them to my garage sales as well. Mid-May I also had a garage sale for Jackie, actually straight out of her garage in the alley of her apartment complex. I sat on a couch out in the sun talking to customers as they came and went. I kept myself busy and made extra cash here and there when I could, which allowed me to go out with friends and to see wonderful live music.

I quit my job with the little girl one day after her mom had neglected to come home on time for the nth time too many, which made me late yet again for an appointment. When I told Steve's parents that I was going to move, they decided to let me go precisely two weeks later; they got scared and wanted to set up someone new to work that summer through the fall and onward. I lost my dependable income so quickly and scrambled to find something for the summer.

Instagram: May 19, 2015: In a ton of pain, but excited about continual big decisions and my new life ahead in the fall. I was gonna store stuff here in MN, but have   decided to sell more and just pack a truck when I go in September.

Instagram: May 21, 2015: I am working on painting brighter days and continuing to walk by faith, only God knows, grace, strength, faith, courage, thank God for good friends.

In the summer of 2015 I was back on the bandwagon, trying to date more again. It was nicer out, I had more free time on the weekends, and was willing to squeeze in more dates, as they usually didn't go beyond thirty to sixty minutes at a coffee shop or Liquor Lyle's before I'd call it quits and go home. I had a few dates that were quite odd -- they definitely were not what they had advertised. I tried Tinder and found some really neat people to talk to, but they just weren't very put together. They didn't have jobs, cars, lived with their parents or had recently gotten out of relationships. I was an educated adult woman with my own house, job, car, former marriage and knew what I wanted. That didn't seem to scare them away, but made them run to me, which was not welcomed. I had tried Match.com during the winter and had failed miserably; the commercials lied, in my experience. My friend Zoe told me, "Grayson did you a disservice, by treating you so well," at which I laughed. I wanted to find that again and knew someone great was out there.

Somehow my self-worth in regard to men decreased. I knew I was an amazing person, but was so desperate for someone to like me, that I lost sight of reasonable expectations. I guess I felt I needed to know that I was ok, for that to be reinforced because I was so lonely despite my strength in character and will to keep going and fighting. At the same time, dating was great and fascinating, as I was able to see myself through someone else's eyes. I was funnier than I'd ever been, was able to work, take care of my home and animals and still go out and meet new people. There definitely were a few times I wished I could turn off my sarcasm and the zaniness, but I kept going and going like the Energizer Bunny. My friend Vera told me years later that I just kept dating to try to find the right person and even if she'd told me that it was okay to just stop, I'd eventually find someone, I would not have listened as I kept racing on like, "pew pew" with my guns blazing like Yosemite Sam in the Wild West.

I somehow had a zip of energy no matter what time of day it was, yet I was so empty in other ways. I was running a race with no finish line in sight, truly enjoying life but not always being smart. There were times I made questionable choices, but my amazing and forgiving God loved me just the same. I would go to church and be so at peace feeling at home in God's space, that I felt pumped and prepped for another grueling week of working multiple jobs and having tons of garage sales just to survive and keep my house. Sometimes at night after I'd turned off all the lights and gone to bed, I'd get up, turn on the dining room and kitchen light or the living room, and just look around in awe that it was all mine. My beloved house of my dreams, with its retro cabinets, original stove from 1956 and coved ceiling that I busted my butt to pay for, was all mine.

Instagram: June 6, 2015: Somewhere Another Life & Love & Adventures Are Waiting for Me. Life. Love.

Instagram: June 11, 2015: I started working with a super disabled kid exactly a week ago. He is 17, mentally 2, Autistic, non-verbal and has epilepsy (so I have to literally watch him like a hawk as he has several kinds of seizures a day). This is one of the most challenging and rewarding jobs, and physically boundary pushing (he weighs 130 lbs. =quite a daily workout) job that I have ever had. Blessings, love it.

Instagram: June 12, 2015: These peonies are from my back garden…something I won't want to leave behind. I remember Grayson posing proudly by them with a bald head. It's like he was never here sometimes. This 'Blessed," tattoo and my other ones help me more than I can ever say…they remind me of where I was, where I am, and where I'm going.

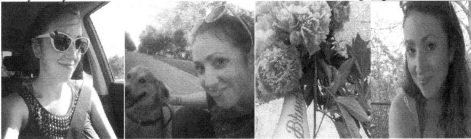

Instagram: June 16, 2015: Serendipity. Good things happen, especially when we don't plan them. Happy Tuesday peeps. Life is short, take chances, laugh, love and live for the moment.

Chapter 37:

Adaptation is Key, Trying to Make it Work Again for Me

Instagram: June 28, 2015: Begin anew & take a breath & let life's serendipitousness lead one foot in front of the other. Truths, leaps of faith, Rachel. Furious lil cinnamon bun, strength, faith, courage.

It was clear that my house wasn't going to sell. I had several showings, and a week after my house went on the market, another home one street over, that had been built around the same year that mine had, had the same square footage and had listed for $20,000 less. There was no way I'd make a profit and be able to afford to move to Maine. I threw in the towel, decided to stay and went to IKEA and Target to switch up a few things to try to make the house a little newer for me. I bought a three-foot by three-foot Aubrey Hepburn canvas for my bedroom, with some fake potted plants, a purple throw rug, candles, some pink and purple storage boxes, and new loud-colored pillow cases for the living room. At Target I bought new runner rugs for the hallway and kitchen, and new kitchen mats. Small things, but big things in the grand scheme of my everyday life, consolations for giving up my dream to move to the beloved seaside town I'd researched online, had apartment- and job- hunted for, and the hours I'd spent pouring over the New England and Portland books I'd bought and knew by heart. I told my pets I was staying and began to unpack under their questioning glances. It was very difficult, but I had to force myself to accept yet another fate I didn't want or ask for, and to use my strengths to carry me forward.

Instagram: July 4, 2015: This weekend I am chicken sitting for the family that I work for while they are out of town. I have to let them out at 7 a.m. and pick up all 7 of them…or should I say catch them, then put them in their house around 8 or 9 p.m. This has been a crazy and silly task.

Instagram: July 6, 2015: Time either rushes by or is snail slow. The path ahead is muddled with who knows what's and who's and where's … but this I know… strength, faith, courage.

Instagram: July 10, 2015: Every weekday I walk 2-3x daily arm in arm, usually slowly, sometimes pulling him- with this sweet, gentle 17 yr old that is mentally 2…praying he does not fall, as we make our way the two miles to the grocery stores to get the items on the list.

His family is strong, kind, funny and full of joy and Faith. It is cool to be a part of their journey.

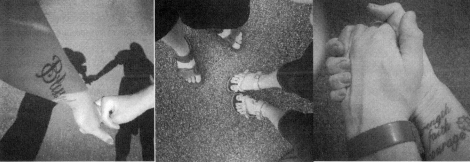

Summer 2015 with the Kiddo I worked with.

That summer I really enjoyed the little things, things I hadn't done or had in a long time like the little pretzel with cheese snack- Combos, or the McDonald's filet of fish with fries and a Coke or Sprite on the way home as a special treat after a long day working with the teen boy. Once I had to dive into the hot tub when he'd had a seizure and attempted to heft him out of it. I was getting my butt kicked daily and took small pleasures in eating ice cubes on blazing hot days, re-watching Friends and laughing 'til I cried or dancing around my house with Rufus, to his old feline annoyance.

I took Greta on endless long walks, going as far as I could before we'd both become tired and I'd have to quit. God kept giving me more strength and energy to keep going when I thought I was toast and breakfast was over.

I fell in love with the movie "Take Me Home," with Sam and Amber Jaegar, as it rang true about one's uncertainties in life, and most importantly as it helped me discover the music of the band Bootstraps. Their self-titled album provided me calm and solace on so many nights as I'd lie and look at my popcorn ceiling above my bed and wonder where I was going in life and what would happen. I'd see roads ahead of me, but never saw anything more than trees on both sides and blue skies above. I enjoyed doing yard work, planting, weeding, and tending to my giant garden along the fence behind my house. I took pride in getting the saw out of my little red shed and cutting branches off my giant trees in the backyard, watering all of my flowerbeds, and playing with my dog in the green grass and hot summer sun, as she smiled and panted.

Instagram: July 18, 2015: A good far away friend of mine that is a single dad with two little kids is having a hard time. He wondered and stated that he doesn't know how to make people happy. I've learned over the years via small and huge losses, friendships and letting go of toxic people in my life: we can only make ourselves happy. Sounds cliché and simple, but we all have to learn it repeatedly in life. It's like trying to water an entire apple tree when you only have enough for your branch. Being authentically you and being proud of how you got from those point A's to B's…when you thought you'd never be able to… is enough! Radiate your own possibilities and positivity and when you're quite blessed, there are some good apples that grow along the tree that lives within us, and beside us. Know that the right ones feel the same way about us. We feel fortunate to have that tandem growth and all we can do is keep growing and take a bite out of good situations that help foster us into decent human beings in our short time here. P.S. Sometimes you will feel more like applesauce, lol, but you're still the apple you were meant to be. That's why there are so many varieties of them that are mostly good!

I found it increasingly harder for people to hear that I was a widow. The looks on their faces were as if I told them I had killed my dog. People just don't know what to say or do, it's always so awkward for them, as they look at you in a horrified way. I'd have to tell them I was okay, I was moving on and was blessed to have had what I had.

I had a really bad date that summer. The guy told me that there was a reason that Grayson was gone and he was there, that it was supposed to happen. Check, please! Dating turned out to be a loss of humanity for myself. I cared for everyone so much and was so burned out by juggling jobs, and hated being so isolated and alone, that I lost respect for myself and just wanted attention, even if it was the wrong kind. I prayed, read my devotional and went to church, but also drank and dated too much and kept looking to fill the gaping void that seemed to grow deeper and wider as each exhausting week went by.

I had found some really quality and nice guys online, or at least they seemed that way, but had to say no when I was asked out on dates, as they were firefighters and policemen. I'd already been widowed once and couldn't risk it again until I was very old. I needed to find an accountant or some sort of desk job guy. When I talked about myself in honest words and truths, several times I was told that I wasn't real, I was a charlatan, too good to be true. I knew I was a really good person and couldn't figure out what was going on. So many times in my life whether with friends or dating- I'd taken in and been drawn to those that would end up sucking the life out of me and/or playing me like the naïve fiddle I was, making me feel like I needed to be there for them.

I dated a really nice tech guy the previous winter for a few weeks. He'd been open and vulnerable with me, then when he saw I was too nice and the real deal, he freaked out and said he was too busy with work. I pined after him for weeks, only to find him back on the same dating app; he'd been on it the whole time according to the date listed on there.

I spent time dating and being friends with a young guy who was a teacher at the school for the autistic child I worked with. He was nine years younger than me, was very mature in many ways, a published author, very articulate and kind, but just didn't have it all together to be a safe relationship for me, either.

I had a few dates with a guy that was nearly seven feet tall. He said he coached the WNBA team here. It turned out he lived with his mom, had no car, and was a volunteer coach who got free tickets to games. Insert face palm here.

Mid-summer I began talking to a local radio station personality that I'd listened to on my way to work, hearing him say how dating was so hard. He seemed smart, funny, and was a single dad. I contacted him via Facebook messenger and he said he wasn't interested, but then after I made him two short videos of me saying, "Hello, Pete, I am Rachel, fancy a beer at a local pub? Come on, come hang out with me," in a British accent, he decided to meet me.

We went to dinner, saw Nick Offerman at a book reading, went to a Black Diet concert of my friend Jonathan's band, and talked daily to each other on messenger. He said he only wanted to be friends, but would message me songs he thought I'd like to hear very early in the morning, shared photos and videos, and his actions didn't quite match his words. I bought last-minute tickets to see the Foo Fighters, as he said he wanted to go. I told him it cost less than it did, as I really wanted to go with him, so I asked for fifty dollars less than what I'd actually paid. I have no idea why I was so desperate to see this guy, but I was. We went to dinner ahead of time, he first picked me up from where I parked in St. Paul, then we sat down at a table and ordered. As we were waiting for our food, he told me that I was the perfect girl, but he was waiting on his ex-girlfriend to want to get back together with him.

I sat there in my new little green and black dress, feeling like an idiot. I should have just left, my car was only a couple blocks away. Instead I stomached the news, went to the concert, drank too much and ended up telling him the tickets were more expensive and I'd hoped he liked me, to his surprise.

I watched Dave Grohl sing the Foo Fighters' amazing hits, "Monkey Wrench," "Everlong," and "Big Me," as this lead singer slid up and down the stage in a king's chair as he'd recently broken his leg, and attempted not to cry. When I'd finally had it and was not able to stay any longer, I went outside and stood crying in the pouring rain as I called Vera. She came to pick me up, I spent the night at her house and was awoken the next day by one of her sweet little dogs licking my arm.

When I went home I took off my dress and threw it on my coffee table. On Monday, Pete talked live on the radio about how awesome the concert was and how he had so much fun. No mention of anything else, of course. I later heard a ripping sound in the living room and found Greta tearing apart the dress I wore to the concert with her teeth. That seemed about right.

My sister Diana kept wondering why I kept attempting to date. She told me "To take time for yourself." All I had pretty much was time to myself. Two out of my three jobs for the past year were children that were living in their own little worlds, and I kept learning about myself the more I dated, anyway. It was almost like an anthropological experiment. I'd get a free dinner or beverage, learn the culture of dating, what I did and didn't want in a companion and move on. Of the fifty-four dates I went on in one and a half years, I dated in fits and starts. Some weeks I'd have two or three dates a week, and sometimes I'd go weeks or a month with no dates. It depended on my interest, energy level around work and if I even cared to get out there and look nice. Even with all the heartache and mistakes I made, I knew I had to forgive these people. We're all just wandering around in life, trying to figure out what we're doing every day, and that requires grace.

Instagram: July 20, 2015: We all walk many paths and are fortunate enough at times to be able to choose which one we take. Paths. Positivity.

Instagram: July 21, 2015: Every day is another blank slate…radiate positivity and smile…it's a gift. Happiness. Positivity. Blessings. Unicorns.

Instagram: July 31, 2015: Sometimes dreams are the worst. I woke up in a sweat with a migraine after dreaming that my late husband was alive on life support and I had to make the crappy decisions all over again. It's been 27 months, thank God. Cancer Sucks. Widow Life. StupidCancer.

Instagram: August 3, 2015: Dreamer: It's always better to be a dreamer than a pessimist, I believe…don't let life's negatives take away the possible positives.

Instagram: August 3, 2015: Keys in the engine, sunglasses on, windows down. As I drive from city blocks to highways then uneven gravel roads…I'm accompanied only by my thoughts and melodies of Crowes of Black, Pumpkins of Smashing and a Purple Prince…Lyrics that I've known for years by heart, flow through my windswept hair and fields of green corn that pops up row after row. I smile, a left side turn up of a near smirk…so pleased as your Aunt Gladys's punch… that I'm me…That I've made it so far in such a small amount of time…two years and a handful of months and although there are still so many uncertainties and I don't know if the lights at the end of the tunnel will be blinking, bright colors or dancing…but I do know ~they're lights just for me.

Instagram: August 9, 2015: Within the rhythm, within the rhyme, the chaos of everyday routines, traffic jams and standing in lines, I find a quiet place in my mind, spaces and corners of Zen, whether it be reading a book for a bit, taking a nap or doing even dreaded job searches again on a rainy Sunday afternoon. This space, this silence, this breathing room…is entirely mine. I look at my collection of art on the walls that surrounds me, a juxtaposition of who I was, where I've been and who I want to be. Photographs and memories of abstracts and things that in my mind hit my soul and bring a smile to my lips…life's individual onomatopoeias. Boom, zap, crash…like my own individual wah wah pedal. These quiet reflections always bring solace in the busyness of this life…a bringing of truths to sly rhetoric. The rain continues to fall and I have thoughts and visions of what the world…so large and un-Rachel discovered holds for me out there…Thoughts on a Sunday.

Instagram: August 11, 2015: Birds chirp, cars speed by. The crickets sing their praises of summer, the sun begins to beat down. My fingers itch, as if I've just been bit...my blood the sweet treat of a mosquito, on a Tuesday. I caught him as he fell, seizure number 1 of the day.

Youth and babyness in his sweet gentle face and inability to speak…such a kind soul is he in his life and demeanor. Each day is a gift…we must live in the present…the past shedding light to who we are…what brought us here and dreams and visions…we should and shall chase. For otherwise, life will be taken for granted...don't let the day waste.

I had tickets to go to Metallagher at the Triple Rock Social Club that I'd gotten when Pete and I were talking, but that blew up, so I ended up going alone. It was a busy day. I'd gone to a craft beer crawl all over Minneapolis and seen Charlie Mars in concert at the Aster Café, both with my friend Addie, then went alone to the concert. I stood in the back of the room sipping a Pabst Blue Ribbon as this Metallica tribute band that did Gallagher antics sang and smashed melons all over the room. Within twenty minutes of them going on stage my tank top had been splattered with fruit juices and I'd been hit pretty good by a chunk of cantaloupe in the leg. I couldn't say I didn't try new things.

Instagram: Aug. 18, 2015: I have 9 days left of summer with this super disabled amazing 17 yr old kid…I reflect: Light the fires, here comes the champ. So quiet is he, as he's non-verbal, but the significance of his presence and what I've learned, comes loud and clear, like a speaker or a guitar amp. Forever this gentle child mentally will always be 2 years old under lock and key…His mind beyond that will never be free…He will probably always pick his nose, someone will have to choose his clothes, he'll be happy on hot days when you get out the garden hose. This experience has been the toughest job I've had yet. Catching him as he falls from seizures, measuring his meals to the gram, cooking and feeding him his so important meals…While my life has been in transit, the move, the house selling that didn't work… I didn't realize how much this job heals. Fore life is about how we see not the "dis" but the "ability." Such a privilege it is in hindsight to take care of someone who cannot, a pleasure…Grayson never believed my parents and I when we told him that-when he was in the depths of illness and fragility…but with my constant laughter and feistiness, those are the memories now that he is gone…however tough it was…that I treasure. The family of this teen take each day with such grace and calm. The harshness of life is true, but their life and adaptedness for others to see, is quite a healing balm. I continue to seek jobs that are tough, helping others, because I know they continue to mold me into a better human. This is true from A to B…It's all there is...kindness, authenticity, and the way I choose to be and see.

In August I had to suck it up, and put an ad online for a roommate. I was having trouble making ends meet, paying my two student loans, car payment, mortgage, etc., and decided to rent out my basement to a young woman. I ended up renting to Carolina who was twenty and wanted to find her first place as an adult. She had a key to come in the side door through my three-season porch, shared the kitchen with me, and had the basement that was seventy feet long, and her own private bathroom with a shower. I only saw her every now and then and we never talked for more than a few minutes, which was nice, as it gave me the space and privacy

I craved, while providing me the income I needed to help pay the mortgage. She only ended up staying until the following June, as I told her that no, in-fact, it was not okay for her and her boyfriend to use my bathroom in that private part of my house, especially after her boyfriend went in and out of there one day, then when I asked him not to, he said "I didn't want to poop in front of Carolina, she would be able to hear me downstairs!" Sigh. My sister Felicity referred to Carolina as "The Lady in the Basement."

Chapter 38:
New Beginnings....I Think

In August and September I interviewed at several companies, this time trying social service agencies again. I felt I was ready to get back in the swing of doing what I'd been trained to do in grad school, and what my heart knew I did best. I'd lie on the couch, staring at the painting on the wall across from me, night after night, looking at the swirl of colors and just pray, knowing that God had a plan, even if I didn't know it.

One afternoon I got a call from a job recruiter at an insurance company. She said that my application to work in the behavioral health department had been accepted and they wanted to interview me. I thought I was going to fall off the couch, as I listened, sitting there sweating in the humid temperatures despite the air conditioning. I had an interview for the following Tuesday, September 8th. I knew in that moment somehow that my life was going to change forever: as the last several years of my life had been wife, widow, now what? It was the same kind of feeling I had when I knew Grayson had cancer, when I knew I had to get a hysterectomy, and when I knew I had to not move away…God had a plan for me…I just had to be patient to figure out what it was.

A week after my interview I received another call from the same recruiter with a job offer. I could not believe it. My life was changing. It had really happened! I was offered a full time, stable job that paid much better than any other social services position I'd had before, along with great health insurance and other benefits. When I called my parents to give them the great news, my dad said, "Rachel, we are so pleased for you. You've been through so many hard times and have handled it all well. I believe great things are going to happen for you in this new life." Felicity, who is a professor of social work and had familiarity with the program and product I'd be working with, was ecstatic for me as well. Diana told me, "I knew you could do it! Good job Buttercup!" and Jack said, "Great news, Rachel!"

I woke up extra early on my first day, wore a tan and brown striped dress with a little green cardigan over it, sandals and a simple necklace. It was September 21st, 2015, fourteen years to the day that I met Grayson. I smiled all the way there, just feeling it and knowing that in this new life of mine that started that day, other big things would happen. I didn't know how I knew it, I just did. I sat in the lobby with two other newbies like myself and waited until my new boss came to get us to show us to our desks.

I followed her into a land of cubicles on a buzzing, busy floor full of bright faces that were all on phone calls. The two-hundred-foot long space was brightly lit by fluorescent lighting, and I was happy to find my cube was all the way at the end of the long room, one block of cubicles from the windows that overlooked the lake below. I was going to be working in cube land. When I stood up I looked across the sea of cubes and felt a 'zing' of belonging somehow. There was a woman in front of me, behind me, and a man to my left. I had a backwards "L"-shaped desk with places to put up my own décor on the small cloth walls, and above those, fourteen-inch-tall glass paneled windows. I had a little "good luck" doll that my friend Sandy had given me years ago that I went to put on my desk, stopping as I remembered that it had a fortune you could write on in the bottom. I took out the little sheet of paper and wrote, "Within the next year I will meet a nice man that will become my boyfriend." It was a random thing to write, but it felt right at the time.

I would spend the next six weeks in training, most of the time downstairs on the first level in the classroom, but would have time for lunch and breaks to set up my desk. My boss gave us a tour of the café, workout room, break room and other relevant places. I had already been welcomed by several people on my team, and when we were in the workout room my boss said, "This is Ethan, he comes to work out on his breaks most days." He smiled and waved, said "Welcome!" then went back to his workout.

That first day I went home feeling happy, a bit overwhelmed after seeing the training I'd receive and intake of knowledge and systems I'd learn in such a short amount of time, yet also thrilled for the stability and new friendships and connections I hoped I'd make.

The next day I had a training to do at my desk computer and as I sat there concentrating on the screen, learning about the organization's mission and ethics, I saw out of the corner of my eye Ethan, the salt and pepper haired guy from the cube right next to mine, get up from his desk and walk over. I looked up as he knelt down on one knee and said in a soft voice, "I know this is going to sound weird, but I have to ask you a question,"…

Epilogue

"Are you afraid of needles?," Ethan asked me, which made me throw my head back, roaring in laughter at the oddness of it all. I didn't even factor in the quiet workforce around me, I just thought what he asked was so funny. Ethan, a Type 1 diabetic eleven years older than me, wanted to make sure that I wasn't afraid or queasy from needles, as he regularly took insulin before he snacked at his desk and I was now his cube-mate on the other side of the window. We got to know each other within thirty-second to a couple-minute segments between calls he received over the next few weeks.

By week three we were talking to each other on work messenger, and by the first week in October we had a lunch that turned into a dinner, an eight-hour unplanned first date. I told myself explicitly not to hug or kiss, even touch him as we said goodbye at our cars, knowing a domino effect would follow if I did, and I wanted to keep my new work life professional and separate from my dating world. I gripped my keychain in my hand, waved and ran to get into my car before my resolve broke, as he was so fun, kind, neat cute, and unlike anyone I'd met in a long time. The next day I texted him to his surprise.

For our second date we went to see Matt Damon in "Martian," after work at the nearby movie theater, grabbing Subway to take into the movie with us. I stealthily paid for the tickets ahead of time and rushed ahead of him to pay for the sandwiches to his dismay and surprise, as he'd paid for everything on our first date. As we were walking back to our cars in the parking lot, I said bye, gave him a quick odd handshake or something like that, then walked away. I then turned around and yelled, "Hey Ethan?," then pointed to him and back at myself, doing the two-fingered eye to eye point gesture, "You and me. This is going to happen!" I ran up to him, gave him a big hug, sliding my arms around his back inside his coat, then smiled and ran back to my car in the evening's dusk.

I had hour long lunches during my training where we met in the lobby, sitting on couches among the amazing jungle of plants and greenery. He came downstairs on his fifteen minute breaks and chatted with me while I ate my lunch, and at times, he threw a pencil on the floor near me, then leaned over to pick it up while giving me a quick kiss on the cheek or head.

We kept our relationship under wraps for nearly four months before telling any of our coworkers. We wanted to remain professional and have boundaries in place, even though our employee handbook specified we were allowed to date. Our coworkers were ecstatic to find out, all having known and loved Ethan for months to years before I had started there. One stated that she knew something must have been going on, based on how I'd thrown almonds over my cube wall for Ethan to catch in his mouth when we had time between calls.

I sent him a "Get to know your cube-mate" survey and learned we had both had major losses in our lives, were big fans of Kiefer Sutherland's "24," and had many of the same tastes and likes in music, such as Metallica, Depeche Mode, Duran Duran, the Cure and so much more.

It turns out that that feeling I had at the Depeche Mode concert in August of 2013…was legit. In that sea of 17,000 people at the Minnesota State Fair, that hot summer night, was Ethan. He'd been at the same show where I'd looked around and knew that somehow, somewhere was the next guy I'd marry.

Ethan told me that for a year plus he would listen to his favorite preachers and sermons on his way to work, and pray aloud and proclaim God's promises, as he asked for God to give him exactly what he needed. He says that he had no idea what these needs looked like, he prayed for a significant other, not knowing if it would be marriage, etc; but definitely needing Christian friends and a significant other that would come into his life to uplift and embrace the family that he and his young daughter Bridget were becoming. He told me that when he got to work each day, he'd do a little wish, asking God to bring him Christian friends, proclaiming good things to come, which ended up bringing two other Christian co-worker friends, aside from myself. When my computer, keyboard and phone were being set up in what would be my cubicle, Ethan says he remembers believing that someone great would end up there next to him, taking it all with a grain of salt, while also laughing at his wishes of what he hoped the Lord could do for him.

As I would chatter to him with stories of people I was going on dates with, he says he remembers thinking no way in the world would this younger woman ever be someone he'd date. He'd told his step-mom about me one night, a couple weeks after meeting me, saying that he'd met someone really neat, that had so much positivity and good energy, that was an exciting addition to his life. He'd hoped I'd be a good friend, but never had any clue what was to come.

Ethan and I bonded over our difficult lives, faith, and inner strength that had kept us going even in the times the world was trying to break us down. Ethan's daughter Bridget, was only four years old when we met. I learned that she'd been abducted from him as an infant, and ever since then the other parent has attempted to control, manipulate and deceive the child and all those that come into contact with her, creating collateral damage that never seems to stop. No matter how discouraging, difficult and exhaustive it all continues to be, God has allowed Ethan and I to grow stronger and wiser as a unit together through these experiences for better or worse.

Little did I know, such a horrific circumstance could result in such an incredible attachment with this little girl, and how it would create such a strong family bond in our little rowboat of three. We are grateful for God being with us through it all, just like His promise in Deuteronomy 31:6 that states, "Be strong and courageous. Do not be afraid or terrified because of them, for the Lord your God goes with you; He will never leave you or forsake you," (New International Version). Bridget is a mini-me that loves the unconditional love,

316

independence and freedom she receives when in our care. Over the years that I've known her, she has blossomed into the intelligent, singing, dancing, silly, fun and wonderful creature that she is today. It's fun watching her become her own person and make more of her own choices, whether it be what she wants to say or do, or making music videos with Greta, our ever patient dog.

Ethan and Bridget have both continued to support me, as they express their love and support of Grayson and my past life journey and continued evolution as a former widow, including asking questions, and understanding there are difficult anniversaries that pop up each year. I have cried a couple times knowing that Ethan and Grayson would have been such good friends and really liked each other, as impossible as that would be here on earth in my situation. The dry wit and ability to be spontaneously silly, as well as selfless kindness and authenticity are what I adore most about them both. I continue to find similarities between the two of them to my surprise, as the years go on.

It's been a rocky road at times due to these co-parenting challenges with the other side; however, we face them with laughter, positivity and gusto from our joint past experiences. I've come to find that God placed Victoria in my life to prepare me for the opposition we face.

One month into my new life, I did have a major life change, just like I'd thought I would, but not in a good way. I had really negative side effects from antibiotics that I took after a dental surgery, that resulted in chronic lifelong gastrointestinal diseases. It took me a year and a half of painful procedures and a hellish of a time being very ill and permanently losing almost thirty pounds, clinic and emergency room visits, and completely changing my eating to the Low FOD Map diet to figure it all out. I had to cut out wheat, gluten, tons of fruits and veggies that are high in gases or fructose, as well as caffeine, carbonation (yes, my beloved Coke), and all alcohol (no more craft beer, or my beloved Stella Artois or Leinenkugel's Cranberry Ginger). I traded in my beer and burritos for lemonade, water, tea and becoming an amazing baker and chef, who makes food to rival most restaurants.

From time to time I do miss a good beer, but I wouldn't trade it for anything in the world for the Hello Kitty and My Little Pony playing times and flavored water I have now. Ethan and I are equally yoked in another way as well, as we both have major health conditions, him with his diabetes, and me with my gastrointestinal issues, which makes life more doable with a partner in crime that knows how important self care is.

One day several months into dating Ethan, when I was looking out the window from where I sat twenty feet away, I saw an eagle swoop down to my eye level in front of my tall office building. It turned its head toward me, then flew away, just as the one had in Alaska. I knew in that moment that Grayson was solidifying my choice in Ethan. I didn't need his permission to move on in any way, but felt a sudden rush of clarity and acceptance that this was it, as tears sprung to my eyes. Ethan would be my other half for the rest of my life. I cannot believe how much God has blessed me, as He stood by me in the storms, and continues to be my guide and life raft when I need Him most.

Ethan and I were married at Emerald Bay in Lake Tahoe, California in October of 2016, just the two of us and the minister we'd hired. He had proposed to me the June before, taking the leap of faith into a positive future with me, putting our years of tears and trauma behind us, and choosing to move forward as the new team that we'd become. We were scheduled to get married on a Friday, flying out the day before on Thursday. I got a call from the minister the Wednesday before, asking if it was okay to move the wedding up a day, as it was slated to rain all day Friday. We knew God was going before us, so trusted this quick change of plans. As Deuteronomy 31:8 states, "The Lord is the one who goes ahead of you; He will be with you. He will not fail you or forsake you. Do not fear or be dismayed," (New International Version). We flew out early Thursday morning and were treated like royalty, as the Southwest Airlines plane crew made us crowns out of pretzel and peanut packages, a veil for me out of toilet paper, and gave us a bottle of champagne. Napkins were passed out to passengers to write marital advice on, which we accepted as we stood at the front of the plane with a hundred passengers smiling and cheering in front of us. We drove two hours to our cottage where we took a nap, then dressed and got ready for our wedding. The minister took a plethora of photos among the yellow fall leaves on the way there, and at the Emerald Bay lookout site before performing the ceremony, handing us the photo memory card and our marriage certificate, then leaving us to take fun pictures at one of the prettiest places I've ever been to, to this day. We went to a CVS with the memory card, walking in the store, in our wedding attire, just perusing the shelves of chips and soda, while waiting for the discs with our forever memories to be saved on. That night around one in the morning we heard a crack of lightning, rain and then the sound of several emergency vehicles' sirens blare in the distance. When we woke the next day on Friday, we found out on the news that there had been a giant fire at Emerald Bay, where we were originally supposed to get married just hours later. God had certainly orchestrated it all, preserving and protecting us, as the road was now closed for several miles around the wedding site, and the other weddings that day would have to be cancelled. Over the next week we took amazing day trips to discover the towns around the lake, perused around the local shopping areas, got up early to see the sunrise at Zephyr Cove, and ate the delicious salmon and grilled veggies I made daily.

When Ethan is asked what it was like to date then marry a widow, he says that when he heard about Grayson from the very beginning of my days on the job, and has said dozens of times since, "I first learned of who Rachel really was by hearing of her life and love for Grayson. I fell in love with her by hearing about her love for her late husband. I, too, love Grayson for that." I believe it's incredible and quite rare to find someone who is so respectful, not threatened and inclusive of my former Rachel 1.0 life. I found my lost mitten when I met Ethan. I'd been able to keep my hand warm by putting it in my jacket pocket and had survived without it, but life was so much better with a pair.

I have received so many serendipitous blessings in this new life of mine, more than I'd ever thought possible. Ethan's family is incredible. His parents divorced when he was little, and both sets of his parents are great. It is a whole other world to be loved, accepted and appreciated by them. It took a while to get used to, after having the past experiences I'd had. I still talk to Grayson's cousins who are excited and supportive of my new life with Ethan and Bridget, and I am very encouraged by the love and support that I receive from Ethan's family of my past life and widow evolution as well. To honor the man who married a widow with a complicated past, I had a large cursive "E" tattooed on the inside of my right arm, an inch below "strength, faith, courage." Of course as soon as Bridget saw it, she was upset that I hadn't gotten a "B" for her. Maybe one day, we'll see.

I still have some PTSD from time to time when I think of everything I went through. I have dreams that Grayson has no idea who I am when I show up at our house or old apartment, but have to be rational when I wake, knowing it was just a dream. I miss Grayson's goofy laugh, dances and the kind soul he was, and I feel so sorry for everything he went through. He used to make fun of me when I lost the TV remotes in the blankets that were wrapped around me. I still do that all the time and think of him chuckling at me. Whenever I have stomach issues and need to lie down, I hear him telling me, "Lay on your left side Rachie, it will help."

He told my sister Diana when she asked him what his New Year's resolution was one year, "Well, I am going to fill up the bathtub with milk, pour in a box of alphabet cereal and eat my way to the answer!" That is the Grayson I choose to remember and treasure. Cancer may have torn down his body and wore down his spirit in the end, but it cannot change the years of love, laughter and life I had with him.

When I think back on the girl who went through everything in this book…I cannot believe she faced and tackled so many fires and wars and still came out on the other side. She was so strong and had such a hard time, and most of the time all these years later, it's hard to believe she was me.

Being a widow feels like being isolated in a snow storm with nothing surrounding you but whiteness, blowing winds and cold. Even in a sea of friends and family, you're so isolated and feel so desperate. Your other half is forever gone and all the involuntary, knee-jerk reactions or actions you had for years to get your partner a beverage when you got one, to ask a question or to tell them something, is all of a sudden so obsolete. It's just you. You. You. You. Starting from scratch. It's haunting and so unfamiliar and foreign. But it is doable.

Some days I think that if I didn't have "Grayson" tattooed on my wrist, I'd never believe it happened. Even as I type this very line, it feels like my mind is gaslighting me, trying to convince me that it all never happened, making me think I am crazy for questioning I went through the whole thing! It was so hard and so much work, and I've moved past and beyond it with God's grace, but man was it a tough time. I didn't think I'd make it and I'm here to say that I did! Just like Darius Rucker's song "This," everything has brought me to the path I am on.

I wish I could have taken away Grayson's pain and everything he had to endure, and of course wish he didn't have to die, but I wouldn't change anything in the world for how this experience has crafted me into the person I am today. Cancer and widowhood, as awful as they both are, have gifted me with experience and knowledge that has lit a fire within me to help others who are walking in the same shoes I was in, all those years ago.

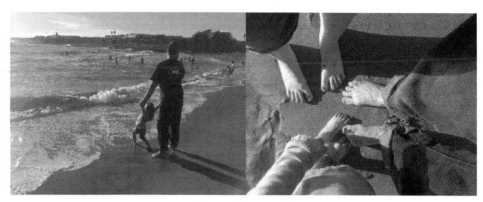

Prayers Answered.

Extras:

Music/TV While Writing, Wife, Widow, Now What?:

I wrote this book either in silence inside or out on my deck under an umbrella in the beauty of nature, or while I was watching Parks and Recreation or Will and Grace, or listening to a few artists. I was transfixed by Andrew Belle's music, especially the "Black Bear" album and the song, "Pieces." I also wrote while streaming COVID-19 at-home video concerts of Pete Yorn and Melissa Etheridge, and to the CDs of Dawes, Cat Stevens, Bootstraps, Ben Howard and Bill Withers.

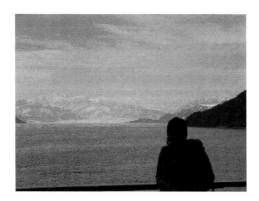

My Favorite Cancer Resources of All Time:

Social Media:

- CaringBridge: https://www.caringbridge.org
- Facebook, Instagram.

Health Information:

- The American Cancer Society: https://www.cancer.org
- The Leukemia and Lymphoma Society: https://www.lls.org
- Be the Match: https://bethematch.org
- National Cancer Institute: https://www.cancer.gov/about-cancer/understanding/what-is-cancer
- CDC: Center for Disease Control and Prevention: https://www.cdc.gov/cancer/index.htm

Survivorship: Resources for the Cancer Survivor:

- Cancer.net: Survivorship: https://www.cancer.net/survivorship/what-survivorship

- National Coalition for Cancer Survivorship:

https://www.canceradvocacy.org (This organization offers a really neat pamphlet and CD/DVD packet you can get for free in the mail about the cancer process and survivorship)
- American Cancer Society: https://www.cancer.org/treatment/survivorship-during-and-after-treatment.html
- Your Cancer Story: http://www.yourcancerstory.com/survivorship

Widows/Widowers Resources:
- Hope for Widows Foundation:
  https://hopeforwidows.org/resources/widows/
- A list of several resources for widows and widowers"
  https://www.sfmadvisorgroup.com/widow-and-widower-resources
- Meetup.com Widow and Widower Support Groups:
  https://www.meetup.com/topics/widows-and-widowers-support-group/
- National Widowers Org: https://nationalwidowers.org/support-groups/
- Article on finding support groups: https://www.joincake.com/blog/widow-support-groups/

Info/Shopping:
- Stupid Cancer: https://stupidcancer.org (Info)
o Stupid Cancer Store: https://stupidcancerstore.org
- Stand Up to Cancer: (Info and store) https://standuptocancer.org/
o Stand Up to Cancer Store: https://www.shopsu2c.org/store

- Comfport: https://comfport.com/ (My friend Connor that is a cancer survivor, along with his brother make shirts that have little pockets on the chest that open to fit ports that are implanted on the chest. Each time two shirts are purchased, one shirt is donated to a cancer patient in need. Beanies and ball caps are also for sale as well.)
- Cool Cancer Shirts and Clothing:
  https://www.spreadshirt.com/shop/clothing/t-shirts/cancer-survivor/
- Cancer Gifts: https://www.cancergifts.com

Publications: Free!
- Cure: Cancer Updates –Research and Education
  https://www.curetoday.com/subscription
- Cancer Today Magazine: https://www.cancertodaymag.com
- Conquer: The Patient Voice: https://conquer-magazine.com

Books I Found Helpful:

- "Geography of Loss: Embrace What Is, Honor What Was, Love What Will Be."-Patti Digh
- "Transform Your Loss: Your Guide to Strength and Hope." Ligia M. Houben
- "Mars and Venus Starting Over: A Practical Guide for Finding Love Again, After a Painful Breakup, Divorce, or the Loss of a Loved One." John Gray, Ph.D. (This has 101 ways to work on healing, that I found really helpful!)
- "From We to Me: Embracing Life Again After the Death or Divorce of a Spouse." Susan J. Zonnebelt-Smeenge, RN. Ed.D., Robert C. De Vries, DMin, Ph.D.
- "A Grief Observed." C.S. Lewis
- "Happily Even After: A Guide to Getting Through (and Beyond) the Grief of Widowhood" Carole Brody Fleet
- "Widows Wear Stilettos: A Practical and Emotional Guide for the Young Widow." Carole Brody Fleet.
- "Jesus Lives" and "Jesus Calling," Sarah Young.
- "Streams in the Desert" L.B. Cowman
- "Walk in a Relaxed Manner: Life Lessons from the Camino." Joyce Rupp
- "The Gifts of Imperfection." Berne Brown, Ph.D., L.M.S.W.
- "The Tao of Inner Peace." Diane Dreher
- "The Sunflower: On the Possibilities and Limits of Forgiveness." Simon Wiesenthal
- "Tao Te Ching." Lao Tzu
- "The Daily Zoo: Keeping the Doctor at Bay with a Drawing a Day, Vol 1." Chris Ayers
- "The Daily Zoo: Keeping the Doctor at Bay with a Drawing a Day, Vol 2, Year 2." Chris Ayers
- "Picture Your Life After Cancer." The New York Times and the American Cancer Society

Made in the USA
Monee, IL
12 October 2020

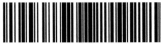